REPRESENTING INFIRMITY

This volume is the first in-depth analysis of how infirm bodies were represented in Italy from *c.* 1400 to 1650. Through original contributions and methodologies, it addresses the fundamental yet undiscussed relationship between images and representations in medical, religious, and literary texts.

Looking beyond the modern category of 'disease' and viewing infirmity in Galenic humoral terms, each chapter explores which infirmities were depicted in visual culture, in what context, why, and when. By exploring the works of artists such as Caravaggio, Leonardo, and Michelangelo, this study considers the idealized body altered by diseases, including leprosy, plague, goitre, and cancer. In doing so, the relationship between medical treatment and the depiction of infirmities through miracle cures is also revealed. The broad chronological approach demonstrates how and why such representations change, both over time and across different forms of media. Collectively, the chapters explain how the development of knowledge of the workings and structure of the body was reflected in changed ideas and representations of the metaphorical, allegorical, and symbolic meanings of infirmity and disease.

The interdisciplinary approach makes this study the perfect resource for both students and specialists of the history of art, medicine and religion, and social and intellectual history across Renaissance Europe.

John Henderson, Professor of Italian Renaissance History, Department of History, Classics and Archaeology, Birkbeck, University of London. His most recent books include *The Renaissance Hospital: Healing the Body and Healing the Soul* (2006) and *Florence under Siege: Surviving Plague in an Early Modern City* (2019).

Fredrika Jacobs, Professor Emerita, Virginia Commonwealth University. She is the author of *Defining the Renaissance 'Virtuosa': Women Artists and the Language of Art History and Criticism*, *The Living Image in the Renaissance*, and *Votive Panels and Popular Piety in Early Modern Italy*. Her current project is '10 objects + a shadow'.

Jonathan K. Nelson, Teaching Professor, Syracuse University Florence. His books include *The Patron's Payoff: Conspicuous Commissions in Italian Renaissance Art* (with Richard Zeckhauser), *Bad Reception: Negative Reactions to Italian Renaissance Art* (co-editor; forthcoming), and monographic studies of Leonardo da Vinci, Filippino Lippi (with Patrizia Zambrano), Michelangelo, Plautilla Nelli, and Robert Mapplethorpe.

The Body in the City

Series Editors: Peter Howard and John Henderson
*Institute for Religion & Critical Inquiry, Australian Catholic University, Australia;
Birkbeck, University of London, UK.*

This series aims to intersect and to energise two strands in historical studies: the pre-modern city as an historical subject (encompassing political institutions, rituals, built environments, religious activities, etc.) and histories of the pre-modern body with their debates about how bodies are shaped by discourse and context. The series will highlight approaches which emphasize the vernacular as revealed by new sources and novel approaches to them. While there are numerous studies of the body in history, this series will explore critically and in innovative ways the relationship between bodies and environments. This will allow scholars involved to analyse how particular spaces, locations, and physical *milieux* affect understandings of the body and govern responses to particular problems. The multi-disciplinary approach to the topic places the series at the leading edge of its field.

In this series:

Plague and the City
Edited by Lukas Engelmann, John Henderson and Christos Lynteris

Gaspare Tagliacozzi and Early Modern Surgery
Faces, Men, and Pain
Paolo Savoia

Popular Politics in an Aristocratic Republic
Political Conflict and Social Contestation in Late Medieval and Early Modern Venice
Edited by Maartje Van Gelder and Claire Judde De Larivière

Representing Infirmity
Diseased Bodies in Renaissance Italy
Edited by John Henderson, Fredrika Jacobs, and Jonathan K. Nelson

For more information about this series, please visit: www.routledge.com/The-Body-in-the-City/book-series/BOCY

REPRESENTING INFIRMITY

Diseased Bodies in Renaissance Italy

Edited by John Henderson, Fredrika Jacobs,
and Jonathan K. Nelson

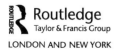

Routledge
Taylor & Francis Group

LONDON AND NEW YORK

First published 2021
by Routledge
2 Park Square, Milton Park, Abingdon, Oxon OX14 4RN

and by Routledge
52 Vanderbilt Avenue, New York, NY 10017

Routledge is an imprint of the Taylor & Francis Group, an informa business

British Library Cataloguing-in-Publication Data
A catalogue record for this book is available from the British Library

Library of Congress Cataloging-in-Publication Data
Names: Representing Infirmity: Diseased Bodies in Renaissance and Early
   Modern Italy (Conference) (2017 : Prato, Italy), author. | Henderson,
   John, 1949 June 12– editor. | Jacobs, Fredrika Herman, editor. |
   Nelson, Jonathan K., editor.
Title: Representing infirmity : diseased bodies in Renaissance Italy /
   edited by John Henderson, Fredrika Jacobs and Jonathan K. Nelson.
Description: Abingdon, Oxon ; New York : Routledge, 2021. | Series:
   The body in the city | Includes bibliographical references and index.
Contents: Approaches to the representation of infirmity. Cancer in
   Michelangelo's Night / Jonathan K. Nelson — Institutions and
   visualising illness. The friar as medico / Diana Bullen Presciutti —
   Disease and treatment. Artistic representations of goitre in early modern
   Italian art / Danielle Carrabino — Saints and miraculous healing.
   Infirmity in votive culture / Fredrika Jacobs.
Identifiers: LCCN 2020024938 | ISBN 9780367470203 (paperback) |
   ISBN 9780367470210 (hardback) | ISBN 9781003032885 (ebook)
Subjects: LCSH: Sick in art. | People with disabilities in art. | Diseases in
   art. | Art and society—Italy—History.
Classification: LCC N8243.S5 R47 2017 | DDC 700/.453561—dc23 LC
   record available at https://lccn.loc.gov/2020024938

ISBN: 978-0-367-47021-0 (hbk)
ISBN: 978-0-367-47020-3 (pbk)
ISBN: 978-1-003-03288-5 (ebk)

Typeset in Bembo
by Apex CoVantage, LLC

CONTENTS

FIGURES

CONTRIBUTORS

Maggie Bell, Assistant Curator, Norton Simon Museum of Art. She is curating two exhibitions, *The Expressive Body: Memory, Devotion, Desire (1400–1750)* (2020) and *Doing Without: Representations of Need, Greed and Sacrifice* (2021). Her forthcoming articles include 'Health as Harmony: The Pellegrinaio Frescos of Santa Maria della Scala' (2020).

Danielle Carrabino, Curator of Painting and Sculpture, Smith College Museum of Art. Her current exhibition projects include "SCMA Then\Now\Next" and an exhibition on polychrome wooden sculpture from the fourteenth to the seventeenth century. She is also completing her manuscript on Caravaggio in Sicily.

John Henderson, Professor of Italian Renaissance History, Department of History, Classics, and Archaeology, Birkbeck, University of London. His most recent books include *The Renaissance Hospital: Healing the Body and Healing the Soul* (2006) and *Florence under Siege: Surviving Plague in an Early Modern City* (2019).

Peter Howard, Professor and Director of the Institute for Religion and Critical Inquiry at Australian Catholic University. He has published widely on the Florentine Renaissance and medieval sermon studies, including books titled *Creating Magnificence in Renaissance Florence* (2012) and *Experiencing Religion in Renaissance Florence* (2021).

Fredrika Jacobs, Professor Emerita, Virginia Commonwealth University. She is the author of *Defining the Renaissance 'Virtuosa': Women Artists and the Language of Art History and Criticism, The Living Image in the Renaissance,* and *Votive Panels and Popular Piety in Early Modern Italy.* Her current project is '10 objects + a shadow'.

Jenni Kuuliala, Senior Research Fellow, Centre of Excellence in the History of Experiences, Tampere University. She is the author of *Childhood Disability and Social Integration in the Middle Ages: Constructions of Impairments in Thirteenth- and Fourteenth-Century Canonization Processes* (2016) and *Saints, Infirmity, and Community in the Late Middle Ages* (2020).

Jonathan K. Nelson, Teaching Professor, Syracuse University Florence. His books include *The Patron's Payoff: Conspicuous Commissions in Italian Renaissance Art* (with Richard Zeckhauser), *Bad Reception: Negative Reactions to Italian Renaissance Art* (co-editor; forthcoming), and monographic studies of Leonardo da Vinci, Filippino Lippi (with Patrizia Zambrano), Michelangelo, Plautilla Nelli, and Robert Mapplethorpe.

Diana Bullen Presciutti, Senior Lecturer of Art History, University of Essex. She is the author of *Visual Cultures of Foundling Care in Renaissance Italy* (2015) and the editor of *Space, Place, and Motion: Locating Confraternities in the Late Medieval and Early Modern City* (2017).

Paolo Savoia, Assistant Professor of the History of Science, University of Bologna. He specializes in the history of the body and knowledge. His most recent publications include *Gaspare Tagliacozzi and Early Modern Surgery: Faces, Men, and Pain* (2019) and 'Cheesemaking in the Scientific Revolution' (*Nuncius*, 2019).

Michael Stolberg, Chair of History of Medicine, University of Würzburg, Germany. His most recent monograph is *A History of Palliative Care 1500–1970: Concepts, Practices and Ethical Challenges.* With De Gruyter, he will soon publish *Learned Physicians and Ordinary Medical Practice in the Renaissance.*

Evelyn Welch, Professor of Renaissance Studies, King's College London, is a Wellcome Trust Senior Investigator. She is the author of *Shopping in the Renaissance* (2005) and *Making and Marketing Medicine in Renaissance Florence* (with James Shaw, 2007) and the editor of *Fashioning the Early Modern* (2017).

PREFACE

This volume grew out of a project born in a café in Cambridge, Massachusetts, on April Fool's Day, 2016. Jonathan K. Nelson met John Henderson to propose an idea he had just discussed with Fredrika Jacobs: an interdisciplinary workshop on how disease was depicted in early modern Italy. Little did we realize how topical this subject would become, precisely four years later, with the emergence of Covid-19. Each country where we are based—Italy, the UK, and USA—has seen both similar and different reactions to the crisis, whether in the form of government policies or the ways in which individuals have adjusted their lives to containment and quarantine. These themes are echoed in measures to cope with plague in Renaissance Italy, which provided the template for later public health policies, as reflected in the first volume in this 'Body in the City' series. *Plague and the City* (2019) examined reactions to plague between the Middle Ages and the early twentieth century. This topic is also explored in the chapter by John Henderson in the present book, where authors address the ways of representing infirmity in Renaissance Italy.

As we are editing this volume, Covid-19 is conceptualized in quite similar visual terms around the world and brought into our homes on the news and social media. In the past, however, there was a great range in how different diseases were represented, depending in part on the medium and context. This theme provided the focus for our workshop, 'Representing Disease in Italy (ca. 1350–ca. 1650)', held at the Monash University Centre in Prato on 14 December 2016. This brought together historians of art and of medicine for complementary explorations of what turned out to be a surprisingly understudied topic. The event led to a genuinely interdisciplinary meetings of minds at a conference, 'Representing Infirmity: Diseased Bodies in Renaissance and Early Modern Italy', also held at the Monash University Centre in Prato, on 13–15 December 2017. The shift in the titles from 'disease' to 'infirmity' reflects the development in our thinking. The original concentration on 'disease' at the workshop limited us to more modern nosological definitions, whereas the term 'infirmity' at the conference was wide enough to embrace broader humoral concepts. Physicians and the general public in the early modern period often saw diseases as collections of symptoms, which fail to fit within our modern neater definitions.

The chapters in this volume, which developed out of those given at the conference, represent the first analysis of how infirm and diseased bodies were represented in Italy from the early 1400s through *c.* 1650. Many individual studies by historians of art and medicine address specific aspects of this subject, yet there has never been an attempt to define or explore the broader topic. Moreover, most studies interpret Renaissance images and texts through the lens of current notions about disease, often based on retrospective diagnoses. The chapters in this volume take a different analytical tack, viewing 'infirmity' in humoral terms within a contemporary Galenic framework and cultural practices. Individual chapters explore which infirmities were depicted, in what context, why, and when. Specific examples consider the idealized body altered by disease and the relationship between the depiction of infirmities through miracle cures and by medical treatment. Authors also examine how and why these representations change across media and over time. The interdisciplinary approach of the volume and the range of specialists allow the book to address the fundamental, but hitherto undiscussed, relationship between these images and those in medical, religious, and other texts. Finally, it explores how the development of greater knowledge of the workings and structure of the body in this period was reflected in changing ideas and representations of the metaphorical, allegorical, and symbolic meanings of infirmity and disease.

The volume is divided into four main sections, moving from (1) methodological considerations to (2) how institutions visualized illness, (3) the treatment of disease, and (4) the role of saints and miraculous healing. The first section considers approaches to the representation of infirmity in three different mediums: sculpture, text, and painting. Jonathan K. Nelson examines the possible identification of cancer in sculpture through discussion of Michelangelo's *Night*. The physical signs of cancer in the breast of this marble statue force us to reconsider a series of widely held views, from the artist's reputed ignorance of female anatomy to the modern fascination with medical diagnoses of art. This suggests that Michelangelo made a conscious decision to represent the symptoms of a specific infirmity, though he may also have associated *Night* with Melancholy, a condition that Renaissance texts often linked to cancer. Peter Howard then examines the striking role of metaphor and the language of infirmity in sermons, focusing on the complex interplay between spiritual and bodily health at a fundamental conceptual level. The metaphors of infirmity, health, and healing were more than figurative or ornamental; the preacher's art was to engage with the particulars of their hearers' lives, which included struggles with illness and infirmity. In the third chapter, John Henderson discusses visual representation of infirmity in early modern Florence in relation to the last epidemic of plague to afflict the city. In addition to providing the first overall survey of paintings commissioned during the seventeenth-century plague, he aims to raise wider questions about how disease was represented. Accordingly,

Henderson asks in what ways did the medical and religious imperatives of the period determine how infirmity was shown in the art commissioned in the 1630s, and how and why did artists represent sickness and infirmity and bodily suffering more generally?

The second section examines institutional influence, asking to what extent patrons determined the way illness was visualized. Maggie Bell analyses the extraordinary fifteenth-century fresco-cycle painted in the central male ward, the *pellegrinaio*, of the Hospital of Santa Maria della Scala in Siena. Examining compositional structure and figure placement, she shows how the role of the hospital determined the ways in which poverty and infirmity were represented to underline the vital Christian charitable imperative of the institution and staff. Diana Bullen Presciutti explores the ways in which religion and medicine combined within the context of the Franciscan Order in Italy. She focuses on an illustration depicting St Francis of Assisi and his companions caring for victims of leprosy in a late-fifteenth-century manuscript, *La Franceschina*. Her analysis reveals how the image, with an unusually strong emphasis on the disfiguring symptoms of disease, negotiates the relationship between leprous bodies and ideal Observant Franciscan behaviour.

The third section turns to representations of disease and treatment. Evelyn Welch examines two engravings which depict cupping, based on a fresco by Giulio Romano, by considering how sixteenth-century viewers perceived their own bodies and those of others. She focuses on one of the central questions addressed by this volume, namely how the shifting humours and blockages of the diseased body were imagined by artists. Paolo Savoia discusses early modern surgery within the wider cultural imagery of pain and suffering. He begins by focusing on two illustrations in Giovanni Andrea Della Croce's manual of surgery (1583): one represents a Christian soldier undergoing battlefield surgery in the aftermath of the battle of Lepanto, and the other depicts an Ottoman enduring the same ordeal. He then expands his discussion by analysing these images in relation to representations of martyrdom and discourses on the necessary braveness and moral strength of patients. More broadly, Savoia looks at and beyond the epistemic function of images in the history of early modern science and medicine. The third chapter in this section, by Danielle Carrabino, examines the representation of goitre in early modern Italian art within the contexts of humoral definitions and contemporary cultural contexts. Once again, the complexity of contemporary representation of infirmity is addressed. Looking at various examples that include Caravaggio's *Crucifixion of St Andrew* and the modelled figures at the Sacro Monte of Varallo, she discusses how goitre carried different meanings—from moral corruption and poverty to humility and piety—according to the function and significance of the works of art in which they appear. In each case, the representation of goitre sought to elicit responses of empathy and wonder in the viewer.

The final section addresses the relationship between religion and medicine through an examination of representations of saints and miraculous healing. Fredrika Jacobs begins with an analysis of Giovanni Lanfranco's *St Luke Healing the Dropsical Child*. Then, focusing on a case study comprising seventeen votive panel paintings from the Neapolitan Sanctuary of the Madonna dell'Arco, she addresses the way in which infirmity was represented in sixteenth- and seventeenth-century votive culture. Most unusually, the seventeen panels under consideration show the votary symptomatically and in some cases attended by a doctor or a priest, the physicians of body and soul, respectively. The question about how much these paintings disclose about the therapeutic landscape of early modern Italy is examined within the contexts of votive culture and the medical discourse. Jenni Kuuliala examines the portrayal of illness and impairment in selected works representing the life and miracles of St Carlo Borromeo from the cycle of paintings in the Duomo of Milan. Contemporary written records of the depicted events, which include canonization proceedings, allow Kuuliala to make a comparison between visual and written representations of miraculously cured bodies. She analyses how the physical and emotional sides of infirmity were portrayed, considers which elements of the written miracle narrative were selected for visualization, and examines how depicted reactions were used to highlight the message of the painting.

The volume is rounded off by an Epilogue by Michael Stolberg, the respondent at the conference, who examines the themes of the chapters of this book within the wider context of the history of medicine in early modern Europe. He returns to one of the main themes addressed in the volume: the necessity to examine representations of illness and disease through contemporary medical understanding of health and sickness. In this way Stolberg explores how these case studies and methodologies provide points of departure for research in the field. If there is one thing that the editors have learnt through the process, which began with those discussions in Cambridge, Massachusetts, and ended with the intercontinental editing of this volume, it is that this field is still in its early stage of development. It is the collective hope of both editors and contributors of the volume that this book will stimulate continued discussion and lead to further interdisciplinary studies.

We are very grateful to the Monash Centre in Prato and its staff, and especially Dr Cecilia Hewett, its Director, who graciously hosted and supported financially both the 2016 workshop and the 2017 conference; all the participants at both events; and above all Associate Professor Peter Howard, who was a co-organizer of both events, and was at the time Director of the Centre for Medieval and Renaissance Studies and Deputy Dean of the Faculty of Arts, Monash University, Melbourne. A generous grant from the Samuel H. Kress Foundation provided funding for graduate students at the conference and helped to defer costs of the colour photography.

John Henderson, Fredrika Jacobs, Jonathan K. Nelson

PART I

Approaches to the representation of infirmity

1

CANCER IN MICHELANGELO'S *NIGHT*. AN ANALYTICAL FRAMEWORK FOR RETROSPECTIVE DIAGNOSES

Jonathan K. Nelson

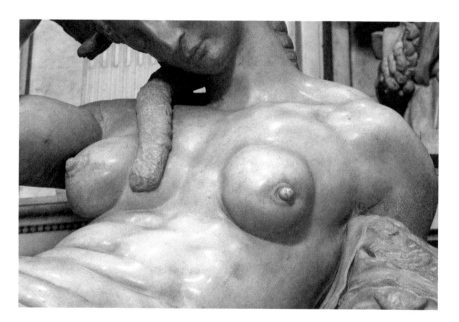

FIGURE 1.1 Michelangelo Buonarroti, *Night*, detail

Source: Gianni Trambusti, with the concession of the Ministero per i beni culturali—Museo Nazionale del Bargello

The uses and abuses of retrospective diagnoses

The lump on the left breast of the *Night* (Figure 1.1), a marble sculpture carved by Michelangelo in the 1520s, forces us to reconsider a series of widely held views, from the artist's reputed ignorance of female anatomy to the modern fascination with medical diagnoses of art.[1] Before turning to the sculpture, the first section considers some methodological problems posed by retrospective diagnoses through art. As discussed in the second section, the breast of the *Night* shows the physical signs of advanced cancer, and it is portrayed in such a way to suggest that Michelangelo made a conscious decision to represent an infirmity. This all-too-human element alludes to death, an appropriate subject for the decoration of the Medici mausoleum in the Church of San Lorenzo, Florence, known since the sixteenth century as the New Sacristy. Moreover, early sources often refer to cancer as gnawing into flesh, and this metaphor complements perfectly Michelangelo's overall conceit for the tomb: 'time devours all things'. The third section presents the hypothesis that Michelangelo associated *Night* with the melancholic temperament, given that doctors then believed that the disease of melancholia could lead to cancer. The poses and body types of the four allegorical statues in the New Sacristy—*Night* and *Day* on the tomb of Duke Giuliano (Figure 1.2), and *Dawn* and *Dusk* on the tomb of Duke Lorenzo (Figure 1.3)—seem to reflect the four canonical temperaments.

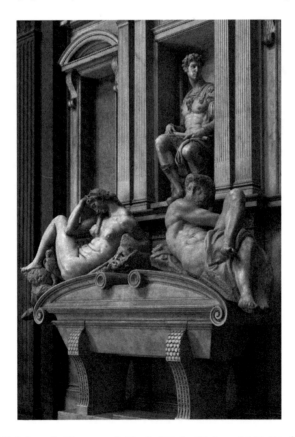

FIGURE 1.2 Michelangelo Buonarroti, *Tomb of Duke Giuliano de' Medici*, detail

Source: Gianni Trambusti, with the concession of the Ministero per i beni culturali—Museo Nazionale del Bargello

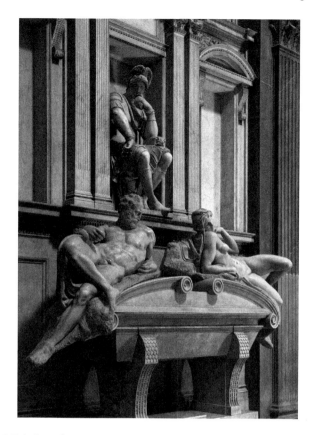

FIGURE 1.3 Michelangelo Buonarroti, *Tomb of Duke Lorenzo de' Medici*, detail

Source: Gianni Trambusti, with the concession of the Ministero per i beni culturali—Museo Nazionale del Bargello

Over the last three decades, medical journals have regularly included articles by physicians attempting to discover various diseases represented in paintings and sculptures.[2] About twenty years ago, James Stark and I published one such study in the *New England Journal of Medicine*, 'The Breasts of *Night*: Michelangelo as Oncologist'.[3] Publications of this type attract little interest among historians of art or medicine. Specialists of paintings and sculptures generally ignore the research by physicians because of their unconvincing visual analyses of art. Another objection to this type of retroactive diagnose, especially for historians of medicine, is the lack of good data. Nevertheless, all can agree that modern physicians are trained and experienced in carrying out visual examinations. Surely some of the doctors who examine paintings and sculptures can make valuable observations for historical research. Many art historians, for example, now accept the proposal that Raphael represented the possessed boy in the *Transfiguration* (Vatican City) with the physical signs of epilepsy.[4]

Though an article from 2018 in *The Lancet Oncology*, titled, 'Earliest evidence of malignant breast cancer in Renaissance paintings', presents a valuable insight about the left breast depicted in Michele Tosini's *Night*, as discussed in the following section, it also makes the erroneous claim that the painting shows 'an irritated region surrounding the areola-nipple'.[5] Photographs seem to support this observation, but direct observation reveals only a shadow, created in part with red pigment. The authors also identified a tumour in the left breast of the *Allegory of Fortitude* (Figure 1.4), painted in about 1560 by Maso da San Friano. Their discussion of the 'large bulge' reveals a more serious misreading of Renaissance art. The representation of a debilitating disease in an allegory of strength should have set off some

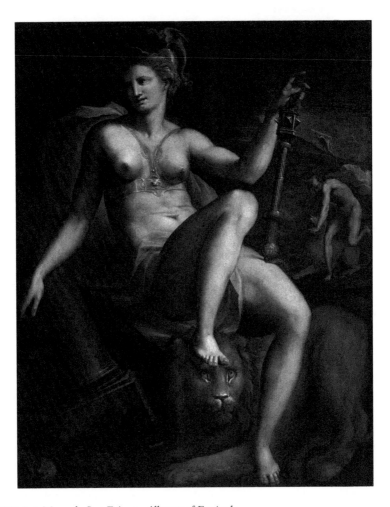

FIGURE 1.4 Maso da San Friano, *Allegory of Fortitude*

Source: With the concession of the Ministero per i beni culturali—Galleria dell'Accademia

warning signs. In reality, Maso first painted a smaller breast and then enlarged it; over time, the uppermost paint layer became more transparent, revealing the original version below. From afar, this might be confused with a lump, but up close, it looks as if the smaller breast is enclosed within a sphere of flesh-coloured glass[6] (Figure 1.5). The methodological problem with the analyses of both paintings is obvious. The authors, all oncologists, did not know how to evaluate the visual evidence and did not consult a specialist in Renaissance art. One can only imagine how physicians would react if an art historian published conclusions about the unusual physical aspect of a patient, based on the examination of a single radiograph, without speaking with a doctor or technician. The oncologists' study of the *Fortitude* is said to be part of a larger project aimed at 'training the eye of medical

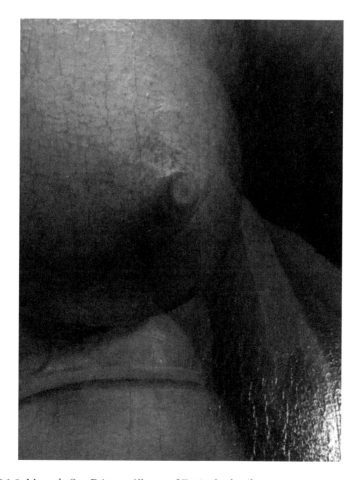

FIGURE 1.5 Maso da San Friano, *Allegory of Fortitude*, detail

Source: Rossella Lari, with the concession of the Ministero per i beni culturali—Galleria dell'Accademia

students'.[7] This would transform the painting into a dangerous didactic tool, given that Maso did not depict a tumour.

Painters and sculptors from the fifteenth and sixteenth centuries rarely depict serious illness or wounds in large-scale works, except for images of plague and leprosy victims. Far more typical is the highly stylized wound of Christ in Michelangelo's *Pietà* (Vatican City). The artist and the educated viewers of his works were certainly familiar with Pliny the Elder, who addressed the topic of representing infirmity. In *Natural History* (34. 19. 59), he observed that a bronze sculpture by Pythagoras of Reggio depicting a lame man, presumably Philoctetes, 'actually makes people looking at it feel a pain from his ulcer in their own leg'.[8] Rather than follow this ancient example, Michelangelo and his contemporaries probably agreed with a view expressed by Plutarch, on the need for suitable imagery: 'We avoid a man who is sickly or covered with sores as a disagreeable sight, but enjoy seeing Aristophon's *Philoctetes* or Silanion's *Jocasta*.'[9] For Plutarch, the painting and sculpture, now both lost, evinced the beauty of representing what is fitting and suitable. A comparable sense of decorum led the sculptor Giammaria Mosca, working in the 1520s, to represent Philoctetes without physical imperfections (Figure 1.6), though

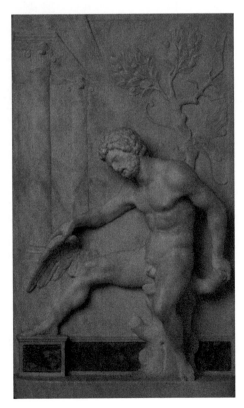

FIGURE 1.6 Giammaria Mosca, *Philoctetes*

Source: © Victoria and Albert Museum, London

the inscription of his marble relief reads: 'This Poentian hero suffers from the Lernaean wound'.[10] Infirmity, it seems, was better suited for words than images. Understandably, art historians remain sceptical about claims that Renaissance works include graphic representations of diseases.

Historians of medicine are suspicious about diagnoses based on a single image, especially one that does not provide information deemed essential for identifying diseases. For example, medical texts from antiquity through the seventeenth century regularly use the term 'cancer' to describe a range of unnatural swellings. Over the last twenty years, studies by Luke Demaitre, Alanna Skuse, and Michael Stolberg have documented how the concept of cancer was constructed in pre-modern Europe.[11] The disease 'was associated primarily with the breast and the uterus, with putrid, contagious secretions, and a pervasive impurity or contamination of the humours'.[12] Among other physical signs identified by Gabriele Falloppio, the sixteenth-century physician still noted for his study of the female reproductive system, are a 'hard tumour', a 'rather ashen colour', and 'sharp and piercing' heat.[13] Naturally, a white marble statue cannot directly communicate the smell, feel, colour, or temperature of a tumour.

Medical historians have also addressed the incommensurability of Renaissance and modern models of disease.[14] Notions about how the body (mis)functions have changed so radically over the centuries that we cannot simply overlay our modern understandings on the past. The main risk of presentism is not that one winds up with the wrong answer. Rather, the investigation itself reconfirms the widespread misconception that modern categories can be imposed on the past. For millennia, and throughout the early modern period, learned and popular authors agreed that infirmities could be traced to the corruption or impeded flow of one or more of the four essential humours circulating throughout the body: black bile, yellow bile, phlegm, and blood.[15] The predominance of one humour determined the temperament and complexion of an individual.[16] All pre-modern authors agreed that cancer was caused by a congestion of black bile, a condition never mentioned by physicians today, so just what does it mean for a modern-day doctor to detect 'cancer' in a Renaissance work?

Scholars faced with the potential representation of an infirmity in early modern art can start with a few basic questions. These are the very same ones that art historians typically ask themselves when exploring the viability and significance of a reputed ancient source. When modern scholars argue that Michelangelo or Raphael created a figure based on an antique statue, they employ at least three types of inquiries, focusing on the original appearance, context, and associations of the source. First, what did the work look like at the time: for example, was it fragmentary, restored, or pigmented? Second, when and where did the artist see the source? Third, how was the source identified in the artist's day, and what meanings did it carry? This analytical framework allows us to evaluate the validity of another type of reputed visual source: a woman with lump in her breast, now identified as a cancerous tumour. Medical journals often present the diagnosis of a painted or sculpted figure as an endpoint for research, but historians of art and medicine can use these hypotheses as points of departure for exploring the visual and cultural world of artists and their audiences.

Cancer in the *Night*

With these problems in mind we can enter the New Sacristy, where Michelangelo carved the *Night* as the first of four representations of Times of Day.[17] Though some rough details of the *Night* remain ambiguous, such as the unidentifiable plants at her feet, the sculpture is more complete than the *Day*, *Dawn*, or *Dusk*. Michelangelo considered the *Night* finished enough to polish it. To indicate that the figure represents night-time, a highly unusual subject for the period, the artist depicted her as sleeping. For this statue only, Michelangelo also included several attributes: a nocturnal bird, the owl, under *Night*'s leg; a moon and star on her diadem; and a mask under her arm. Not surprisingly, neither the breast nor the attributes are mentioned in the many written sixteenth-century responses to the sculpture. Following literary conventions, authors celebrated the beauty of the statue, with special praise for its pose. Already in Michelangelo's lifetime, the *Night* became a canonical figure for study in the art academies of Florence and Perugia.[18]

Three anomalies in the left breast of the *Night* were first noted by Stark: an obvious bulge to the breast contour medial to the nipple, a swollen nipple-areola complex, and an area of skin retraction on both sides.[19] In a living woman, these signs would indicate a large tumour, involving either the nipple itself or the lymphatics immediately below, and causing tethering and retraction of the skin on the opposite side of the nipple.[20] A dozen oncologists have concurred with this diagnosis of the *Night*.[21] The most prominent specialist, Gianni Bonadonna, identified the prominent tumour as 'T4b' in the standard staging system.[22] The lone dissenting voice was published by a surgeon who noted only one indentation.[23] An undergraduate student of computer science has clarified this detail.[24] Working from a three-dimensional scan of the statue, May Allen measured the indentations on both sides of the nipple. By sharpening the shadows, these features became even more evident. The presence of two distinct troughs, flanking the nipple, demonstrates that Michelangelo intended to carve these indentations. The question is why, but art historians have not addressed Stark's diagnosis.[25] In an extremely influential survey of Italian Renaissance art, first published in 1969, Frederick Hartt identified the *Night* as a mother, 'whose abdomen and breasts are distorted by childbirth and lactation', and this view still predominates in scholarly literature on the statue.[26] Hartt's interpretation must now be questioned, given that the left breast shows the physical signs of disease. Though nursing could lead to a swollen nipple, it would not cause a lump or skin retraction.

Modern viewers often mention that female breasts in Michelangelo's works look odd, though not for the reasons first mentioned by Stark. Like many of his Florentine contemporaries, Michelangelo usually shows breasts as 'freestanding', without the axillary tail of breast tissue that smooths the transition to the pectoral muscles.[27] But in striking contrast to contemporary norms, Michelangelo also shows the *Night* as unusually muscular. Taken together, these two points give many observers today the impression that female breasts were attached to a powerful male torso, though the hips clearly signal the body as female.[28] In any case, only the left breast of *Night* has what oncologists today identify as the physical signs of breast cancer. Most sixteenth-century copies and variations of the *Night*, in prints, drawings, paintings, and sculptures, correct the bulge, swelling, and retraction in the left breast. In contrast, a painting of *Night* by Michele Tosini (Rome, Galleria Colonna, Figure 1.7), from about 1560, includes all three anomalies.[29] They are not visible in the right breast, or in any of the other female figures sculpted, painted, and drawn by either Michelangelo or Tosini.

The questions typically asked about visual sources for Renaissance art help us evaluate Stark's retrospective diagnosis of the marble *Night*. First, we can inquire about when and where Michelangelo observed a breast tumour. It is extremely unlikely that he saw a drawing, print, painting, or sculpture with the fatal combination of a lump, swelling, and retraction. On the rare occasions that breast cancer appears in ancient, medieval, or early modern art, the images show only a lump, and none of these works exhibit the degree of accuracy found in the *Night*.[30] Michelangelo must have seen the tumour in a female body, and most probably in a living woman who was seated or standing. Though a large breast tumour would remain visible in a cadaver, the rapid loss of turgidity would make it very difficult to observe a swollen nipple and the skin retraction on both sides, especially in a supine body.

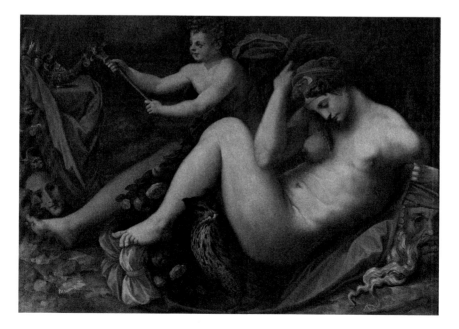

FIGURE 1.7 Michele Tosini, *Allegory of the Night*, c. 1560

Source: © Heritage Image Partnership Ltd/Alamy Stock Photo

Perhaps the artist's visual source was a female model, though we cannot determine when Michelangelo saw her. This could have been a few days or even several decades before carving the *Night*. Unfortunately, too many people still believe the old chestnut about Michelangelo not having access to female nudes. In a popular monograph on Michelangelo, Howard Hibbard wrote about the *Night* that 'her breasts, used and spent, became unwanted appendages, attached in an unanatomical fashion, and betraying Michelangelo's lack of interest in or even familiarity with the female nude'.[31] On the contrary, the left breast of the *Night* reveals the artist's knowledge about a specific detail he must have seen in a female body. Some scholars assume that Michelangelo based the entire figure of the *Night* on a man because one study for the left arm evidently reflects a male model.[32] Nevertheless, as the most famous artist of his day, Michelangelo had the same access to female models as his male contemporaries, such as Raphael and Lorenzo Lotto.[33] Pietro Aretino wrote that Sebastiano del Piombo used a prostitute as his model for various religious figures, and perhaps this was a common practice for artists.[34] In his autobiography, Benvenuto Cellini described in detail how in the 1520s his maidservant became his lover and model.[35] In his *Lives of the Artists*, Giorgio Vasari explained that the best way to acquire skill in drawing was 'to sketch men and women from life'.[36] Most scholars rightly ascribe to Michelangelo the study of a nude girl, seemingly drawn from life, for the *Entombment* (London).[37] At some point before he completed the *Night*, Michelangelo evidently saw another female figure, and perhaps a model, with the physical signs of breast cancer.

Michelangelo also carried out dissections, according to his contemporaries Vasari and Asciano Condivi, and perhaps he observed tumours in this context.[38] Modern scholars usually assume that Michelangelo dissected only male bodies, though one contemporary stated that Leonardo da Vinci had 'carried out dissections of more than 30 bodies, between male and female, of every age'.[39] Renaissance artists rarely if ever wielded a scalpel when they 'did an anatomy', much as they did not hold a trowel when they made buildings, but artists regularly made sketches at dissections.[40] At universities, guests were invited to attend these events; here they could see male, and more infrequently female, cadavers with all their imperfections.[41] The academic study of medicine focused primarily on male anatomy. The dissection of a woman appears in the celebrated frontispiece of Andreas Vesalius's *De humani corporis fabrica* (1543), but he does not discuss the female breast, and Alessandro Achillini mentions it only in passing in his *Anatomical Notes* (1520).[42] Vesalius aimed to describe a universal body, and anatomy textbooks do not show anomalies, such as deformities, injuries, or disease.[43] Of course, these were familiar to doctors from post-mortems that, at least since the fifteenth century, were regularly preformed in homes. When examining female corpses, doctors gave special attention to the reproductive system, including the breasts. At some point before he made the *Night*, Michelangelo probably witnessed the examination of a woman's corpse, and most probably, any features out of the ordinary would have caught his attention.

Turning to the second question in the analytical framework, when Michelangelo saw a breast tumour, what appearance did it have? On the one hand, if the woman was still alive, her tumour might have appeared just as we see in the *Night*, with the three anomalous features. If Michelangelo was in contact with the woman, he might have seen the development of her disease. Given the absence of effective treatment, the size of the tumour would have increased. On the other hand, if Michelangelo had studied the corpse of a woman who had died of cancer, she probably had multiple tumours. Some of these might have ulcerated, which presented artists with an easily recognizable sign of infirmity. Nevertheless, and in spite of the antique example of Pythagoras's *Lame Man*, neither Michelangelo nor Tosini ever represent open wounds in their works.

The recent article in *The Lancet Oncology* rightly noted that Tosini painted the left breast of his *Night* with a retracted nipple, a key detail that is not present in Michelangelo's marble.[44] The painter must have observed this feature in a living woman, presumably one with an advanced cancer. First, Tosini associated the appearance of the woman's tumour with the left breast of Michelangelo's statue. Second, the painter decided to elaborate on his artistic prototype, in order to clarify the representation of the disease. Significantly, most of the physical signs noted by modern oncologists in representations of *Night* by Michelangelo and Tosini are not discussed by pre-modern physicians. Renaissance texts did not provide a point of departure for the artists, and they did not set out to show a textbook example of cancer. Rather, both Michelangelo and Tosini decided to reproduce in art several of the physical signs they had personally observed in a woman.

Turning now to the third question about artists' sources, how was the lump in a woman's breast identified in the mid-sixteenth century? Michelangelo knew that the left breast he carved in the *Night* was different from every other he had seen in ancient and modern art. For modern oncologists, the details in Tosini's painting confirm the diagnosis of 'a malignant neoplasia'.[45] Though Renaissance artists would not have used modern terms, both Tosini and Michelangelo probably knew that their models were very ill. They would have identified the lump in the *Night* as a malady and probably called it 'cancer', the general term used for unnatural swellings. Some physical signs of the disease were well known in their day, when the Italian terms *cancro* and *cancaro* appear regularly in letters, stories, treatises, and convent records.[46] In one of their most famous miracles, Saints Cosmas and Damian amputated and replaced the ulcerated leg of a man, often described as cancerous.[47] These two doctors (*medici*) were the patron saints of the Medici family, and statues of them appear prominently in the New Sacristy. Among the many cures attributed to the Medici saints, there were even two cases of breast cancer.[48] These miraculous cures have no obvious bearing on the representation of breast cancer in the *Night* but help indicate that knowledge about the disease was widespread. In *City of God*, Augustine of Hippo even referred to 'cancer of the breast, a thing which doctors say cannot be cured by any kind of treatment.'[49]

How does the appearance of cancer fit into a broader understanding of the New Sacristy? We must first consider the most reliable interpretation of the tomb of Giuliano, provided by Michelangelo's friend and former student. According to Condivi, in his 1553 biography of the artist, the supine figures represent 'Day and

Night and, collectively, Time which consumes all'.[50] This concept corresponds perfectly to the first line of the poetic verses that Michelangelo penned on a sheet of drawings relating to the ducal tombs. Here the artist gives voice to his sculptures: 'Day and Night speak and say: "We with our swift course led Duke Giuliano to his death"'.[51] The enigmatic text then states that the duke took his revenge on Day and Night by shutting their eyes, thus depriving them of light. Michelangelo translated this concept into stone. In contrast to all of his other sculptures, Michelangelo did not indicate pupils in the figures of *Duke Giuliano*, *Duke Lorenzo*, *Day*, *Dusk*, and *Dawn*. These figures cannot see, and *Night* sleeps with closed eyes.[52] The uncarved eyes captured the essential nature of an infirmity. In a similar way, the poet Poliziano, whom Michelangelo knew well, invented the literary figure of 'Fever', daughter of the Night.[53] She holds a burning torch and snow, a literary allusion to the sensations of hot and cold experienced by the sick. In the New Sacristy, Michelangelo created a marmoreal allusion to blindness.

In the tomb of Duke Giuliano, Michelangelo represented sightless eyes and a lump on the breast of *Night*. To understand the latter, we can begin with two proposals, both firmly grounded in the visual and literary evidence, then move on to a couple of more speculative hypotheses. First, the artist linked the infirmity with night-time. In four sonnets dedicated to this theme, written immediately after he stopped working on the New Sacristy, Michelangelo gave a range of meanings to the night, from positive to neutral to negative.[54] As a result, scholars have selected different poems to defend their own interpretations of the *Night*. In a funerary chapel, combined with the sombre expression of the sleeping figure, the lump on the breast suggests that Michelangelo made an association between the end of the day and the end of life. This sculpted detail, clearly visible and intentional, represents an imperfection, more appropriate for the representation of a mortal figure than for a goddess or an allegory. Gods, with their perfect bodies, are eternal. The imperfection in the *Night* signals infirmity, and thus mortality. Though centuries had passed since Augustine, cancer remained 'firmly established in the popular consciousness as a cruel and fatal disease.'[55]

Second, early sources insist on the way that cancer eats into the surrounding flesh.[56] Since antiquity, and throughout the early modern period, the most common association with the disease was its corrosive quality.[57] In 1387, for example, the papal physician said that when cancer 'breaks out onto the surface of the breast and starts to ulcerate, [patients] die within a year or a year and a half, from the flesh being gnawed away.'[58] The perceived nature of cancer complements the central idea of the tomb, that Time consumes all, as expressed by Condivi. In the same passage, Condivi added a detail presumably provided by Michelangelo himself, given that the biographer never visited the chapel. In the tomb, Michelangelo had originally intended to carve a mouse, because 'this little creature is forever gnawing and consuming, just as time devours all things'.[59] He never included this feature but depicted *Night* as suffering from a consuming disease. She appears at the feet of Giuliano, who died after a long illness, as Michelangelo probably knew. One doctor described the Duke as 'exhausted and consumed', though of course he does not appear this way in the heroic sculpture.[60] To express, in a funerary chapel, the concept that time devours all things, Michelangelo included the physical signs of cancer, which devours all of its victims. In life, Night and Day ruled over the Duke, but now that Giuliano is dead, and transformed into a statue, they are subject to his revenge. Art, personified by the sculpture depicting Giuliano, triumphs over the powerful forces of Nature, represented by the Times of Day.[61]

Though this interpretation corresponds to the words written by Michelangelo and Condivi, and to the placement of the figures in the tomb, Michelangelo's powerful image of *Night* hardly indicates a consuming disease. As Pietro Aretino said of Michelangelo's *Venus*, she evinces 'the muscles of the male in the body of the female'.[62] For this artist, and throughout his career, muscles imply active movement: Michelangelo's powerful figures, both male and female, express agency.[63] His musclewomen might act for good, like Mary in the *Doni Tondo* (Florence), or for evil, like Eve in the *Temptation* on the Sistine Chapel (Vatican City). As we read in Michelangelo's own notes, the rapid movements of *Day* and *Night* caused the early death of Duke Giuliano. Though their robust body types do not express infirmity, many scientific texts expressed 'a profound discomfort with displaced gender attributes', such as one finds in masculine females.[64] Soranus of Ephesus, one of the most authoritative ancient medical sources on women, stated that 'the majority of those not menstruating are rather robust, like mannish and sterile women.'[65] He did not see this as problematic, but many authors from Michelangelo's day stated that the cessation of monthly periods could lead to severe illnesses, including cancer.[66] Doctors warned women suffering from cancer about the urgent need to restore menstruation and to avoid strenuous exercise.[67] Perhaps some early observers of the *Night* saw 'the muscles of the male in the body of the female' as potentially dangerous. Moreover, though her body does not convey illness, the lump in her breast certainly does.

Tosini clearly understood that the left breast of the *Night* exhibits a disease, given that he elaborated on this very feature in his painted copy. We can only wonder how many early observers noticed this detail and how they might have interpreted it, especially when seen in an otherwise powerful body. Already in the sixteenth century, Michelangelo was criticized for the cryptic features in his works. The protagonist of Ludovico Dolce's *Aretino* (1577) attacks Michelangelo because he 'does not want anyone to understand his inventions, apart from a small number of intellectuals'.[68] Hubert Günther probably exaggerates when he argues that Michelangelo was not very interested in having his iconography understood by viewers, given that he does not supply many iconographic clues,[69] but the New Sacristy offers a striking example of this phenomenon. The set of four figures representing the Times of Day is entirely unprecedented. The *Night* includes attributes, but as for the *Dawn*, *Day*, and *Dusk*, Raffaello Borghini has Bernardo Vecchietti say in *Il Riposo* (1584) that 'if the names that Michelangelo had for them were not already known, I do not know that any . . . would be able to be recognized'.[70] Vecchietti may have commissioned the four reduced versions of the Times of Day, recently attributed to Giambologna. In these alabaster copies, the artist reproduced the odd indentations on the breast of the *Night* and added attributions to the other three statuettes.[71] Of course, Michelangelo's works in the New Sacristy are unfinished, but even his completed works often included features that defy simple explanations. Condivi wrote about Michelangelo's Vatican *Pietà* that 'some object to the mother as being too young in relation to the Son'.[72] Here, as in the *Night*, the physical features of a tomb statue defy the expectations of Renaissance and modern observers.

Today we think of cancer as a hidden disease. In the opening of her celebrated study *Illness as Metaphor*, Susan Sontag wrote that cancer 'fills the role of an illness experienced as a ruthless, secret invasion'.[73] Often there are no clear physical signs on the body surface of the destruction below, and so we learn about cancer from sophisticated examinations and then take treatment which reduces or eliminates tumours. In Michelangelo's day, however, the disease was identified only when it advanced enough to leave physical signs that one could see or feel.[74] All medical sources concurred on 'the unanimous and categorical verdict, that "confirmed" or advanced malignancies were incurable'.[75] The diagnosis of cancer was often interpreted as a death sentence, and Michelangelo provided observers of the *Night* the three signs necessary to identify the disease.

Cancer and melancholy

Michelangelo, Tosini, and their contemporaries must have asked themselves why a woman would have a lump on her breast. The standard explanation, and not only from doctors, was an accumulation of black bile. The excess of this humour indicated melancholy, according to popular and scholarly texts in the medieval and early modern period. Since antiquity, innumerable medical and literary sources have explored the four temperaments, each related to one of the humours: choleric, sanguine, phlegmatic, and melancholic. Modern scholars of the Renaissance often associate melancholy with inspiration and the dark moods of creative geniuses. This view was already promoted in the late fifteenth century by the philosopher Marsilio Ficino, the son of a physician.[76] According to Vasari, Michelangelo depicted a melancholic figure on the Sistine ceiling: the prophet Jeramiah. When he worked in the New Sacristy, Michelangelo certainly had his own melancholy on his mind. In a letter of 1525, we learn that he had attended a dinner party 'from which I had great pleasure, because I came a little out of my melancholy'; during the same period, Paolo Giovio referred to Michelangelo as a melancholic in his *Life* of the artist.[77]

Learned doctors at the time distinguished between two related conditions with similar names. On the one hand, an excess of black bile led to the melancholic temperament; those suffering from this condition, like Michelangelo, were known as (complexionate) melancholics. On the other hand, corrupt or burnt black bile led to the disease of melancholia, which could result in cancer. According to Avicenna, among the most respected medical authorities throughout the sixteenth century and beyond, cancer is 'a melancholic aposteme caused by black bile that is burned by choleric matter'.[78] In Michelangelo's day, Falloppio explained that the pain from a tumour was caused by 'an acrid, malignant exhalation derived from the melancholy matter, which begins to putrefy'.[79] These sources derive from Galen's seminal chapter on 'Diseases of the Black Bile'. Here the Greek physician explained that according to Hippocrates, a depressive mood renders patients melancholic; the disease of melancholia 'comes from worry and grief combined'.[80] According to many early modern texts, 'complexionate melancholics were deemed to be especially susceptible to the disease of melancholy.'[81] All agreed that melancholy afflicted both the body and the soul. Michelangelo, known for his admiration of Dante, could have read about this in Cristoforo Landino's annotated edition of the *Divine Comedy*, published in Florence in 1481: 'Given that the melancholic humour is the excrement of the blood, we understand the Sluggish to be stuck in the slime, that is, in sadness and melancholy'.[82] Pre-modern case reports on cancer often noted that negative emotions 'made the humoral flow stagnate and impeded the natural secretions'.[83]

This overlap between the temperament and disease of melancholy leads to my first speculative hypothesis about the New Sacristy. Michelangelo included the representation of a breast tumour in the *Night* because he associated the abnormal growth with the melancholic temperament. If we see the *Night* as a melancholic, many details about the statue fall into place. Vasari described this funerary figure as exhibiting 'not only the stillness of one sleeping, but the pain and melancholy (*malinconia*) of one who has lost a great and honoured possession'.[84] In Renaissance art, melancholy is often represented by a figure with a downcast gaze, head in hand.[85] Michelangelo might have even seen the most famous representation of Melancholy, an engraving by Albrecht Dürer, which was created just a few years before the *Night*. In the New Sacristy, Michelangelo included a prominent but rather mysterious mask under the left arm of *Night*, quite close to the diseased breast. Perhaps this refers to nightmares, which were often associated with the melancholic temperament.[86] The frightening mask, downcast gaze, head-in-hand gesture, and breast tumour might all work together to indicate the melancholic nature of the *Night*. Of course, Michelangelo could have depicted the melancholy temperament in a positive light, as he had already done in the Sistine Chapel. In the New Sacristy, however, the artist evidently decided that the female figure should express 'pain and melancholy'. But how to show these qualities in a sleeping figure? Perhaps Michelangelo based the pose of the *Night* on the melancholic female figures who represent conquered cities on ancient coins.[87] The figure of *Night*, according to Vasari, appears in the state of mourning.[88] Many period sources included worries and sadness among the extrinsic causes of cancer, itself caused by a blockage of black bile.[89] Perhaps Michelangelo wanted to suggest a link between the *Night*'s melancholy, caused by the death of Duke Giuliano, and the infirm stagnation of humoral flow, expressed by a lump in her breast.

The association between *Night* and melancholy contributes to a new reading of the two ducal tombs. For each, Michelangelo planned two allegorical Times of Day and conceived of these as a series of contrasts in genders, poses, and ages.

In the tomb of Duke Giuliano de' Medici, the powerful male figure of *Day* turns towards the viewer and reclines on a sarcophagus near the older figure of *Night*. In the tomb of Duke Lorenzo de' Medici, the awakening and youthful *Dawn* rises from her bed, and the older, enervated *Dusk* descends towards the ground. My second speculative hypothesis is that the set of four temperaments offered Michelangelo a point of departure for the appropriate body types and poses exhibited by the four reclining figures. Certainly, the temperaments were associated with four well-established characteristics, as well as the four times of day, four ages of man, and four seasons. Already in the Sistine Chapel, four of the prophets and sibyls seated on the easternmost section of the vault reflect the four humoral types, as observed by Piers Britton.[90] Daniel, in his prime, is choleric, the elderly Persian sibyl is phlegmatic; the mature Jeremiah is melancholic; and the youthful Libyan sibyl is sanguine. Britton argues convincingly that many Renaissance figures exhibit these four types, in a wide variety of contexts, and occasionally, as in the Sistine Chapel, within the same work.

In their fundamental study of melancholia, Raymond Klibansky, Erwin Panofsky, and Fritz Saxl presented one set of traditional associations for the four temperaments: youth with sanguine, prime with choleric, middle age with melancholic, and old age with phlegmatic.[91] Elsewhere in the volume, in a footnote, they also made a very tentative proposal about Michelangelo's Times of Day, based in part on the gender of the sculpted figures: *Dawn* is sanguine, *Day* is choleric, *Dusk* is melancholic, and *Night* is phlegmatic.[92] Nevertheless, Michelangelo clearly represented *Night* as younger than *Dusk*, but older than both *Dawn* and *Day*. If we use the apparent age of the Times of Day as a key factor in determining their temperaments, just as it was for Britton's identification for prophets and sibyls in the Sistine Chapel, we arrive at a new set of identifications. Youth is sanguine *Dawn*, a statue which reflects her harmonious nature. Prime is choleric *Day*, whose powerful body and twisting pose seem to indicate an irascible nature. Middle age is melancholic *Night*, who appears to be mourning, a state that indicates her gloomy nature. Old age is phlegmatic *Dusk*, whose tired body evinces his lethargic nature. Michelangelo created four very different poses and moods for the four Times of Day. These map perfectly on the four temperaments, and thus the four main natures and humoral types.

In 1999, after Stark wrote to Katharine Park about his initial observations about the *Night*, the renowned historian of medicine asked, 'How does a modern diagnosis of breast cancer help or not help us to understand mid sixteenth-century ideas of diseases of the breast?'[93] Two decades later, we have a few answers. The tumour in the *Night* may help identify a melancholy temperament. This would indicate a conflation in the understanding of the disease and temperament of melancholy during the period and underline the importance of emotional states for the Renaissance conception of cancer. Even if readers reject the proposed linkage between the *Night* and melancholy, all can see the lump in her left breast. In the mid-sixteenth century, Tosini studied it as well, and to judge from his painted copy of Michelangelo's *Night*, he considered this imperfection to be a tumour. Tosini added a detail, the retracted nipple, found in cancer patients but not in the original sculpture. As a symbol of consuming disease, the tumour in Michelangelo's *Night* reinforces the message of the tomb, as described by his student Condivi: Time consumes all. This interpretation complements the recent research of Christian Kleinbub on how the gestures and appearance of several figures by Michelangelo reflect the artist's understanding of internal organs.[94] In the *Night*, Michelangelo sought to establish a balance between two goals. On the one hand, he aimed to create an extraordinarily idealized body, one described by his contemporaries as beautiful. On the other hand, Michelangelo wanted to indicate an imperfection, the lump, that some original observers in the Medici funerary chapel could identify with a fatal illness. The artist's decision to represent a tumour in order to express a symbolic message enriches our understanding of sixteenth-century views about diseases. An analysis of the *Night* also indicates the potential use of retrospective diagnoses. These much-maligned studies by physicians can help historians of both art and medicine to better understand the visual sources used by past authors and artists.

Notes

1   I am most grateful to Dr James Stark, oncologist, for teaching me about breast cancer, and to the many Renaissance scholars who provided extensive comments on drafts for this paper: Monica Azzolini, Silvia Catitti, Victor Coonin, Christian Kleinbub, John Paoletti, Sharon Strocchia, and Michael Stolberg.

2   For two surveys of such studies in relation to Italian Renaissance art, see Gorkey, 'Medical issues'; and Strauss and Marzo-Ortega, 'Michelangelo and medicine'.

3   Stark and Nelson, 'The breasts of "Night"'. The title is inaccurate: though Stark is an oncologist, the artist was not.

4   Bendersky, 'Remarks on Raphael's *Transfiguration*'.

5   Bianucci and others, 'Earliest evidence'. Their conclusions reached a much great public thanks to many online articles, including Daley, 'Earliest images'; and Traverso, 'Earliest depiction'.

6   For these observations I thank Rossella Lari, paintings conservator at Galleria dell'Accademia (Florence), who noted that similar revisions appear throughout Maso's *Fortitude*, such as where he broadened the torso.

7   Interview with two authors, Raffaella Bianucci and Antonio Perciaccante, in Rikken, 'Researchers find evidence'.

8   Pliny, *Natural History*, 170–71. The term *ulceris* was translated as *malore* by Lorenzo Ghiberti, *I commentarii*, 61 (1. 6. 27), and not included in Cristoforo Landino's translation: Pliny, *Historia naturale* [373].

9   Plutarch, 'On the study of poetry', 198 (18c). In *Quaestiones convivales* (5. 1. 2), he explained that in the bronze statue *Jocasta*, the artist added silver to create the appearance of someone on the verge of death.

10 For four versions of the relief, often attributed to Antonio Lombardo, see Schulz, *Giammaria Mosca*, 65–67, 239–42, without reference to Plutarch.

11 See Demaitre, 'Medieval notions of cancer'; Skuse, *Constructions of Cancer*; and Stolberg, 'Metaphors and images of cancer'. For earlier studies, see Rather, *Genesis of Cancer*; and De Moulin, *A Short History*.

12 Stolberg, 'Metaphors and images of cancer', 74.

13 As translated and discussed in Rather, *Genesis of Cancer*, 18. Similarly, the prominent medieval French surgeon Guy de Chauliac, described 'a hard, round, veined, darkish, fast-growing, restless, warm, and painful tumour'; as quoted in Demaitre, 'Medieval notions of cancer', 611.

14 Arrizabalaga, 'Problematizing retrospective diagnosis'.
15 For the importance of flow, including specific reference to breast cancer, see Pomata, 'The obstructed body'.
16 For temperaments and complexions, see Groebner, *Who Are You?*, 119–25.
17 For discussion, documentation, and extensive bibliography, see Nelson, 'Poetry in stone'.
18 For drawings and prints made in Florence, see Rosenberg, 'Artists as beholders'; for a plaster copy by Vincenzo Danti in Perugia (which shows the anomalies in the breast); see Marta Onali in Conforti, in *Vasari*, 188.
19 Stark and Nelson, 'The breasts of "Night"'. In 1983, Rosenzweig, 'Disease in art', described the appearance of the left and right breasts as 'typical of an advanced carcinoma', but this reference to both mammary glands led Pluchinotta, *I secoli della senologia*, 22, to question his diagnosis. For a reference to the 'tumorous (?)' breasts of the *Night*, see Howard, 'Eros, empathy, expectation', 90, and 116 note 97, without reference to the above-mentioned studies.
20 Bickley and Hoekelman, *Bates' guide*, 352; Stark in Bland and Copeland, *The Breast*, ii (with reference to the *Night*).
21 Gros, 'Cancer ou laideur?'; and Bianucci and others, 'Earliest evidence'. The diagnosis was accepted by Daniela Berni, in a paper given at the conference *La diagnostica invasiva in senologia: dalla citologia alla chirugia* (Florence, 13–14 October 2000), in letters sent in 2000 to the *New England Journal of Medicine* by Giovanni Bonadonna, Jonathan L. Meakins, Roland M. Strauss, and Helena Marzo-Ortega, and in a letter sent to the author in 2007 by Luigi Cataliotti, former president of the Italian Society of Senology.
22 Gianni Bonadonna, letter to the author, 2007. He published the statue as an example of breast cancer in *La cura possibile*, 109.
23 Landor, 'The question of breast cancer'. He also argued that the lump is not large and that other figures in the chapel have oddly shaped breasts, but one of his examples is the breastplate of Duke Giuliano.
24 Allen, 'The left breast'.
25 The one exception is a chapter on the *Night* co-authored by an oncologist and an art historian (my former student); see Arena and Bastianich Manuali, *Reflections of the Breast*, 57–70, esp. 66: 'Her left breast appears to be afflicted with signs of malignancy, signs that are glaring clear to oncologists visiting the New Sacristy'.
26 Hartt and Wilkins, *History of Italian Renaissance Art*, 554. For similar views, see Balas, *Michelangelo's Medici Chapel*, 69; Campbell, 'Fare una Cosa Morta', 609; and Ruvoldt, 'Michelangelo's dream', 98–99.
27 For artistic representations of female breasts, see Yalom, *History of the Breast*; Pluchinotta, *Incanto*; and Ashton, *Interpreting Breast Iconography*.
28 See Nelson, 'The Florentine *Venus*'.
29 See the entry by Jonathan K. Nelson in Falletti and Nelson, *Venere e Amore*, 167.
30 See Arena and Bastianich Manuali, *Reflections of the Breast*; Pluchinotta, *I secoli della senologia*. For an unconvincing identification of breast cancer in Raphael, see Espinel, 'La Fornarina', and the dissenting opinion by Baum, 'La Fornarina'; both authors are physicians.
31 Hibbard, *Michelangelo*, 191.
32 See, for example, Even, 'Heroine as hero'.
33 Bernstein, 'The female model'.
34 Aretino, *Sei giornate*, 311.
35 For a discussion of Caterina, Cellini's model and mistress, see Vickers, 'The mistress in the masterpiece'.
36 Vasari, *Le vite*, I, 114.
37 For the drawing (Paris, Louvre, n. 726), see Hirst, *Michelangelo*, 63–64.
38 For discussion, see Jacobs, '(Dis)Assembling: Marsyas', esp. 440–41; Ciardi, *Il corpo trasparente*, 2000.
39 For this passage, written by Antonio de Beatis in 1517, see Nelson, *Leonardo*, 17.
40 See Jacobs, '(Dis)Assembling: Marsyas'; and Azzolini, 'Exploring generation'.
41 Park, *Secrets of Women*, 211–15; and Park, 'Holy autopsies'.

42 Park, *Secrets of Women*, 161–221.

43 Siraisi, 'Vesalius'; Carlino, *Books of the Body*. For Vesalius on women's bodies, see Park, *Secrets of Women*, esp. 219–21.

44 Bianucci and others, 'Earliest evidence', 167.

45 As quoted in Rikken, 'Researchers find evidence'.

46 Owens, 'The Cloister', documents how frequently references to breast cancer appear in chronicles kept by nuns, e.g. in Riccoboni, *Life and Death*, 96.

47 Spicer, 'European Perceptions', 44–45.

48 Festugiere, *Sts. Come et Damien*, 100–03. A fifteenth-century Florentine booklet mentions the cancer miracles but does not refer to the location of the disease in the body; see Giannarelli, *Cosma e Damiano*, 183.

49 Augustine, *City of God*, 220–21.

50 Condivi, *Life of Michelangelo*, 67.

51 The text continues: 'And it is only just that he has his revenge for this, as he does. And the revenge is this: that we, having brought about his death, he, thus dead, has deprived us of light and, with closed eyes, has sealed our own, which no longer shine upon the earth. What might he have done with us, if he had continued to live?' For the Italian text, see Buonarroti, *Rime*, 24; for discussion, see Nelson, 'Poetry in stone'.

52 Gilbert, 'Texts and contexts', 404.

53 For this 1473 elegy, see Perosa, 'Febris'.

54 For dating and discussion, see Nelson, 'Poetry in stone'; and Residori, 'Michelangelo e la notte'.

55 Skuse, *Constructions of Cancer*, 115; for a similar view, see Demaitre, 'Medieval notions of cancer', 630.

56 Stolberg, 'Metaphors and images of cancer', 57–59.

57 Skuse, *Constructions of Cancer*, esp. 61–73 (chap. 3: 'It Is, Say Some, of a Ravenous Nature': Zoomorphic Images of Cancer).

58 See Jean of Tournemire, quoted in Wallis, *Medieval Medicine*, 345.

59 Condivi, *Life of Michelangelo*, 67; Panofsky, 'The Mouse'.

60 For the letter of 1515, see Pieraccini, *La stirpe de'Medici*, I, 222. Another contemporary wrote that Giuliano appeared 'la maninconia al naturale'; for the 1511 letter, see Schwarzenberg, 'Glovis', 165 n. 92. No contemporaries suggested that Giuliano died of cancer.

61 For this interpretation, see Campeggiani, 'La "vendetta" del duca Giuliano', followed by Nelson, 'Poetry in stone', 464.

62 For the quote, see discussion in Jacobs, 'Aretino and Michelangelo', 59, 63; and Nelson, 'Florentine *Venus*', 38–39.

63 For Michelangelo's muscular women, see Nelson, 'Poetry in stone', 467–69.

64 Cadden, *Meaning of Sex Differences*, 212.

65 Soranus, *Gynecology*, 26; for discussion, see Green, *The Transmission of Ancient Theories*, 29–30, 93.

66 Stolberg, 'A woman's hell', 406, 411.

67 Skuse, *Constructions of Cancer*, 48, 101, 182 n. 28.

68 Dolce, *Aretino*, 167. I thank Diletta Gamberini for this reference.

69 Günther, 'Michelangelo's works in the eyes of his contemporaries', 71–75.

70 Borghini, *Il Riposo*, 66.

71 Rosenberg, 'Michelangelo's new sacristy', 38–55. The left breast of the *Night* is oddly shaped, but from reproductions, it is not clear if there is a lump. The same is true of the cast after Tribolo's lost model of this figure; see Kryza-Gersch in Koja and Kryza-Gersch, *Shadows of Time*, 160–61, cat. no. 16.

72 Condivi, *Life of Michelangelo*, 24.

73 Sontag, *Illness as Metaphor*, 5.

74 Though some early modern sources mention 'occult' or 'hidden' cancer, they usually refer to a tumour that could be felt below the surface of the skin; see Stolberg, 'Metaphors and Images of Cancer', 56 n. 25; Demaitre, 'Medieval notions of cancer', 616–17; and Wallis, *Medieval Medicine*, 345.

75 Demaitre, 'Medieval notions of cancer', 638.
76 See the classic study by Klibansky, Panofsky, and Saxl, *Saturn and Melancholy*; and Radden, *The Nature of Melancholy*, 88–94.
77 For both quotes, and discussion, see Britton, 'Mio malinchonico'. On Michelangelo as a 'Divine Melancholic', also see Hetherington, *Melancholy Figures*, 28–76.
78 Demaitre, 'Medieval notions of cancer', 612. In a well-known medical text, John of Gaddesden defined cancer as 'a melancholic disease which causes a tumour'; see Demaitre, 'Medieval notions of cancer', 618 n. 36. This volume was republished in Pavia in 1492, in an edition aimed at medical students. On the linkage between black bile, melancholy, and cancer, also see Skuse, *Constructions of Cancer*, 31–36, 99–100.
79 See Rather, *Genesis of Cancer*, 18.
80 As translated and discussed in Radden, *The Nature of Melancholy*, 67, 68.
81 Gowland, 'The problem of early modern melancholy', 98.
82 Cited from the commentary to *Inferno* (7. 123), as found in the Dartmouth Dante Project.
83 Stolberg, 'Metaphors and Images of Cancer', 62. By way of example, he cited the account of a woman whose sadness led to the development of a fatal breast cancer.
84 Vasari, *Vite*, vi, 58, 'conoscendosi non solo la quiete di chi dorme, ma il dolore e la malinconia chi chi perde cosa onorata e grande'. In his otherwise invaluable essay on '(Hu)moral Exemplars', Britton incorrectly states (184) that 'Vasari did not comment on the mood or complexion of the figure of Night'. He also errs (186) in affirming that 'Vasari explicitly describes the figure of Dawn . . . as melancholy'; in reality Vasari wrote that she can 'free the soul of melancholy' (fare uscire il maninconico dell'animo).
85 Ceccarelli Pellegrino, 'Iconografie "Malinconiche"'.
86 The mask has been associated with nightmares but not with melancholy; for the mask, see Paoletti, 'Michelangelo's masks', and Dempsey, *Inventing the Renaissance Putto*, 220–23.
87 See Ward, *Hidden in Plain Sight*, 74, though I do not find his political interpretation convincing. For citations of these captive figures in Italian Renaissance art, see Giuliano, 'Germania capta'.
88 Schiesari, *Gendering of Melancholia*, 12, argues that the frequent representation of the melancholia temperament by a female figure 'functions as a metaphor of male sorrow'.
89 Demaitre, 'Medieval notions of cancer', 619.
90 Britton, 'The four humors', 27–28.
91 Klibansky, Panofsky, and Saxl, *Saturn and Melancholy*, 10–11.
92 Klibansky, Panofsky, and Saxl, *Saturn and Melancholy*, 369–70 note 304. They explained that 'Steinmann's suggestion of equating Michelangelo's Hours of the Day with the temperaments can be maintained, if at all, by following the traditional literary correlation of the hours of the day with the four humours'. Steinmann, *Das Geheimnis der Medicigraeber*, had identified *Night* with sanguine, *Dawn* with melancholic, *Day* with choleric, and *Dusk* with phlegmatic.
93 Letter of Katharine Park to James Stark, 1999.
94 See Kleinbub, *Michelangelo's Inner Anatomies*, e.g. his excellent chapter on Michelangelo's *Venus and Cupid*, 83–102.

Bibliography

Primary sources

Aretino, Pietro, *Sei giornate. . . .*, ed., Giovanni Aquilecchia (Bari: Laterza, 1969).
Augustine, *City of God*, vol. 7, books 21–22, trans., William M. Green (Cambridge, MA: Harvard University Press, 1972).
Bocchi, Francesco, *The Beauties of the City of Florence: A Guidebook of 1591*, ed. and trans., Thomas Frangenberg and Robert Williams (London: Harvey Miller Publishers, 2006).

Borghini, Raffaello, *Il Riposo*, ed. and trans., Lloyd H. Ellis (Toronto: University of Toronto Press, 2007).

Buonarroti, Michelangelo, *Rime*, ed., Matteo Residori (Milan: Oscar Mondadori, 1998).

Condivi, Ascanio, *The Life of Michelangelo*, trans., Alice S. Wohl, ed., Hellmut Wohl, 2nd edn (University Park, PA: Pennsylvania State University Press, 1999).

[Dolce, Ludovico] in Roskill, Mark W., *Dolce's Aretino and Venetian Art Theory of the Cinquecento* (New York: New York University Press, 1968).

Ghiberti, Lorenzo, *I commentarii: biblioteca nazionale centrale di Firenze, II, I, 333*, ed., Lorenzo Bartoli (Florence: Giunti, 1998).

Pliny the Elder, *Historia naturale di C. Plinio Secondo: tradocta di lingua latina in fiorentina per Christophoro Landino fiorentino al Serenissimo Ferdinando Re di Napoli*, trans., Cristoforo Landino (Venice: Nicolas Jenson, 1476).

Pliny the Elder, *Natural History*, vol. 9, books 33–35, trans., H. Rackham (Cambridge, MA: Harvard University Press, 1952).

Plutarch, 'On the study of poetry', trans., D. A. Russell, in D. A. Russell and Michael Winterbottom (eds), *Classical Literary Criticism* (Oxford and New York: Oxford University Press, 1998), 192–216.

Riccoboni, Bartolomea, *Life and Death in a Venetian Convent: The Chronicle and Necrology of Corpus Domini, 1395–1436*, ed. and trans., Daniel Bornstein (Chicago: Chicago University Press, 2000).

Soranus' Gynecology, trans., Owsei Temkin (Baltimore: Johns Hopkins University Press, 1991).

Vasari, Giorgio, *Le vite de' più eccellenti pittori scultori e architettori: nelle redazioni del 1550 e 1568*, ed., Rosanna Bettarini and Paola Barocchi, 11 vols (Florence: Sansoni and SPES, 1966–97).

Secondary sources

Allen, May, 'The left breast of Michelangelo's statue of Night' (online project for 'The Science of Art', Stanford University, 7 February 2001), https://graphics.stanford.edu/courses/cs99d-01/projects/breast-of-night/breast-of-night.htm.

Arena, Francis and Tanya Bastianich Manuali, *Reflections of the Breast: Breast Cancer in Art through the Centuries* (New York: Brick Tower Press, 2013).

Arrizabalaga, Jon, 'Problematizing retrospective diagnosis in the history of disease', *Asclepio*, 54, 1 (2002), 51–70.

Ashton, Anne M., *Interpreting Breast Iconography in Italian Art 1250–1600* (unpublished PhD dissertation, University of St. Andrews, 2006).

Azzolini, Monica, 'Exploring Generation: A Context to Leonardo's Anatomies of the Female and Male Bodies', in Alessandro Nova and Domenico Laurenza (eds), *Leonardo da Vinci's Anatomical World: Language, Context and 'Disegno'* (Venice: Marsilio Editore, 2011), 79–97.

Balas, Edith, *Michelangelo's Medici Chapel: A New Interpretation* (Philadelphia: American Philosophical Society, 1995).

Baum, Michael, 'La Fornarina does not have breast cancer', *The Journal of Surgery*, 2, 1 (2004), 48–49.

Bendersky, Gordon, 'Remarks on Raphael's *Transfiguration*', *Source: Notes in the History of Art*, 14, 4 (1995), 18–25.

Bernstein, Joanne G., 'The female model and the Renaissance Nude: Dürer, Giorgione, and Raphael', *Artibus et Historiae*, 13, 26 (1992), 49–63.

Bianucci, Raffaella and others, 'Earliest evidence of malignant breast cancer in Renaissance paintings', *The Lancet. Oncology*, 19, 2 (2018), 166–67.

Bickley, Lynn S. and Robert A. Hoekelman, *Bates' Guide to Physical Examination and History Taking*, 7th edn (Philadelphia, New York, Baltimore: Lippincott, 1999).

Bland, Kirby I. and Edward M. Copeland (eds), *The Breast: Comprehensive Management of Benign and Malignant Disorders*, 4th edn, 2 vols (Philadelphia: Elsevier, 2009).

Bonadonna, Gianni, *La cura possibile: nascita e progressi dell'oncologia* (Milan: Raffaello Cortina, 2001).

Britton, Piers Dominic, 'The four humors on the Sistine Chapel Ceiling', *Source. Notes in the History of Art*, 21, 3 (2002), 26–31.

Britton, Piers Dominic, '(Hu)moral Exemplars: Type and Temperament in Cinquecento Painting', in Jean A. Givens, Karen M. Reeds, and Alain Touwaide (eds), *Visualizing Medieval Medicine and Natural History, 1200–1550* (Aldershot and Burlington: Ashgate, 2006), 177–204.

Britton, Piers Dominic, '"Mio malinchonico, o vero . . . mio pazzo": Michelangelo, Vasari, and the problem of artists. Melancholy in Sixteenth-century Italy', *The Sixteenth Century Journal*, 34 (2003), 653–75.

Cadden, Joan, *Meanings of Sex Difference in the Middle Ages: Medicine, Science, and Culture* (Cambridge and New York: Cambridge University Press, 1995).

Campbell, Stephen J., '"Fare una Cosa Morta Parer Viva": Michelangelo, Rosso, and the (un)divinity of art', *Art Bulletin*, 84 (2002), 596–620.

Campeggiani, Ida, 'La "vendetta" del duca Giuliano: ipotesi michelangiolesche', *Humanistica*, 6, 2 (2011), 87–94.

Carlino, Andrea, *Books of the Body: Anatomical Ritual and Renaissance Learning*, trans., John Tedeschi and Anne C. Tedeschi (Chicago: University of Chicago Press, 1999).

Ceccarelli Pellegrino, Alba, 'Iconografie "Malinconiche" dell immaginario rinascimentale', in Luisa Rotondi Secchi Tarugi (ed.), *Malinconia ed allegrezza nel Rinascimento* (Milan: Nuovi orizzonti, 1999), 129–58.

Ciardi, Roberto Paolo, *Il corpo trasparente: modalità di iconografia anatomica in Michelangelo* (Florence: Olschki, 2000).

Conforti, Claudia, ed., *Vasari, gli Uffizi e il duca* (Florence: Giunti, 2011).

Daley, Jason, 'Earliest images of breast cancer found in Renaissance paintings', *Smithsonian Magazine* (2 March 2018), www.smithsonianmag.com/smart-news/ealiest-images-breast-cancer-found-renaissance-paintings-180968325/.

Demaitre, Luke E., 'Medieval notions of cancer: malignancy and metaphor', *Bulletin of the History of Medicine*, 72, 4 (1998), 609–37.

De Moulin, Daniel, *A Short History of Breast Cancer* (Boston: Martinus Nijhoff, 1983).

Dempsey, Charles, *Inventing the Renaissance Putto* (Chapel Hill: University of North Carolina Press, 2001).

Espinel, Carlos H., 'La Fornarina: breast cancer or not?', *The Lancet*, 361, 9363 (2003), 1130–32.

Even, Yael, 'The heroine as hero in Michelangelo's art', *Woman's Art Journal*, 11, 1 (1990), 29–33.

Falletti, Franca and Jonathan K. Nelson, eds, *Venere e Amore. Michelangelo e la nuova bellezza ideale/Venus and Cupid. Michelangelo and the New Ideal of Beauty* (Florence: Giunti, 2002).

Festugiere, André-Jean, *Ste. Thècle, Sts. Come et Damien, Sts. Cyr et Jean* (Paris: Saint Georges, 1971).

Frangenberg, Thomas and Robert Williams, eds, *The Beholder: The Experience of Art in Early Modern Europe* (Aldershot: Ashgate, 2006).

Giannarelli, Elena, ed., *Cosma e Damiano dall'Oriente a Firenze* (Florence: Meridiana, 2002).

Gilbert, Creighton, 'Texts and contexts of the Medici Chapel', *Art Quarterly*, 34, 4 (1971), 391–409.

Giuliano, Antonio, 'Germania capta', *Xenia*, 16 (1988), 101–14.

Gorkey, Sefik, 'Medical Issues in Italian Frescoes', in Luciana Caenazzo, Lucia Mariani, and Renzo Pegoraro (eds), *Medical Humanities: Italian Perspectives* (Padua: CLEUP, 2015), 43–53.

Gowland, Angus, 'The problem of early modern melancholy', *Past & Present*, 191 (2006), 77–120.

Green, Monica Helen, *The Transmission of Ancient Theories of Female Physiology and Disease through the Early Middle Ages* (unpublished PhD dissertation, Princeton University, 1985).

Groebner, Valentin, *Who Are You?: Identification, Deception, and Surveillance in Early Modern Europe*, trans., Mark Kyburz and John Peck (New York: Zone Books, 2007).

Gros, Dominique, 'Cancer ou laideur? L'énigme du sein gauche de La Nuit par Michel-Ange', *Oncologie*, 8, 7 (2006), 696–700.

Günther, Hubertus, 'Michelangelo's works in the eyes of his contemporaries', in Frangenberg and Williams, *The Beholder*, 53–86.

Hartt, Frederick and David G. Wilkins, *History of Italian Renaissance Art: Painting, Sculpture, Architecture*, 7th edn (Upper Saddle River: Pearson Prentice Hall, 2007 [1st edn, 1969]).

Hetherington, Anna, *Melancholy Figures: From Bosch to Titian* (unpublished PhD dissertation, Columbia University, 2013).

Hibbard, Howard, *Michelangelo* (New York: Penguin Books, 1985).

Hirst, Michael, *Michelangelo and His Drawings* (New Haven and London: Yale University Press, 1988).

Howard, Seymour, 'Eros, empathy, expectation, ascription, and breasts of Michelangelo (A prolegomenon on polymorphism and creativity)', *Artibus et Historiae*, 22, 44 (2001), 79–118.

Jacobs, Fredrika H., 'Aretino and Michelangelo, Dolce and Titian: *Femmina, Masculo, Grazia*', *Art Bulletin*, 72, 1 (2000), 51–67.

Jacobs, Fredrika H., '(Dis)Assembling: Marsyas, Michelangelo, and the Accademia Del Disegno', *Art Bulletin*, 84, 3 (2002), 426–48.

Kleinbub, Christian K., *Michelangelo's Inner Anatomies* (University Park, PA: Penn State University Press, 2020).

Klibansky, Raymond, Erwin Panofsky, and Fritz Saxl, *Saturn and Melancholy: Studies in the History of Natural Philosophy Religion and Art* (New York: Basic Books, 1964).

Koja, Stephan and Claudia Kryza-Gersch, eds, *Shadows of Time: Giambologna, Michelangelo and the Medici Chapel* (Munich: Hirmer, 2018).

Landor, John, 'The question of breast cancer in Michelangelo's *Night*', *Source: Notes in the History of Art*, 25, 4 (2006), 27–29.

Nelson, Jonathan K., 'The Florentine *Venus and Cupid*: a heroic female nude and the power of love', in Falletti and Nelson, *Venere e Amore*, 26–63.

Nelson, Jonathan K., *Leonardo e la reinvenzione della figura femminile: Leda, Lisa e Maria* (Florence: Giunti, 2007).

Nelson, Jonathan K., 'Poetry in stone: Michelangelo's Ducal Tombs in the New Sacristy', in Robert W. Gaston and Louis A. Waldman (eds), *San Lorenzo: A Florentine Church* (Florence: Villa I Tatti, The Harvard University Center for Italian Renaissance Studies, 2017), 450–80.

Owens, Sarah E., 'The cloister as therapeutic space: breast cancer narratives in the early modern world', *Literature and Medicine*, 30, 2 (2012), 319–38.

Panofsky, Erwin, 'The mouse that Michelangelo failed to carve', in Lucy Freeman Sandler (ed.), *Essays in Memory of Karl Lehmann* (New York: Institute of Fine Arts, 1964), 242–51.

Paoletti, John T., 'Michelangelo's masks', *Art Bulletin*, 74, 3 (1992), 423–40.

Park, Katharine, 'Holy autopsies: saintly bodies and medical expertise, 1300–1600', in Julia L. Hairston and Walter Stephens (eds), *The Body in Early Modern Italy* (Baltimore: Johns Hopkins University Press, 2010), 61–73.

Park, Katharine, *Secrets of Women: Gender, Generation, and the Origins of Human Dissection* (New York: Zone Books, 2006).

Perosa, Alessandro, 'Febris: a poetic myth created by Poliziano', *Journal of the Warburg and Courtauld Institutes*, 9 (1946), 74–95.

Pieraccini, Gaetano, *La stirpe de'Medici di Cafaggiolo. Saggio di ricerce sulla trasmissione ereditaria dei caratteri biologici*, 3 vols (Florence: Nardini, 1986 [1st edn, 1924–25]).

Pluchinotta, Alfonso Maria, ed., *Incanto e anatomia del seno* (Milan: Charta Edizioni, 1997).

Pluchinotta, Alfonso Maria, *I secoli della senologia dal bisturi al farmaco* (Milan: Zeneca, 1995).

Pomata, Gianna, 'The obstructed body: popular images of sickness and healing', in *Contracting a Cure: Patients, Healers, and the Law in Early Modern Bologna*, trans., Gianna Pomata (Baltimore: Johns Hopkins University Press, 1998), 129–39.

Radden, Jennifer, ed., *The Nature of Melancholy: From Aristotle to Kristeva* (Oxford: Oxford University Press, 2001).

Rather, L. J., *The Genesis of Cancer: A Study in the History of Ideas* (Baltimore: Johns Hopkins University Press, 1978).

Residori, Matteo, '"E a me consegnaro il tempo bruno": Michelangelo e la notte', in Paolo Grossi and Matteo Residori (eds), *Michelangelo: Poeta e artista* (Paris: Istituto italiano di cultura, 2005), 103–23.

Rikken, Maarten, 'Researchers find evidence of breast cancer in Renaissance paintings', *ResearchGate* (13 February 2018), www.researchgate.net/blog/post/researchers-find-evidence-of-breast-cancer-in-renaissance-paintings.

Rosenberg, Raphael, 'Artists as beholders: drawing after sculptures as a medium and source for the experience of art', in Frangenberg and Williams, *The Beholder*, 103–22.

Rosenberg, Raphael, 'Michelangelo's New Sacristy and Vecchietti's Criticism of the Missing Attributes of the Times of the Day', in Koja and Kryza-Gersch, *Shadows of Time*, 38–55.

Rosenzweig, William, 'Disease in art: a case for carcinoma of the breast in Michelangelo's La *Notte*', *Paleopathol Newsletter* [Richmond, Va. Paleopathology Club], 41 (1983), 8–11.

Ruvoldt, Maria, 'Michelangelo's dream', *The Art Bulletin*, 85, 1 (2003), 86–113.

Schiesari, Jiuliana, *The Gendering of Melancholia: Feminism, Psychoanalysis, and the Symbolics of Loss in Renaissance Literature* (Ithaca: Cornell University Press, 1992).

Schulz, Anne Markham, *Giammaria Mosca called Padovano: A Renaissance Sculptor in Italy and Poland* (University Park, PA: Pennsylvania State University Press, 1998).

Schwarzenberg, Erkinger, 'Glovis, impresa di Giuliano de' Medici', *Mitteilungen des Kunsthistorischen Institutes in Florenz*, 39, 1 (1995), 140–66.

Siraisi, Nancy, 'Vesalius and human diversity in De *humani corporis fabrica*', *Journal of the Warburg and Courtauld Institutes*, 57 (1994), 60–88.

Skuse, Alanna, *Constructions of Cancer in Early Modern England: Ravenous Natures* (London: Palgrave Macmillan UK), 2015.

Sontag, Susan, *Illness as Metaphor* (New York: Farrar, Straus and Giroux, 1978).

Spicer, Joaneath, 'European Perceptions of Blackness as Reflected in the Visual Arts', in Joaneath Spicer (ed.), *Revealing the African Presence in Renaissance Europe* (Baltimore: Walters Art Museum, 2012), 36–60.

Stark, James J. and Jonathan K. Nelson, 'The breasts of "Night": Michelangelo as oncologist', *New England Journal of Medicine*, 343, 21 (2000), 1577–78.

Steinmann, Ernst, *Das Geheimnis der Medicigraeber Michel Angelos* (Leipzig: Hiersemann, 1907).

Stolberg, Michael, 'Metaphors and images of cancer in early modern Europe', *Bulletin of the History of Medicine*, 88, 1 (2014), 48–74.

Stolberg, Michael, 'A woman's hell? Medical perceptions of menopause in pre-industrial Europe', *Bulletin of the History of Medicine*, 73 (1999), 408–28.

Strauss, Roland M. and Helena Marzo-Ortega, 'Michelangelo and medicine', *Journal of the Royal Society of Medicine*, 95, 10 (2002), 514–15.

Traverso, Vittoria 'The earliest depiction of breast cancer, in Renaissance paintings', *Atlasobscura* (28 February 2018), www.atlasobscura.com/articles/breast-cancer-renaissance-paintings.

Vickers, Nancy, 'The Mistress in the Masterpiece', in Nancy K. Miller (ed.), *The Poetics of Gender* (New York: Columbia University Press, 1986), 19–41.

Wallis, Faith, ed., *Medieval Medicine: A Reader* (Toronto: University of Toronto Press, 2010).

Ward, James O., *Hidden in Plain Sight: Covert Criticism of the Medici in Renaissance Florence* (New York: Peter Lang, 2019).

Yalom, Marilyn, *A History of the Breast* (New York: Ballantine Books, 1997).

2

THE LANGUAGE OF MEDICINE IN RENAISSANCE PREACHING

Peter Howard

Introduction

Health, infirmity, and healing were intertwined in the theological and devotional language—textual, visual and oral—of fifteenth-century Florence. In the Brancacci Chapel of the Church of the Carmine, for example, the dramatic, innovative rendering of the scenes from St Peter's life both drew the imagined devotees into a narrative which reached back into biblical history and also effectively connected them to the present with familiar local figures, current clothing, and Florentine streetscapes. Noteworthy is the prominence given to scenes that represent infirmity and healing: the healing of the cripple in Jerusalem and the raising of Tabitha from the dead in Joppa (Masolino); and Peter healing the sick with his shadow (Masaccio).[1] These representations are juxtaposed with the visual images of Peter preaching: in Jerusalem on the day of Pentecost, in Rome, and in Antioch.[2]

In terms of texts—written or 'oral' (often the artefacts that presaged sermons or remained after their delivery)—it is striking the degree to which medical metaphors and language abounded.[3] This is not surprising in a world where sickness, death, and plague were constant companions and they appear frequently in the *exempla* that were derived from the Bible—the constant companion of not just preachers but also thinkers (including humanists) in the period.[4] Indeed, a survey of the biblical text by way of a concordance, the usual recourse of preachers in the period when developing a sermon, indicates the extensive array of such metaphors: sixty-three occurrences of variations on *infirmitas* (infirmity), fifty-five of *peste* (plague), seventy-six of *lepra* (leprosy), and numerous occurrences of forms of *claudus* (lame). *Curare*—in the sense 'to heal'—occurs 114 times.

Images like the frescoes of the Brancacci Chapel or those illustrating the miracles of preacher-saints, as we will see, provide access to a 'medicalized culture'.

They allow us to attempt to see with a 'period eye' and to hear 'with a period ear' and not only to trace how infirmity was represented at that time but also to probe the culture more deeply. I draw attention to the prominent role of the language and metaphors of infirmity in fifteenth-century Florence by examining their appearance and use in sermons from the period.[5] There the stark reality of physical illness meant that it was readily harnessed for discourses of meaning or persuasion and gives us access to a theological understanding of experience. My contribution to 'representing infirmities' argues that there was a complex interplay between spiritual and bodily health. The way they interconnected, moreover, was not simply at the level of rhetorical ploy but at a fundamental conceptual and cognitive level. In other words, the metaphors of infirmity, health, and healing were more than merely figurative or ornamental. They shaped thinking and perception.

I begin with a discussion of a way of thinking about metaphor and language in the period before turning to the 'health and well-being' dimension of the culture of preaching on the basis of the sermon culture of fifteenth-century Florence.

Illness and metaphor

In her *Illness as Metaphor* (1978), Susan Sontag urges resistance of the idea of illness as metaphorical thinking as avoiding the reality of illness and infirmity. Her enquiry, however, serves conversely to sharpen our focus on the role of metaphors of illness in historical discourse where they imbue sometimes banal social perception with new urgency. As Sontag bluntly notes:

> Everyone who is born holds dual citizenship, in the kingdom of the well and in the kingdom of the sick. Although we all prefer to use only the good passport, sooner or later each of us is obliged, at least for a spell, to identify ourselves as citizens of that other place.[6]

Inhabitants of Renaissance Florence, in these terms, were as likely to identify with the kingdom of the sick and so with the threat of mortality, rather than with the kingdom of the well. The wealthy merchant Giovanni Rucellai, for example, remarks in his diary (*zibaldone*) that 'every person knows his own infirmities and the privations of his own body', including how to maintain health and happiness in the world, and the dispositions and inclinations to different moral and emotional behaviours predicated on the different humours.[7] For Florentines (and early moderns in general) the earthly and the heavenly worlds were perceived as permeable, without the fixed boundaries that developed in later centuries. But how did they put language on the experience, and to what degree did that language confront or hide the realities to which metaphors points?

As a way of thinking about language and metaphor in the period, along with the world to which language gives access, Stephen Greenblatt's formulation provides a helpful approach. Florentines in the fifteenth century, profoundly aware as they were of the power of language, would have found his formulation perspicacious:

> In any culture there is a general symbolic economy made up of the myriad signs that excite human desire, fear and aggression. Through their ability to construct resonant stories, their command of effective imagery, and above all their sensitivity to the greatest collective creation of any culture—language— literary artists are skilled at manipulating this economy.[8]

If this paragraph were to be re-written and 'preachers' and/or 'painters' included with 'literary artists', we not only valorize the importance of language in relation to culture but also have some idea of what preachers and artists in this period were trying to achieve: to communicate a transformative message by being attentive to texts and language, by telling compelling stories (what they referred to as *exempla*), and by creating metaphors and images that gripped the imagination and lingered in the mind. This accords with how *exempla* were described by Humbert of Romans towards the very beginning of the period characterized by the preaching of the friars: they were found by people to be 'more moving than mere words; they are also easier to grasp and make a deeper impression on the memory, and many people find them more enjoyable to listen to, so that the sheer pleasure of them attracts some people to come to sermons'.[9]

In addition, *exempla* functioned as more than illustrative anecdotes; they also served to structure and render immediate what might otherwise be remote and obscure. An *exemplum*, or string of *exempla*, could bear the weight of a discourse of complex ideas, making them accessible and memorable.[10] Moreover, they added human weight to what could seem abstract and remote by stirring the emotions, persuading, praising or blaming, imprinting on the memory—all different aspects of the rhetorical art.[11] They were to be remembered and in a sense anchored the different parts of a sermon for the hearer.

The *exemplum* was the key device which allowed the preacher to adjust spontaneously to the mood, needs, and expectations of hearers clustered around the pulpit. The autograph sermon texts of Antoninus of Florence, for instance, show just how porous and adaptable sermons were. They include such strategically placed self-instructions as: 'Descend to the practical with examples and conclude as soon as possible etcetera', or 'elaborate the subject matter and come down to the particulars and practicalities and conclude as soon as possible'.[12] This provided the framework for inserting the sort of metaphors associated with health and well-being in the period.

This approach also had implications for the way in which the texts of sermons connect to society, especially in terms of the medical metaphors which are our concern here. In what way and to what extent can a sermon be said to relate to a particular world? Mark Pattison, in the mid-nineteenth century, was cautious: 'The pulpit does not mould the forms into which religious thought in any age runs, it simply accommodates itself to those that exist. For this reason, because they must follow and cannot lead, sermons are the surest index of prevailing religious feeling of their age'.[13] The notion of 'accommodation' is more mitigated in an exemplary study of Bernardino of Siena as a preacher of peace, which concludes with a concise articulation of the problem of how sermons relate to the worlds which produce them: '[Bernardino's] preaching did not mirror social reality, but did identify pervasive cultural patterns and the hopes and fears which surrounded them'.[14] Preachers can be seen as both reflecting and responding to influences which were making themselves felt or noticed within the particular society. But because preachers thought and articulated their discourse self-consciously on or around fragments of scriptural texts, what they spoke was often articulated through codes which were commonly understood within the culture in question, and so meaning could often turn on the counterpoint of biblical types and biblical phraseology. The medium itself was often a part of the message. This could often mean that there was a gap between what the preacher intended to convey and what he was taken to mean by his audience, especially since, in a Wittgensteinian way, the preacher could not control chains of associations set off in the minds of hearers.[15] Mention of 'infirmity', 'health', 'illness', 'doctor', and 'plagues' could spark a train of associations. Such metaphors—as individual words or embedded in *exempla*—did not simply refer or illustrate but worked actively in the minds of both speaker and listener. In short, the language of preachers functioned both as mirror and agent and helps us understand the way in which religion and the experience of infirmity and well-being intermingled in the period.

The preacher as physician to the body politic

These *exempla* were embedded in a broader public discourse. To understand the importance of the sermon in the medieval and early modern period, one first has to firmly resist modern expectations, in order to appreciate the degree to which preaching gives access to the linguistic, and therefore conceptual and cultural capital (to adopt Bourdieu's phrase) of the city.[16] Preaching was anything but peripheral. A claim for its centrality is grounded in an expansive understanding of the role of sermons in fifteenth-century Florentine society, where preachers produced theologies that meshed with the constantly changing circumstances of the urban environment—political, social, and cultural. The paradigmatic humanist Leon Battista Alberti, for example, wrote of citizens flocking to piazzas to hear preachers and to be enticed by them 'to denounce vice for virtue, and ignorance for an understanding of things noble.'[17]

Approaching the representation of infirmity through the language of the preacher has a methodological point. It provides one way of liberating 'infirmity' and related words which may be enveloped in our own contemporary usage and our own culture's assumptions—as highlighted by Sontag. In a society in which 'all their activities, every day, are saturated with religion' (to borrow from Lucien Febvre), sermons hold out the possibility of allowing us to catch the particular weight and emanation of a word in its precise historical context.[18] They allow us to begin to wrench words free from their later accretions and, in terms of the theme under discussion here, to explore how Christian attitudes towards the body, infirmity, and disease were beginning to change in this seminal age at the cusp of the late medieval and early modern worlds.

The link between societal expectations and an understanding of the role of the preacher in caring for the good of the body politic, expressed in medicalized language, is well illustrated by a text penned by Poggio Bracciolini, dated *c.* 1427. This sophisticated bibliophile, historian, social critic, papal secretary, and eventual chancellor of Florence had a complex attitude to the friars that were so much a part of the city's social and religious life: for him, in one of his accounts, in their theatricality, they resembled apes more than preachers.[19] Preachers are criticized, too, in *De avaritia*, his incisive perception of the social and moral forces surrounding wealth and its importance for the city. The treatise starts in a general way, criticizing contemporary preachers for their failure in the social world of the Italian city, with his interlocutors discussing how they are more concerned with 'the plaudits of the crowd', rather than being concerned with 'troubled souls' and the real concerns of the populace.[20]

His text illustrates the significant role of sickness as metaphor in the period and how the figure of the physician translated to the role of the preacher in relation to the social body of the city.

[Cencio:]	. . . we still can't find a single person who has been the least improved by the effect of their sermons. This is so for one reason especially, namely, that they do not adapt their words to curing the infirmities that vex our minds. . . . If they were to imitate the method of good physicians, all their labour would bear some fruit. For when doctors are summoned to sick people, they carefully examine the nature of the person and the power of the disease so that they may more correctly effect a cure. But these preachers who are charged with the salvation of souls—unless they diligently scrutinize and examine in what way each person is infected with vice and furnish them aid—can talk long and hard, and still they will not be able to help any more than an ignorant physician can cure a disease.[21]
[Bartolomeo:]	. . . avarice and lust. . . . These are, so to speak, the two cruellest plagues that infect the human race. They never really leave anyone unstained, and since they require the gravest remedies, they are never easily cured.[22]
[Bartolomeo, quoting Vergil:]	'. . . nor any fiercer plague of divine wrath'[. . . .] Thus, if you will consider carefully what I have just

said, you will judge that avaricious monsters of the human race, who should be removed from among us and dispersed elsewhere like the filthiest refuse of the cities, so that they will neither sicken us with their stench nor infect us with their contagion.[23]

Here, the skill and practice of the physician function to highlight the role and necessary skill of the preacher and sermon in relation to the body politic and the salvation of souls. The language of disease, illness, contagion, and plague pervades the text and gives it its power. The expectation here is that preachers would identify and remedy the cankers of the individual soul and thereby society at large. Implied is the relationship between the individual souls of citizens and the good of the whole and the role of the preacher in identifying and remedying the disease.

Preaching and the preacher as doctor

Bracciolini's text implies failure. Contrary to his claim, skilled preachers—and Florence had hundreds of them across the fifteenth century as contemporary records attest—did adapt their words to curing the infirmities that vexed their hearers' minds. The body served as a powerful metaphor for Florentine society in the theological thinking of preachers in the period. For Antoninus, a figure central to the preaching and theological culture of fifteenth-century Florence, the ancient image of 'the body' was fundamental and expressed the meaning and values of communal existence amid changing circumstances, including the therapeutic function of preacher and confessor.[24] The metaphor, grounded in his reading of both St Paul's letter to the church at Corinth and the letter to the Emperor Trajan attributed to Plutarch, had the power to connote a rich conceptual complexity encompassing both the ecclesiastical world and the ordering of society as a whole.[25] Preachers and 'honest clerics' were central to providing for 'the direction, consolation and physical needs of the citizens'—meaning the body corporate of the republic as a whole.[26]

The language of the body and, and by extension, of the doctor provides a way of accessing an understanding of how in the period intervention in the spiritual world was by way of the body—the site of spiritual well-being or ailment. The boundary between the bodily and the spiritual was porous. The type of 'honest cleric' referred to in the preceding quotation was well summed up six decades later by Erasmus: a priest that was 'honest, an expert in law and an authority on the Holy Scriptures, among other things', could, 'like an expert doctor . . . collect the symptoms of the disease [of sin], yet to be diagnosed, thereby eradicating sin'.[27] Writing more than five decades earlier, Antoninus included an entire section on the 'priest as doctor' when writing on the vocation of doctors and their failings. Here he affirms that 'the doctor of the soul is the priest' and that 'the medicine of the spirit is penance and the other sacraments'.[28] As a doctor, the priest applies medicine to the infirm or dying. Just as the doctor of the physical body itself, if he is able, cures by means that are agreeable and gentle (*per suavia et levia*), so also does the priest. And like the doctor who, when it is necessary, cauterizes with iron and the like, so too does the priest resort to harsh measures. Antoninus, therefore, transfers the idea from the bodily to the spiritual at a conceptual and cognitive level. Spiritual doctors, by means of the medicine of penance and confession, do not just heal the infirm but can revive those dead in sin. This is not their own doing, however; it is a result of the power of God: the grace of God revives by means of the sacrament of confession. And for that reason, it should be a guiding principle for the doctors of the body that when they visit the sick, before they attempt to initiate a cure, they summon the doctors of souls, that is, priests, for making confession. In so doing they would be providing better for health of the soul and of the body. And while many infirmities are incurable for physicians of bodies however much they do, by means of the spiritual doctor and spiritual medicine, all lethargy is cured, and as often as happens so many times.[29] In this mode of thought, health, infirmity, and healing were intertwined with the theological and devotional pastoral and medical practice of the day. Doctor-priests were considered as necessary as physicians for curing infirmity.[30]

Such modes of integrating the languages of medicine and theology applied to both the individual body and the social body as a whole. Antoninus himself was celebrated in a *laude* as someone who 'healed the clergy, and kept the city from corruption' and as a saintly intercessor: 'You who now dwell in heaven, please send grace to our city, save it from war, famine, and all the things harmful to feeble mankind, so that a righteous mind may thrive in a healthy body'.[31] Powerful preachers could effect the miraculous healing of the body. As contemporary records attest, the famous preachers in this period were also popular 'santi' (saints) and 'beati' (blessed), as Ida Magli, in a path-breaking study, once pointed out.[32] Correlative to such reputations were attestations to their miracle-working powers in relation to the sick and infirm. For example, an entire section of the canonization testimonies of Antoninus was devoted to the miracle-working powers, both in life and also by way of relics associated with him after his death, including handkerchiefs and a walking stick. Those who touched his body during the days before it was placed in a tomb were healed; for example, Matteo di Giovanni de' Ciacchi, a woolworker with a withered right arm, was healed when he placed it on Antoninus's hands.[33]

These associations between the holiness of famous preachers and healing infirmities extend to Bernardino da Siena, Bernardino da Feltre, Beato Alberto da Sarteano, Beato Giacomo della Marca, S. Antonio da Padova, Beato Giovanni da Capistrano, and S. Vincent Ferrer. The link between 'holy preacher' and miraculous healing is characteristic of the testimonies gathered for canonization proceedings and was often translated into visual representations—visual mnemonics of this understanding, as we find in the iconography of Antoninus and Bernardino.[34]

Infirmity could be turned to support a preacher in his art. He could use a self-representation of infirmity as a rhetorical ploy to identify himself with his hearers and to make his audience complicit in his own right and authority to be heard. The advent of a preaching based more on the epideictic mode favoured by humanist orators facilitated this rhetorical development. The process of the articulation and the affirmation of identity involved a reciprocal recognition between both preacher and audience, a recognition and awareness invariably reflected in the proem of sermon texts. Fra Bartolomeo Rimbertini, humanist and accomplished rhetorician and regarded as the greatest preacher of his day (though neglected in the historiography), in a sermon before Pius II and the papal court began with an epideictic flourish of self-praise as one well equipped to 'paint' (*depingere*) with words. For our theme of representation of infirmities, it is his adroit juxtaposition of his own physical state that serves to beg the tolerance of his hearers: his already grey head, his furrowed brow (though, he adds, of a man of honour), his dewlap hanging down, the slowing of blood in his chest, his flagging memory, and an intellect tarnished with rust. The infirmities of age serve to recommend him to his audience.[35]

For preachers who travelled on business for their religious orders, plague and injury were a constant companion. The Augustinian preacher Timotheo Maffei defends his failure to preach according to the expectations of the populace by referring to an injury that has caused lameness and impeded his mobility but also the '[malevolent] summer heat and of the surging plague'.[36] The sacristan's records of the church of San Lorenzo in Florence state occasions when the preachers commissioned by the chapter were indisposed and unable to ascend the pulpit. On one occasion, the sacristan noted that he had to deliver the sermon himself. Another famous Augustinian preacher at Santo Spirito, Francesco Mellino, was known as *Zoppo*—the lame.[37] This means that preachers were continually negotiating, and articulating, the same quotidian issues of health and infirmity as their listeners.

Because the preacher's art was to engage with the particulars of their hearers' lives, illness and infirmity and the threat thereof surface in texts written by preachers. Early on in his preaching career, Antoninus, for instance, warns that it was the vice of *luxuria* that led God to send plagues and illnesses to the Jews.[38] When he comes to his account of his own times in his *Summa historialis*, Antoninus discusses the recurrent outbreaks of plague in the city, in particular the one of 1448–49, during which he administered the sacraments and distributed alms to the poor. In the very next sentence of this account, the plague as event becomes plague the metaphor and the Fraticelli are figured as heretics 'infected with the leprosy of error'.[39] They are contagion to be eradicated for the good of the social and ecclesial body. Florence itself was vigilant in this regard, with only occasional extreme remedies, such as the execution of Giovanni Cani da Montecatini in 1450.[40]

Issues surrounding health and wellness in the period are further revealed in sermon texts which treat medicine and magic. When preaching on superstition, Antoninus's sermon moves from divination to the more ambiguous topic of medicine and magic. People want healing and bodily health, which turns them towards enchantments and superstition. Proper medicine, Antoninus reminds his audience, is effective only by way of nature.[41] Natural magic was generally associated with medicine and was not regarded as involving the invocation of diabolical forces, even though it sought to obtain the services of the celestials to encourage good health. Profane magic, by contrast, was seen to depend on the worship of demons.[42] It is aligned with pride and hints of the sin of Adam and so enters into spheres proper to God: 'it is unlawful because it is mixed with vanity'. He focuses on the operations of specific magical acts, and their implicit origins, not just the outcomes of the diffuse system of common magic that was part and parcel of ordinary life, clerical as well as lay.[43] Antoninus follows Augustine's *De doctrina Christiana* to the effect that all such arts of futile, damaging superstition must be scorned and avoided by Christians since they derive from a destructive compact between men and demons. Even though some people put their trust in enchantments because they seem to work, anything to do with the occult derives from the devil.

> If in such matters there is some untruthfulness or some impressed letter or skin of a foetus (*charta non nata*—unborn skin), or propitious time or mask— all these things are illicit and false and whoever follows superstitions of this kind, if they are clearly brought about by invoking the devil, is clearly a mortal sin, unless however one did not know them to be evil and still followed them.[44]

This last, excusing phrase indicates that the boundaries between black and white magic were not necessarily hard and fast.[45]

Medicalizing preaching with biblical language

It is not surprising that biblical language surrounding infirmity, disease, and healing provided the preacher with a ready set of verbal representations—*exempla*—that tapped into hearers' most significant bodily experiences in order to recover an understanding of their spiritual state and its demands in a way that was easier to grasp and made a deeper impression than merely doctrinal exhortations. Moreover, such language was embedded in a medicalized understanding of the condition of the human race, the conceptualization of which derived from the biblical humus of the culture itself.

When introducing his discussion of the sacraments in his influential *Summa theologica*, Antoninus, as an adept preacher, opens the treatise as he would any of his sermons, with a verse from a Psalm (106. 20): 'He sent his word, and healed them ('sanavit eos'): and delivered them from their destructions'.[46] The text, predictably, is interpreted with a Christological inflection. As with his sermons, Antoninus structures his chapter by fragmenting his biblical theme into three parts and developing an argument around each. Indeed, in view of its structure, the text itself most likely derives from a sermon.[47] In the second part, dilated around 'sanavit eos', which is exegeted to mean 'men who are sick and infirm' ('homines infirmos'), he goes on to say that it is 'the obligation of doctors to cure the sick'. From this it follows, for Antoninus, that because the human race is ill with an incurable disease, the Lord himself came to heal the contrite heart (*ut medere contritus corde*), pointing to a verse of Isaiah (61. 1) and linking it to a key verse in St Matthew's gospel (9. 12), though twisting the meaning slightly: the text 'They that are in health need not a physician, but they that are ill' is exegeted to exclude Christ, who assumed the flesh of the human race, from the contagion of original sin, and who himself therefore had no need of a physician. For Antoninus, quoting Augustine, Christ is the great physician who comes from on high for the whole human race, which is struck down with a great sickness (*magnus aegrotus*). Christ then becomes the Good Samaritan, who looks to the needs of the traveller laid low by robbers and who tends his wounds with oil and wine. These 'humble materials' are then appropriated into a discussion that revolves around the pride of the first parents and how Christ humbled himself as a servant upon a cross (Philippians 2) in punishment for our iniquities. The discussion foregrounds the lowly materials of the sacraments—bread, wine, and oil—which become the sacraments for the health of the soul: 'The most High hath created medicines out of the earth, and a wise man will not abhor them'.[48] The medicines which Christ instituted are the seven sacraments.[49]

The most telling language of representation of infirmity, as a metaphor in the context of Christ who redeems, is leprosy. Reference to leprosy made sermons practical in a variety of ways and added rhetorical force to move hearers to action. Most often leprosy functions as a metaphor for sin. The example of Namaan the leper, washed clean in the Jordan, is not simply an *exemplum* in the preaching of Jesus himself but becomes the metaphor of the purification of the soul. Leprosy stands for the contagion of mortal sin, cleansed by the water of Baptism.[50] In some instances, the example of the baptism of Constantine is drawn in and linked to the baptism of Namaan.[51] In other sermons the account of the lepers taking themselves to the high priest to show that they have been cured is the example for motivating all penitents to take themselves to the priest as proof of their cleansing in confession. Across a range of sermons, leprosy is drawn into preaching on avarice, simony, omission, presumption, and even the nature of the soul itself.

Another preacher, Fra Mariano da Gennezzano, uses a graphic *exemplum* around leprosy to explain why Christ is redeemer of all people. A mother has a certain infection in her body and gives birth not just to one child infected with leprosy but two. She goes to a doctor and begs for medicine so that she will give birth to a child like all others in the world who are healthy. For the human race infected with original sin, 'the medicine is the grace of God coming through the Virgin'.[52] So Christ is her redeemer and the redeemer of all others.[53]

At other times, preachers used examples drawn from biblical accounts of cures to make doctrinal points about the miracle of God acting in the world in much the same way as the biblical text itself does. For example, the Dominican Marcus Petri de Succhiellis, preaching to the nuns at the Monastery of Santa Lucia in Pistoia in 1494, strings together biblical *exempla* from the life of Christ, including cures from leprosy, the lame walking, the blind seeing, to support his exposition in his sermon *De diuinitate et humanitate christi*.[54] In other sermon passages, *exempla* revolve around health and the cure of the ills of the soul and resistance to vice by way of *medicamenta*—the medicines and unguents of the sacraments.[55]

Biblical *exempla* of infirmity were by far the most common amongst the majority of preachers in Florence in the fifteenth century, but they were no less telling or urgent for that amongst citizens equipped to think and interpret the Bible in a sophisticated way from an early age. Bernardino, however, was more inclined to insert *exempla* drawn from 'the documents of life' (*documenta vitae*). In one sermon, for example, leprosy became the metaphor for the contagion of sodomy:

> Mind you that if you associate with a leper, immediately you will get stricken with [that disease] . . . One contaminated person is sufficient to contaminate in one shop a hundred or more people. All it takes is one rotten apple . . . if you go to the coal-seller's shop, you can expect to come away blackened'.[56]

The preacher's message about the perceived social impact of behaviour would not have been lost to his hearers. The sins of the individual body infect the body social.

Health to the body

Antoninus was central to the generation of 'public theology' in Renaissance Florence. Not only did he himself contribute to the culture that was generated from the pulpit with his own voice, one which was particularly powerful by the time he became archbishop of the city, but he also was producing, and having disseminated by way of Vespasiano da Bisticci's bookshop, key texts which were a source of language and ideas for preachers and confessors and of guidance for the city's literate populace.[57] Especially pertinent is his tract on the vocation of physicians (*De statu medicorum*). This belongs to the *de statu* (concerning the way of life) genre of address that had become a mainstay of mendicant preaching. This text gives insight into the medicalized culture of the day and so into the way in which health, infirmity, and healing were intertwined in theological and devotional language. Antoninus's tract evinces attention to a tradition that reached back into the biblical text (as we have seen) but also gestured to the important medical texts that were the medical culture's point of reference.

The introduction to title seven of the third volume of Antoninus's *Summa theologica* itself is constructed on the model of a sermon. The theme, characteristically, is drawn from a psalm, here Psalm 87 verse 11: 'Wilt physicians raise to life, and give praise to thee?'[58] Antoninus responds: 'Just as Glorious God created remedies so he himself is the first author coming forth with skills and medical knowledge', based on another biblical text (Ecclesiasticus 38. 4): 'The most High hath created medicines out of the earth, and a wise man will not abhor them'.[59] His discussion then turns to the 'natural intellect' with which God has illuminated men for investigating herbs and the like and experiencing their effects of the first authors of medicine. Intriguingly, he refers to Apollo, the ancient god of healing, truth, and prophecy, and his son, Aesculapius, the god of medicine, who Hippocrates, Galen, and Avicenna, the ancient writers of the art of medicine, and others thereafter, followed.[60] Applying treatments created by God to the infirm, the physician thus cures the sick as the instrument of God or nature. Antoninus continues his discussion along lines already discussed earlier: holy men are physicians. The gospel writer is addressed thus by St Paul: 'Luke, the most dear physician, saluteth you' (Colossians 4. 14). The importance of physicians for Antoninus is reflected in his reference to Augustine's rule, where it tells the religious that when there is uncertainty about the infirmity of one of the brothers, a physician should be consulted and his counsel followed in so far as they are able.

In this text there is what might be referred to as a 'slippage', and it is evident how ideas of medicine and healing structure thoughts about the purity of the body of the Church. Antoninus recounts the legend of St John the Evangelist in the baths, where he sees his contemporary gnostic heresiarch Cerinthus bathing and so counsels his companions to flee lest they be corrupted by bathing in the same waters as he is an enemy of the truth.[61] He refers his *exemplum* to Gratian's *Decretum*, where it occurs in the course of the discussion on excommunication.[62] What is therefore reflected here is the language of contamination of the social/ecclesial body. The exact relationship that Antoninus envisages this to have with his discussion of physicians seems oblique, except insofar as physicians are committed to truth rather than being its avowed enemies. They have, therefore, an eye to the well-being of the body, both individual and social.

Conclusion: preaching as a therapy of consolation

There was a natural relationship between religion and a sense of medical well-being pervading Renaissance Florentine society. The culture of preaching in Florence in this period was seen to promote the well-being of the body social. It was also to be a means through which the wounds of the social body were healed. The language clustering around such understandings had an affective import beyond just moral exhortation. Alberti envisaged preaching as a public event that ennobled citizens through lofty things that were heard. Leonardo Bruni, the chancellor of Florence in 1429, saw preachers such as Antoninus of Florence as bringing consolation to the urban populace: Rather than countenance Antoninus's transfer to Naples, he sought to have him remain in Florence 'for the consolation of the whole city'.[63] In a similar way, correspondence initiated by 'the magnificent *signoria* of Siena' seeking the services of a famous friar envisages the impact of preaching in the same way: Fra Antonio da Rimini was pleasing to the people, and brought a particular 'consolatio'.[64] This word peppers letters inviting preachers, with phrases like 'how great consolation for our people' ('quantam consolationem populo nostro') and 'in consolation of this city' ('in huius urbis consolatione'). Indeed, important sermons often bear the title 'Consolatio'.[65] This word is to the fore when Antoninus, in the fourth volume of his *Summa*, discusses what a republic should provide for 'the direction, consolation, and physical needs of the citizens'.[66]

Preachers skilled in the art could evoke feelings that loitered even when the words were forgotten or could not be re-expressed. As one Florentine remarked of a preacher towards the end of the 1480s: '[Fra Niccolò] said in his sermon many beautiful, and indeed, very beautiful things which I don't know how to express, nor do I remember exactly'.[67] The emotional impact of preachers' words lingered, healing the wounds of the body social, even when the words themselves were not remembered. So preaching culture itself was seen to be a way of healing the wounds of the social body. The language adopted by preachers was more than metaphoric or analogic. It often served to structure modes of thought, and the preaching event itself often served as a medical-therapeutic instrument by bringing peace and consolation.

For Susan Sontag, illness is not a metaphor, and the most truthful way of regarding illness is to resist metaphoric thinking. For fifteenth-century Florentines, however, the infirmity of the body was a way of accessing and understanding not only the health or otherwise of the soul but also of the self and society at large. Preachers, with their command of the Bible's imagery, re-presented the values and experience of a world where citizenship of the kingdom of infirmity was a stark, ever-present reality but was one which had a theological edge of meaning, linking the meaning of present existence to the passport to the eternal kingdom. It points to a Renaissance devotional world, which promoted the miracle as the ultimate metaphor, and indeed hoped for reality, of healing.

Notes

1 Acts of the Apostles 3. 1–10; 9. 36–43; 5. 15–16.
2 The artist's source for the juxtaposition of images is most likely one of the preacher's habitual resources, viz. Jacopo da Voragine's *Legenda Aurea*, filtered through the *Lectionarium antiquum* of the Carmine. See Howard, 'Womb of memory', 191–94.
3 For the notion of texts as 'oral artefacts', see Howard, *Aquinas and Antoninus*, 8.
4 On lay religious literacy, see Corbellini and Hoogvliet, 'Artisans and religious reading'; Howard, *Experiencing Religion*, chapter 4.
5 This study is much influenced by several of the articles from *Studies in Late Antiquity* 2, 4 (2018), special issue on 'Medical Metaphors in Late Antique Christianity', esp. Mayer, 'Medicine and metaphor'; also see *Journal of Late Antiquity* 8, 2 (2015).
6 Sontag, *Illness as Metaphor*, 3.
7 Rucellai, *Zibaldone*, 83–84, 199 (fols 36vA–36rB, 86rB). He includes the advice of medical counsellors St Fulgentius, Avicenna, and Hippocrates ('principe de' medici'); Rucellai, *Zibaldone*, 149–50 (fols 65vB–66rA).
8 Greenblatt, 'Culture', 230.
9 Humbert of Romans, citing Gregory the Great, in Tugwell, *Early Dominicans*, 373.
10 In some of the sermon texts which have been preserved in manuscript, there are instructions to 'put in an exemplum here'. See Howard, 'Leoni Superbi'. For how *exempla* can carry the meaning of a discourse, see Gecser, Otto, 'Itinerant preaching'.
11 Howard, *Beyond the Written Word*, 114.
12 Florence, Biblioteca Riccardiana, MS 308, fols 124r–125r: 'Descende ad practicas cum exemplis suis et conclude hoc primum etc'; 'Extende materiam et descende ad particularia et practicas et sic conclude primum'. For Antoninus's use of classical *exempla* in Antoninus's sermons, see Howard, 'The remembered past as present exemplar'. In relation to the exigencies of the day, see e.g. Howard, '"You Cannot Sell Liberty"', 219–21.
13 Quoted in D'Avray, *The Death of the Prince*, 203.
14 Polecritti, *Preaching Peace in Renaissance Italy*, 243.
15 See Howard, 'Sermons reflecting upon their world(s)'.
16 See, e.g., Bourdieu, *Language and Symbolic Power*, 61–62.
17 Alberti, *On the Art of Building in Ten Books*, 128.
18 Febvre, *Le problème de l'incroyance*, 370, 'tous les actes, toutes les journées sont comme saturés de religion'.
19 Quoted by Debby, *Renaissance Florence in the Rhetoric of Two Popular Preachers*, 1.

20 Bracciolini, *On Avarice*, 244.

21 Bracciolini, *On Avarice*, 245.

22 Bracciolini, *On Avarice*, 245.

23 Bracciolini, *On Avarice*, 255.

24 The metaphor enabled Antoninus to oscillate between a theological and sociological view of the reality of the society for which he wrote; both sources appear in his resource for preachers, his *Summa theologica*, in the prologue to the third volume. See the general discussion of Le Goff, 'Head or heart? The political understanding of body metaphors in the Middle Ages', 13–26, especially 16–17. Antoninus cites Vincent's *Speculum historiale* (3:26) which, like John of Salisbury, identifies religion with the soul, the Senate with the heart, and so on. Antoninus, *Summa* III. III. I, IX, coll. 172E–173A.

25 See, e.g., Antoninus, *Sermones*, Ricc. 308, fol. 3, '. . . hoc exigit Christi conformitas. Christus enim est caput nostrum et nos sumus membra eius sec. illud Eph. 1: *Ipsum dedit caput super omnem Ecclesiam quae est corpus ipsius*'.

26 Ad consolationem autem reipublicae valent virtuosi. Non enim solum in civitate debet esse directio, quae est per sapientes, sed etiam recta operatio, quae est per amicos Dei. Et ad hoc maxime debet princeps intendere, videlicet ut habeat in civitate religiosos, verbum Dei praedicantes, clericos honestos divina celebrantes, et alios timentes Deum, qui pro populo orent, quum frequenter inveniamus civitates salvatas propter merita aliquorum amicorum Dei. Antoninus, *Summa* IV. II. VI, col. 64B.

27 Erasmus, *Esomologesi*, 24. Quoted by Caravale, *Inquisition in Renaissance Italy*, 78.

28 Antoninus, *Summa* III. VII. I, col. 280C.

29 Antoninus, *Summa* III. VII. I, col. 280D.

30 See Biller and Ziegler, *Religion and Medicine in the Middle Ages*, especially the contributions by Joseph Ziegler (3–14), William J. Courtney (69–76), and Jessalyn Bird (91–108). Cf also discussion of Cavalca's sermon on 'Christus Medicus' in Henderson, *Renaissance Hospital*, 113–17.

31 Verino, *De illustratione Urbis Florentiae*, '*Infectos Cleri mores correxit et Urbis*', 242.

32 Magli, *Gli uomini della penitenza*, 105.

33 See Cornelison, *Art and the Relic Cult of St. Antoninus*, at n. 74.

34 See Polizzotto, 'The making of a saint', 359; Rusconi, 'Predico' in Piazza', esp. 127–29, 173–80; and Henderson, in this volume.

35 Rimbertini, *Sermones*, fol. 69ᵛ: 'Nunc iam cano capite, et arata iugis fronte ad instar bonum pendentibus amento palearibus: Frigidus obstitit circum precordia sanguinis: ita videlicet ut jam mihi, et memoria exciderit, et contracta rubigine hebes factus sit intellectus'.

36 Maffei, *In magnificentiae Cosmi Medicei Florentini detractores libellus*. 'Haec aestatis, pullulantisque pestis malitia, ac uaria [82r] huius meae Praefecturae negocia silentium magisque praedicationem imperare uidentur', 125 (Latin), 140 (English trans).

37 Manetti, *Life of Brunelleschi*, 120–23.

38 Antoninus, *Sermones*, 5ra: 'Item dedit vobis Deus aërem temperatum, et quia usi estis in luxuria, misit vobis Deus pestes et alias infirmitates. Item dedit vobis Deus aërem temperatum, et quia usi estis in luxuria, misit vobis Deus pestes et alias infirmitates'.

39 Antoninus, *Summa historialis*,. xxx. XII, section 3 (Morçay, *Chroniques*, 83): 'Ubi tunc facta inquisitione et processu contra quosdam hereticos, infectos lepra erroris Fraticellorum. . . .'

40 See Howard, 'For the good of the city'.

41 Antoninus, *Sermones*, fol. 46ra-rb: 'Secundum desiderium est sanationis corporalis: propter hoc aliqui vadunt post incantationes et superstitiones; quod est illicitum quia communiter ista habent mixtas vanitates. Et dicit Ps. Odisti omnes observantes vanitates supervacue. Et secundum Augustinum in libro de doctrina christiana et 26 qu. 2 illud: omnes huiusmodi artes nugatoriae et noxiae superstitionis ex quadam pestifera societate hominum et daemonum quasi pacta infidelis et dolosae amicitiae constituta repudiandae sunt et fugiendae a Christianis. Et nota quod quidam confidunt in talibus, quia interdum prosunt eis per experientiam. Sed dicunt doctores, quod potest esse quod

talia habeant efficaciam super his personis quibus fiunt; nam diabolus operatur per viam occultam. Licet ergo habeant efficaciam talia, tamen non est licitum ea facere, nam nec per viam naturalem habent efficaciam, quia in medicina'.

42 The distinction between profane and natural magic was one which would later be invoked by Ficino. See Celenza, 'Late Antiquity and Florentine Platonism', 96.

43 See Bailey, 'Sorcery to witchcraft', 965, 977–78.

44 Antoninus, *Sermones*, 46rb: 'Et nota quod quidam confidunt in talibus, quia interdum prosunt eis per experientiam. Sed dicunt doctores, quod potest esse quod talia habeant efficaciam super his personis quibus fiunt; nam diabolus dyabolus operatur per viam occultam. Licet ergo habeant efficaciam talia, tamen non est licitum ea facere, nam nec per viam naturalem habent efficaciam, quia in medicina fieret mentio de eis, nec per virtutem divinam, quia Deus non est auctor malorum. Si ergo habent efficaciam procedit ex operatione diabolica. Et si in talibus est aliqua vanitas vel character, vel charta non nata, vel in tempore vel in persona haec omnia sunt illicita et vana et qui sequitur huiusmodi superstitiones, si sit manifesta invocatio diaboli, est manifeste peccatum mortale aliter autem non nisi sciat esse malum et tamen sequitur eas'.

45 See, for example, Zambelli, *White Magic, Black Magic in the European Renaissance*, 24–26.

46 'Misit verbum suum, et sanávit eos, et erípuit eos de interitiónibus eórum'. Antoninus, *Summa* III. XIV. I, col. 635.

47 About this aspect of the generation of the 'public theology' generated by preaching, see Howard, *Beyond the Written Word*.

48 Antoninus, *Summa* III. XIV. I, col. 638, quoting Eccles. 38:4 'Altíssimus creávit de terra medicaménta, et vir prudens non abhorrébit illa'.

49 Antoninus, *Summa* III. XIV. I, col. 639: 'Et propter hoc ad eripiendum nos ab his mortibus, instituit instas medicinas septem sacramentorum.

50 Antoninus, *Sermones*, BNCF CS A. 8. 1750, fol. 28va: 'Figura habetur de Naaman dicto. Nam sicut ille septies se lavans in Jordane mundatus est a lepra, sic et tu per confessionem mundaberis. Nam Jordanis dicitur quasi rivus iudicii. Nam in confessione intervenit iudex et testes et accusator etc. Lava ergo te in hoc rivo iudicii septies, i.e. de septem peccatis mortalibus et mundaberis a lepra peccatorum'. Also fol. 28ra: 'Exemplum etiam habetur 4. Reg. 5 de Naaman principe exercitus regis Syriae, qui donec stetit in ira propterea, quia Elisaeus non venit ad eum, remansit semper leprosus, sed postquam assensit consiliis servorum, ut lavaret se in Jordane, mundatus est a lepra'. See as well, fols 22rb, 28rb. On representations of leprosy, also see Presciutti, in this volume.

51 Ricc 308, fol. 5v: 'Exemplum in Christo, qui in florida aetate voluit mori turpissimo genere mortis.

In Constantino vero leproso lepra idolatriae et immunditiarum gentilium expurgatur. Et Christus tantae puritatis fuit, qui peccatum non fecit nec dolus inventus est in ore suo'.

52 'La medicina è la gratia di Dio preveniente all Vergine', in Gutiérrez, *Testi e note su Mariano da Genazzano*, 178.

53 Here Fra Mariano is entering into controverted territory: whether the Virgin was born with or without original sin. See Sebastian, 'The controversy over the immaculate conception from after Scotus to the end of the Eighteenth century', 228–41, esp. 234–38; and Mayberry, 'The controversy over the immaculate conception', 207–24.

54 Succhiellis OP, *Sermones* fols 23r–25r: 'De diuinitate et humanitate christi. (Ad monasterium sancte lucie pistorii 1494) [c23r.] Deus ipse ueniet et saluabit nos. Tunc aperientur oculi cecorum et aures surdorum patebunt. Tunc saliet sicut ceruus claudus et aperta erit lingua mutorum et cetera Jsaia 35. Tu es qui uenturus es. An alium expectamus. Et respondens jhesus ait illis. Euntes renunctiat iohanni qui audisti et uidisti. Ceci uident. Claudi ambulant. Leprosi mundantur Surdi audiunt. Mortui resurgunt. Pauperes euangelizzantur. Mattheus 11. Spiritus domini super me eo quod unxerunt me. Ad anuntiandum mansuetis misit me ut mederer contristes corde et predicarem captiuis indulgentiam et clausis aperitionem ut predicarem annum placabilem domino et diem ultionis deo nostro ut consolarer omnes lugentes ut ponerem fortitudinem lugentibus sion et darem eis coronam pro cinere. Oleum gaudii pro luctu pallium laudis pro spiritu meroris. Jsaia 61. . . .

[23r] Et si non erat deus quis curauit eos qui uexabantur uariis languoribus et demonia eiecere ibi. Si non erat homo quis descendit de monte et que sunt secute turbe mattheus 8 et marcus 1 et luca 5 declara. Et si non esset deus quis curauit leprosum illum dicente sibi domine si uis potest me m.[edicare?] ibi. Si non esset homo quem rogauit centurio pro seruo suo. . . . [24v] Et si non erat deus quis sanauit idropicum qui erat ibi. Si non erat homo quis iuit in ierusalem quando transibat per mediam samariam et galileam Luca 17. Et si non erat deus quis mundauit decem leprosos. Si non erat deus cuius manus fecerunt flagellum et percusserunt uendentes et ementes in templo . . .'. Apart from this quotation, there are multiple examples throughout the sermon.

55 Succhiellis OP, *Sermones* [fol. 43v.]: (Mulier erat in ciuitate peccatrix. Luca 7). . . . Rogabat ihesum quidam phariseus ut manducaret cum illo. Lucas 7. Simon leprosus postea iulianus ab apostulis cenomansis episcopus factus. Et fuit unus de 72 discipulis cuius maria erat neptis et propterea fuit ausa intrare domum eius. Et de isto dicunt istorie quod tres mortuos suscitauit. Sed prius non nominatur propio nomine quod adhuc phariseus qui erant inimici christi necdum conuersus. Sed nec caritate ductus uel fide inuitauit christum sed ad pompam. Quod potest quia prius ea in semetipso despexit eum minus in illum credens. Dum dixit hic si essem propheta. Sequitur. Et ingressus domum pharisei discubuit Jtidem rex ethiopie qui sanctum matheum intefici mandauit leprosus effectus est et miserabiliter mortus est. Jsti. Jtidem magi qui simonem et thadeum persecuti sunt a fulgore de celo in carbones uersi sunt et jsti. Jtidem barnabas maledixit templo et statim corruit et oppressi paganos et jsti. Jtidem mortuo sancto marco grando terribilis et tonitrua et fulgura super paganos eum incedere uolentes cecidit et hec de apostulis dicta sufficient'.

56 Quoted in Mormando, *The Preacher's Demons*, 132.

57 See Howard, *Beyond the Written Word*; Howard, *Creating Magnificence in Renaissance Florence*.

58 Antoninus, *Summa* III. VII. Intro, col. 277: 'Numquid médici suscitábunt, et confitebúntur tibi' Ps 87.

59 Antoninus, *Summa* III. VII. Intro, col. 277: 'Altíssimus creávit de terra medicinam (*sic*. Medicaménta), et vir prudens non abhorrébit illa'. Cf note 55 above.

60 Antoninus, *Summa* III. VII. Intro., col. 277A.

61 The legend appears in Voragine, 'Cap. IX. De sancto Johanne apostolo et evangelista'.

62 Causa XXIV, Quaest. 1 in *Corpus iuris canonici, Part 1: Decretum Magistri Gratiani*, col. 850.

63 Howard, *Beyond the Written Word*, 139.

64 Bulletti, 'Predicazioni senesi'.

65 A collection of sermon transcriptions belonging to Margherita di Tommaso Soderini bears the title 'Consolation of the Sermons of Maestro Marjano Romano of Lent in Santa Maria del Fiore in Florence'. Florence, Biblioteca Nazionale Centrale, MS Magliab. XXXV, 98.

66 Antoninus, *Summa* IV. II. VI, col. 64B: '. . . ut habeat in civitate religiosos, verbum Dei praedicantes, clericos honestos divina celebrantes, et alios timentes Deum, qui pro populo orent, quum frequenter inveniamus civitates salvatas propter merita aliquorum amicorum Dei'. See earlier at n. 26.

67 'Disse in questa predicha molte belle e bellissime chose, le quali io non so dire e non mi richorda'. Florence, Biblioteca Riccardiana, 1186C, fol. 54r, transcribed in Zafarana, 'Per la storia religiosa', 1079.

Bibliography

Primary sources

Unpublished

Antoninus of Florence, *Sermones*, Florence, Biblioteca Nazionale Centrale, MS Conventi soppressi A. 8. 1750.

Antoninus of Florence, *Sermones*, Florence, Biblioteca Riccardiana, MS 308.

Bartholomaeus Lapaccis de Rimbertinis, *Sermones*, Florence, Bibilioteca Nazionale Centrale, MS Conventi soppressi G. I. 646.

Marcus Petri de Succhiellis OP, *Sermones*, Florence, Biblioteca Nazionale Centrale, MS Conventi soppressi I. VII. 4.

Margherita di Tommaso Soderini, 'Chonsolatio della prediche di maestro marjano romano', Florence, Biblioteca Nazionale Centrale, Magliab. XXXV.

Timotheus Maffei. *In magnificentiae Cosmi Medicei Florentini detractores libellous*. Florence, Biblioteca Laurenziana, MS Plut. 47, Cod. 17, fols 78–102.

Published

Alberti, Leon Battista, *On the Art of Building in Ten Books*, trans. Joseph Rykwert, Neil Leach, and Robert Tavernor (Cambridge, MA: MIT Press, 1988).

Antoninus of Florence, *Sancti Antonini Archiepiscopi Florentini Ordinis Praedicatorum Summa Theologica* (Verona: Augustus Caratonius, 1740; repr. Graz: Akademische Druck—Universitäts Verlagsanstalt, 1959).

Bracciolini, Poggio, 'On avarice', in *The Earthly Republic: Italian Humanists on Government and Society*, ed., Benjamin G. Kohl and Ronald G. Witt (Philadelphia: Pennsylvania University Press, 1978), 241–92.

Corpus iuris canonici, Part 1: Decretum Magistri Gratiani, ed., Aemilius Ludwig Richter and Emil A. Friedberg (Leipzig 1879, reprint, Akademische Druck—Universitäts Verlagsanstalt: Graz, 1995).

Maffei, Timotheus, *In magnificentiae Cosmi Medicei Florentini detractores libellous*, ed. and trans., Howard Saalman, *Creating Magnificence in Renaissance Florence*, Appendix 3, 123–50.

Manetti, Antonio di Tuccio, *The Life of Brunelleschi by Antonio di Tuccio Manetti*, introduction, notes and ed., Howard Saalman, English trans. Catherine Engass (University Park and London: Pennsylvania State University Press, 1970).

Rucellai, Giovanni di Pagolo, *Zibaldone*, ed., Gabrielle Battista (Florence: SISMEL Edizioni del Galuzzo, 2013).

Verino, Ugolino, '*De illustratione urbis Florentiae*', in Baldassarri, *Images of Quattrocento Florence: Selected Writings in Literature, History, and Art*, ed., Stefano Ugo Baldassarri and Arielle Saiber (New Haven and London: Yale University Press, 2000), 241–45.

Zafarana, Zelina, 'Per la storia religiosa di Firenze ne Quattrocento: una raccolta privata di prediche', *Studi Medievali*, 3a ser., 9 (1968), 1017–1113.

Secondary sources

Bailey, Michael D., 'Sorcery to witchcraft: clerical conceptions of magic in the Later Middle Ages', *Speculum*, 76 (2001), 960–90.

Biller, Philip and Joseph Ziegler, eds, *Religion and Medicine in the Middle Ages* (Woodbridge, Suffolk: York Medieval Press, 2001).

Bourdieu, Pierre, *Language and Symbolic Power*, ed., John B. Thompson, trans., Gino Raymond and Matthew Adamson (Cambridge, MA: Harvard University Press, 1991).

Bruni, Francesco, *La Città Divisa: le parti e il bene comune da Dante a Guicciardini* (Bologna: Il Mulino, 2003).

Bulletti, Enrico O. M., ed., 'Predicazioni senesi di Frate Antonio da Rimini (Documenti inediti)', *Bullettino Senese di Storia Patria*, 62–63 (1955–1956), 206–12.

Celenza, Christopher, 'Late Antiquity and Florentine Platonism: the 'post-plotinian' Ficino', in Michael J. G. Allen and Valery Rees (eds), *Marsilio Ficino: His Theology, His Philosophy, His Legacy* (Leiden: Brill, 2002), 71–97.

Corbellini, Sabrina and Margriet Hoogvliet, 'Artisans and religious reading in late medieval Italy and Northern France (ca. 1400—ca. 1520)', *Journal of Medieval and Early Modern Studies*, 43 (2013), 521–44.

Cornelison, Sally, *Art and the Relic Cult of St. Antoninus in Renaissance Florence* (London: Routledge, 2017).

D'Avray, David, *The Death of the Prince* (Oxford: Oxford University Press, 1993).

Debby, Nirit Ben-Aryeh, 'Jews and Judaism in the rhetoric of popular preachers: the Florentine sermons of Giovanni Dominici (1356–1419) and Bernardino da Siena (1380–1444)', *Jewish History*, 14 (2000), 175–200.

Debby, Nirit Ben-Aryeh, *Renaissance Florence in the Rhetoric of Two Popular Preachers: Giovanni Dominici (1356–1419) and Bernardino da Siena (1380–1444)* (Turnhout: Brepols, 2001).

Febvre, Lucien, *Le problème de l'incroyance au xvie siècle: la religion de Rabelais* (Paris: Michel, 1962).

Gecser, Otto, 'Itinerant preaching in Late Medieval Central Europe: St John Capistran in Wrocław', *Medieval Sermon Studies*, 47 (2003), 5–20.

Greenblatt, Stephen, 'Culture', in Frank Lentricchia and Thomas McLaughlin (eds), *Critical Terms for Literary Study* (Chicago: Chicago University Press, 1990), 225–49.

Gutiérrez, David, '*Testi e note su Mariano da Genazzano (d. 1498)*', *Analecta Augustiniana*, 32 (1969), 117–204.

Hatty, Suzanne and James Hatty, *The Disordered Body: Epidemic Disease and Cultural Transformation* (Albany: State University of New York Press, 1999).

Henderson, John, *The Renaissance Hospital: Healing the Body and Healing the Soul* (New Haven: Yale University Press, 2006).

Howard, Peter, *Aquinas and Antoninus* (Toronto: Pontifical Institute of Mediaeval Studies, 2013).

Howard, Peter, *Beyond the Written Word: Preaching and Theology in the Florence of Archbishop Antoninus, 1427–1459* (Florence: Leo S. Olschki, 1995).

Howard, Peter, *Creating Magnificence in Renaissance Florence* (Toronto: CMRS, 2012).

Howard, Peter, *Experiencing Religion in Renaissance Florence* (London: Routledge, forthcoming 2020).

Howard, Peter, '"Leoni Superbi" Florentines, Sant' Antonino and his preaching in the Duomo,' in Timothy Verdon and Annalisa Innocenti (eds), *Atti del VII Centenario di S. Maria del Fiore* (Florence: EDIFIR, 2001), 495–509.

Howard, Peter, 'Preaching to the Mobs: Space, Ideas and Persuasion in Renaissance Florence', in Nancy Van Deusen and Lenny Koff (eds), *Mobs* (Leiden: Brill, 2011), 203–04.

Howard, Peter, 'The Remembered Past as Present *Exemplar* in Florentine Renaissance Preaching', in Machtelt Israëls and Louis Waldman (eds), *Renaissance Studies in Honor of Joseph Connors* (Florence: Villa I Tatti, 2013), 2, 221–29.

Howard, Peter, 'Sermons Reflecting upon Their World(s): A Response to Wim Verball, Eve Salisbury, and Emily Michelson' in Georgina Donavin, Cary Nederman, Richard Utz (eds), *Speculum Sermonis: Interdisciplinary Reflections on the Medieval Sermon* (Turnhout: Brepols, 2004), 181–94.

Howard, Peter, '"The womb of memory": Carmelite Liturgy and the Frescoes of the Brancacci Chapel', in Nicholas Eckstein (ed.), *The Brancacci Chapel: Form, Function and Setting*, Villa I Tatti (Series) (Florence: Villa I Tatti, 2007), 177–206.

Howard, Peter, '"You Cannot Sell Liberty for All the Gold There Is': promoting good governance in Early Renaissance Florence,' *Renaissance Studies*, 24 (2010), 207–33.

Le Goff, Jacques, 'Head or heart? The political understanding of body metaphors in the Middle Ages', in Michel Feher and others (eds), *Fragments for a History of the Human Body* (New York: Zone, 1989), 3, 13–26.

Magli, Ida, *Gli uomini della penitenza: lineamenti antropologici del medioevo italiano* (Milan: Garzanti, 1967).

Mayberry, Nancy, 'The controversy over the immaculate conception in medieval and Renaissance art, literature and society', *Journal of Medieval and Renaissance Studies*, 21 (1991), 207–24.

Mayer, Wendy, 'Medicine and metaphor in Late Antiquity: how some recent shifts are changing the field', *Studies in Late Antiquity*, 2 (2018), 440–63.

Polecritti, Cynthia, *Preaching Peace in Renaissance Italy: Bernardino of Siena and His Audience* (Washington, DC: Catholic University of America Press, 2000).

Polizzotto, Lorenzo, 'The making of a saint: the canonization of St. Antonino, 1516–1523', *Journal of Medieval and Renaissance Studies*, 22 (1992), 353–81.

Rusconi, Roberto, '"Predico' in Piazza": politica e predicaizone Nell'Umbria del '400', in Roberto Rusconi (ed.), *Immagini dei predicatori e della predicazione in Italia all fine del Medioevo* (Spoleto: Fondazione Centro Italiano di Studi Sull'Alto Medioevo, 2016), 141–85.

Sebastian, Wenceslaus, 'The controversy over the immaculate conception from after Scotus to the end of the Eighteenth Century', in Edward D. O'Connor (ed.), *The Dogma of the Immaculate Conception: History and Significance* (Notre Dame, IN: University of Notre Dame Press, 1958), 228–41.

Sontag, Susan, *Illness as Metaphor* (Harmondsworth: Penguin, 1983).

Tugwell, Simon OP, ed. and intro., *Early Dominicans: Selected Writings* (New York: Paulist Press, 1982).

Zambelli, Paola, *White Magic, Black Magic in the European Renaissance: Ficino, Pico, Della Porta to Trithemius, Agrippa, and Bruno* (Leiden: Brill, 2007).

3

REPRESENTING INFIRMITY IN EARLY MODERN FLORENCE

John Henderson

Introduction

The visual representation of infirmity and disease in early modern Italy has until recently tended to have been studied through simplistic models of retrospective diagnosis imposed on to evidence produced many centuries earlier for purposes other than that of modern medical science. The main problem with these approaches is that they have often failed to take into account different conventions and symbolic systems of representation. This has been compounded by assumptions that past disease categories coincide with our own, though these beliefs may have been shaken somewhat by the recent vigorous debates about the identity of plague, the most lethal epidemic to have hit pre-industrial Europe.[1]

Plague, and to a lesser extent leprosy, has tended to dominate the discussion by historians of the representation of disease in medieval and early modern Italy.[2] In comparison, few studies deal with other major epidemics of the time, such as the Great Pox, smallpox, or endemic diseases, such as malaria or even influenza. This may be partly because the signs and symptoms of plague, and above all the bubo, have been seen as the most readily recognizable when viewed through the optic of a post-Yersinian world, following the discovery of the cause of plague by the French scientist Alexandre Yersin.[3] However, it must also be remembered that the ontological concept of disease only gradually emerged in medieval and Renaissance Europe. In other words, the vast majority of sicknesses were seen as collections of symptoms, rather than specific diseases, thus presenting considerable problems of representation and, for us, of interpretation.

The other obvious imperative to consider when approaching this subject is the context in which a particular work of art was produced and how it reflected the purpose for which it was painted or sculpted. The vast majority of images associated with plague were produced for religious contexts, whether imploring the intervention of a particular patron saint for the mitigation of an epidemic or, and this was often linked, reflecting the terrible impact of plague on a city. Well-known representations of these scenes range from the later fourteenth to the mid-seventeenth century and beyond. One of the best known is the Florentine triptych of *Saint Sebastian* by Giovanni del Biondo of *c.* 1375 (Opera del Duomo, Florence).[4] While the central image shows the saint shot full of arrows, in one of the surrounding panels, the dead and dying are strewn across the urban landscape, with people collapsed in houses and streets, while a nun is placed in a bier ready for burial. On the left-hand side there is a group of well-dressed men and women imploring Sebastian and Mary to intervene with the vengeful God punishing the city for its sins. Though the artist may have been referring to the plague of Pavia in 680, Florentines would have seen their own city represented here; the presence of holy protectors would have provided a significance over and above the specific time and place.[5]

Even more dramatic images date from 300 years later during the two major seventeenth-century plague epidemics of 1629–33 and 1656–57. These include Guido Reni's processional standard, the *Pallione del Voto* of 1630 (Pinacoteca Nazionale di Bologna).[6] It was commissioned by the Bolognese city government to be carried through the streets in late December as part of the Reggimento's vow to the Madonna of the Rosary, in which they asked for her intercession and in return promised to provide collective acts of piety.[7] The canvas is divided into three sections, with the top part showing the Madonna and Child seated on clouds; underneath were the city's patron saints praying for her intercession. A small section at the bottom shows a scene outside the city walls during the epidemic, the well-ordered transport of the sick and dead. Seen together, the banner demonstrates the power of faith and the success of Bologna's policies to manage the epidemic.[8] Another equally famous image shows the opposite: Domenico Gargiulo's depiction of the plague in Naples in 1656 is a horrendous scene of hundreds of corpses and the dying in a large piazza, Largo Mercatello, joined together in a deadly struggle with death, painted between 1656 and 1660 (Museo Nazionale di San Martino, Naples).[9] A few coffins were being deployed, but emphasis is placed above all on the indignity of large numbers of abandoned semi-clad corpses left for all to see in a public space. The living try desperately to cope with the dead, but the confusion is emphasized by the upturned cart in the left-hand foreground, from which bodies tumble out. As is the case with other plague images of the time, this is a votive picture and therefore includes the divine presence of the Virgin Mary seated on a cloud. While Reni's *Palliotto* shows the Madonna full of grace and the Christ as a child blessing through His gaze, Gargiulo represents Christ as an adult and Mary, in her role of interceding for the people, desperately trying to dissuade her irate son from destroying the city's population. The two methods of representing the dangers of plague in Bologna and Naples coincidentally reflected relative levels of mortality, 24 per cent compared with 50 per cent.[10]

These painted scenes, along with countless others associated with plague, reflect the close association between the individual's sick body and the body of the city;

the ire of God was thus visited on all inhabitants to punish their collective sins. Participation in processions and private repentance were prescribed to deflect God's anger, as were personal and communal prayers to patron saints to mitigate the effect of the epidemic once it had arrived. But how far were the painters or patrons of these images interested in depicting the symptoms of disease? Both Giovanni del Biondo and Domenico Gargiulo simply showed pale dead bodies, which had collapsed and expired on the spot; even in the case of the Neapolitan scene, while many of the bodies were semi-nude, this did not lead the painter to depict a wide range of buboes and other symptoms associated with plague. The aim in these two paintings, as in the case of the scene at the bottom of Guido Reni's banner, was to show the impact of plague on the sick body of the city rather than its effect on the individual body and to demonstrate personal and civic reactions to the crisis.

The votive chapels and churches commissioned by individuals, families, and cities in gratitude for their recovery from an epidemic also provided the context for a wide range of works of art representing sickness and infirmity. This chapter will explore this theme through iconographic evidence deriving from early modern Florence and its surroundings. While plague imagery for late medieval Tuscany is well-known, the topic remains understudied for early modern Florence, especially when compared with other Italian cities, such as Milan, Rome, and Naples.[11] The aim here will also be to move beyond plague and to raise wider questions about how infirmity and bodily suffering were represented through the twin themes of medicine and religion. How far were specific, readily identified attributes of particular sicknesses shown, given, on the one hand, contemporary humoral understanding of disease as a collection of symptoms, and, on the other, that the role of the vast majority of these images was devotional?

Representing plague in the seventeenth century

Italy saw the return of plague with considerable severity in the seventeenth century, with two main episodes. The first, between 1629 and 1633, affected northern and central Italy from Milan to Florence, while the second, in 1656–57, principally impacted the southern part of the peninsula, most famously Rome and Naples, though it was also carried north to Genoa and the Ligurian coast. Many of these city states adopted similar secular measures to combat the epidemic, based largely on disinfection, quarantine, and isolation. Meanwhile, the Church aimed to enlist the advocacy of a series of local saints to persuade God to divert the punitive arrows of disease elsewhere through the organization of religious processions and the veneration of shrines. All this led as well to the commissioning by Church, State, and individuals of a wide range of votive churches, chapels, and altarpieces and statues, which shared common themes but also reflected regional variations. The Tuscan capital will be examined within a wider geographical context to assess the points of similarity and difference in the representation of infirmity.

Before concentrating on the few representations of plague which appeared in Florence in this period, it is necessary to outline the physical symptoms recorded by contemporaries to see how they might have been reflected visually in art. Dr Antonio Pellicini, who wrote a treatise on plague at the request of the Florentine College of Physicians in November 1630, provided an outline of the main signs:[12]

> there appear sometimes on the skin, not just unusual spots (*macchie*), and different types of petechia, but also boils, and horrible pustules, not less evident in the visible watery vescicles, than in their odious blackness and the legitimate form of malign carbuncles; and also swelling further outside the lymph nodes (*emuntorii*), commonly called 'gavoccioli' or buboes.

The most vivid depiction of a plague bubo in Florence in this period was in a fresco painted by Pietro Dandini for the cloister of Sant'Antonino in the Observant Dominican church and convent of San Marco (Figure 3.1).[13] It is shown clearly as a raised dark-brown swelling under the left arm of the prostrate sick man at the centre of the composition, one of the usual sites of infection. While he appears semi-clad, to his left a fully dressed woman has collapsed on the ground, appealing for the spiritual salvation offered by Antonino. If the woman's appearance does not demonstrate obvious swellings or signs, her pale face and evident weakness may reflect other symptoms mentioned by Pellicini—'the most acute and fevers, with a putrifying mass of humours and . . . excessive headache'.[14]

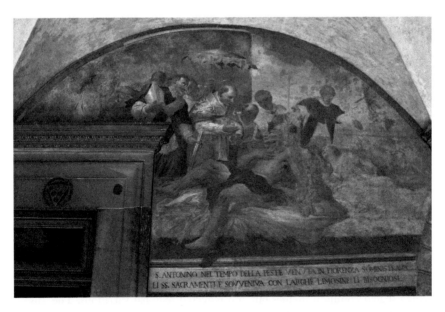

FIGURE 3.1 Pietro Dandini, *Sant' Antonino Visiting the Sick during the Plague of Florence, 1448–9* (1693)

Source: Maggie Bell with the concession of the Museo di S. Marco, Ministero per i beni e le attività culturali, Polo museale della Toscana

When Dandini painted his fresco of Sant'Antonino visiting the sick in 1693, his contribution to the decoration of the cloister represented the culmination of an almost century-long process. Starting in the late sixteenth century, many of the leading Tuscan painters of the period adorned lunettes with the major episodes in the life and miracles of the Florentine Archbishop. As in these other images, the aim of this lunette was the glorification of Antonino's saintly actions, so the depiction of symptoms of the plague was subservient to the main message of saintly charity and penitence. Most probably this was an historical re-creation of a bubo; it is unlikely that Dandini would have seen a plague victim, since he was born in 1646/7 and he spent the first ten years of his life in Florence, which had remained free from plague since 1633. He would probably have copied the symptoms of plague from pictures or prints he had seen as a young man in northern Italy; he had spent two years studying in Venice, from where he visited other cities, among which were Bologna, Modena, and Parma.[15] This influence is confirmed by the disposition of the figures in Dandini's fresco. They reflect the iconography, more common in northern Italian imagery than that of Tuscany, of San Carlo Borromeo carrying and administering the viaticum to those dying from plague, who were shown in the open air as he passed through the streets. Like Borromeo, Sant'Antonino, during the Florentine epidemic of 1448–49, was seen as protected by God through the sanctity of his charitable mission, underlining the strength of spiritual medicine.[16]

Dandini's Sant'Antonino is a striking image by an important artist associated closely with the Tuscan grand-ducal court. It would appear, however, to be in contrast to the more general conclusions of art historians who have examined plague art in early modern Italy. It has been argued, for example, by Christine Boeckl that by the seventeenth century, there were fewer direct pictorial representations of the symptoms of plague on the human body in Italy, with emphasis shifting away from exclusive concentration on suffering and towards the efficaciousness of healing.[17] Sheila Barker has detected a similar shift in seventeenth-century Rome, reflected, for example, in Giovanni Battista Vanni's *St. Sebastian Being Treated by Irene and Companions* for the Florentine confraternity of San Giovanni dei Fiorentini (1630–32).[18]

Various reasons have been put forward for this perceived shift, both religious and medical, but above all it is due to the influence of the Council of Trent. The increased Tridentine emphasis on the role of the sacraments as the true path to salvation is seen as having led to greater stress on representations of saintly persons carrying the Host to the sick and dying. These scenes also underlined Christian charity, reflecting the role of the new Orders in tending to the desperately sick, especially the Jesuits, Camilliani, San Giovanni di Dio, and the Capuchins.[19] If the depiction of the nursing of the sick underlines the importance of male religious orders, the representation of Irene and her companions also reminds us of the vital role of female nursing staff, who worked voluntarily in hospitals across Italy and elsewhere in Europe. While saints, such as Catherine of Siena and Elizabeth of Hungary, made their names in nursing the sick poor, the large numbers of women who belonged to Third Orders or subscribed to the Rule of St Augustine and performed so many duties in medieval and early modern hospitals, from nursing to feeding the sick and, as reflected in Irene's role, performed minor surgical operations and administered herbal remedies.[20]

The greater stress placed on representations of treatment is thus seen as complementary and parallel to the renewed emphasis on the sacraments.[21] The emphasis in iconography away from more traditional themes of plague arrows raining down on individuals and cities led to more commissions reflecting the cure of the soul and the body. The use of physical medicines can be seen in the growth in the number of pictures of Tobias curing his father's blindness, or the Good Samaritan tending to the sick traveller, and the growing popularity of the depiction of a scene following the attempted martyrdom of St Sebastian. Instead of being represented as pierced with arrows, he was shown with St Irene and her assistants treating his wounded body.[22] In all these contexts, it has been argued that the physical manifestation of disease thus assumed less importance than the acts of care and cure.[23]

Given the fiercely independent nature of Italian politics and the different local artistic traditions, it is worth asking if these newer themes in plague iconography were adopted generally across the peninsula. In Venice and the Veneto, for example, the attempted first martyrdom of St Sebastian continued to be an important theme in the post-Tridentine period.[24] San Rocco also remained important, appearing in his traditional guise, revealing his bubo, alongside other saints imploring for the intercession of the Virgin for the cessation of an epidemic. A boost to his visual presence was provided by the foundation of the Scuola di San Rocco, with Jacopo Tintoretto's lavish canvases for the confraternity's meeting hall painted between 1564 and 1588.[25] A century later, a particularly dramatic image was provided by Antonio Zanchi's enormous canvas of the *Plague in Venice in 1630*, which was finished for the staircase of the Scuola di San Rocco in 1666.[26] It depicts the semi-nude abandoned bodies of the sick and dead being piled unceremoniously into boats to be taken off to Lazaretti for treatment or burial. The corpses were clearly identified as plague victims by the prominent black buboes on exposed parts of their body, as on the man in the right panel, whose corpse is being manhandled from the bridge down into a boat in the canal underneath.

Visual representation of plagues in seventeenth-century Florence

This wider discussion helps us to assess how far the iconography of plague and other epidemic diseases in Florence fits the picture traced for other parts of seventeenth-century Italy. Tuscany was unusual compared with Lombardy and the Veneto because it had not experienced plague for a century; the last episode to have affected Florence was in the 1520s, while other cities, particularly in the north of Italy, had suffered from severe outbreaks in the mid-1570s.[27] The epidemic of plague in Florence, which began in summer 1630, lasted for about twelve months, and returned briefly a year later, leading to the death of about 12 per cent of the population of Florence's estimated 75,000.[28] As I have outlined in some detail elsewhere, both religious and secular measures taken by Church and State in Florence had much in common with those adopted by other Italian states. These measures included cordons sanitaire, the inspection and disinfection of houses, the establishment of special plague pits and Lazaretti, along with the imposition of protective measures during religious processions and the celebration of mass within churches, the quarantining of the city's population, and the use of portative altars that were erected in streets throughout the city.[29]

The central nodes of processions were the Cathedral, the Servite church of Santissima Annunziata, and the Dominican church of San Marco. These events were organized by the Church in conjunction with and the approval of the governing regime and the Health Board. Key to this collaboration was Grand Duke Ferdinand II and members of his family and court, who participated in the processions.[30] The churches of Santissima Annunziata and San Marco attracted the most significant artistic patronage in these years, reflecting the local popularity of the relics of Sant'Antonino at the latter and the miraculous shrine at the former.[31] As in Rome during the 1656–57 plague, the Florentine epidemic had a clear impact on the pattern of commissions stemming from private and institutional patrons.[32] Members of the grand-ducal family were prominent among those who paid for a range of artistic commissions. In 1632, the year after the epidemic, they enriched the chapel of the Madonna with valuable silver votive objects and commissioned the architect Matteo Nigetti to reconstruct the Sagrestia of the Madonna,[33] which housed Jacopo Vignali's large altarpiece, *The Madonna and Saints*, including Gregorio Thaumaturgus, a healer and worker of miracles, and Valentino, a protector against plague.[34]

During these years a series of artists, including Vignali, were commissioned to paint a number of images of Sebastian in Florence and its immediate surroundings. It was, above all, the first attempted martyrdom that continued to be popular, far out-numbering representations of his actual martyrdom. For example, Vincenzo Dandini's altarpiece of this subject, originally commissioned in the late 1630s for the Compagnia di San Sebastiano in the parish church of San Mauro a Signa, shows Sebastian tied to a crucifix, pierced by arrows shot by a series of archers who surround him, and small streams of bright red blood are shown issuing from his wounds.[35] In the early 1640s, Vignali's pupil, Carlo Dolci, painted a *St Sebastian* which shows his youthful body before his first martyrdom, untouched by wounds, holding arrows in his left hand.[36]

As Giovanni Pagliarulo has shown in his important study, Jacopo Vignali (1592–1664) remained the pre-eminent painter in Florence of scenes and saints linked to natural disasters in these years, and patrons often turned to him when choosing to depict Sebastian during the plague epidemics of 1630–33.[37] Two altarpieces of St Sebastian were commissioned for churches outside the city. Just to the north, at Montughi, in the church of San Martino, Sebastian was shown in a crucifixion scene in the company of a number of saints, including Carlo Borromeo, Filippo Neri, and Antonino (1631).[38] Better known was his *Madonna and Saints*, commissioned by the abbot of the Abbey of San Bartolomeo at Badia a Ripoli towards the end of 1630. It was to be placed in the chapel dedicated to St Sebastian, which had been built one hundred years earlier during the previous epidemic of plague in Florence. Among the saintly figures imploring the Virgin and Child for their intercession were Sebastian, Rocco, Giovanni Gualberto, and Thomas; the latter was included as the personal patron saint of Abbot Davanzati. While Sebastian was shown tied to a tree in the traditional iconography, what makes this image somewhat different was that instead of his body being pierced with arrows, there were a series of bleeding wounds in his neck, arm, and right-hand side, after the arrows had been removed, possibly a reference to the broader theme of his treatment.[39] Another altarpiece including Sebastian was commissioned in 1634 from Lorenzo Lippi as an ex-voto in thanks for the community of Ronta in the Mugello escaping plague.[40] The Madonna and Child are seated on a cloud, adored by Saints Rocco, Sebastian, Anthony of Padua, and two local patron saints, Michele and Donato, with the parish church in the background.[41] The young St Sebastian gazes in adoration at the Virgin, seemingly unaware of the two arrows which pierce his body.

San Rocco had remained an established presence in the Florentine area, as reflected in Vignali's altarpiece for the Badia a Ripoli and Cesare Dandini's *Assumption of the Virgin* in Santissima Annunziata, both dating from late 1630 to early 1631.[42] In both paintings San Rocco is shown kneeling and either looking or pointing upwards to the Virgin, carrying his staff and sometimes accompanied by his dog. The plague bubo is discretely represented on his leg: at Santissima Annunziata there is a slight swelling below his left knee, at Ronta there is a small blemish on the skin above his right-hand knee, both of which were closer to the earlier stages of the disease than when the bubo is full blown, as in Dandini's fresco in San Marco.

Carlo Borromeo was the other plague saint who became increasingly important from the later sixteenth century, although he was much less common in Tuscany than in northern Italy, particularly in the Milanese area, where he had been archbishop and made his name tending to the sick during the epidemic of 1575–76, reflected in the well-known series of paintings, the *Quadroni* in Milan cathedral, discussed by Jenni Kuuliala in this volume.[43] Andrea Commodi had apparently been commissioned *c.* 1636 to paint the altarpiece *San Carlo Borromeo Praying for the Cessation of the Plague* for the church of San Carlo dei Barnabiti in Florence.[44] Commodi's painting has not survived, but in three previous versions, Borromeo is shown kneeling in front of a large ebonized crucifix mounted on an altar for the cessation of the plague in Milan. In the background there is a desolate scene populated with dead or dying figures, with emphasis placed on the white nude corpses of the plague-stricken. As in the case of the Neapolitan altarpiece by Domenico Gargiulo, the aim was to emphasize the act of abandonment, rather than visualize a close depiction of symptoms.[45]

The most detailed surviving representation of the impact of the plague on the Florentine urban landscape, attributed to Luigi Baccio del Bianco and painted some time before 1657, also provides little in the way of detailed symptoms (Figure 3.2).[46] There are scenes of the sick and dead being taken to hospital or carried for burial

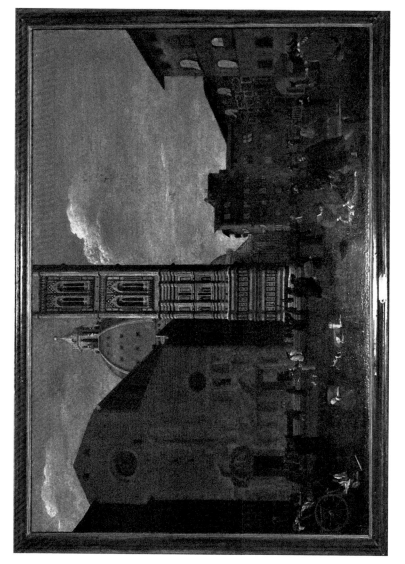

FIGURE 3.2 Luigi Baccio del Bianco, *The Plague in Florence in 1630* (pre-1657)

Source: Venerabile Arciconfraternita della Misericordia di Firenze

in covered biers, underlining the vital role of members of the Archconfraternity of the Misericordia, who carried the sick to Lazaretti and the dead to plague pits. The presence of plague is alluded to in a number of other ways, including the man dressed in black in the middle foreground, who is holding his nose to avoid breathing in the corrupt vapours associated with the disease, and in the left-hand corner the upturned cart belonging to the fumigators, who have allowed possessions belonging to the sick to cascade onto the ground. The only figure in the picture who is very evidently sick is the pale, well-dressed man in the centre foreground, who had collapsed in the street and over whom a physician bends, feeling his pulse for vital signs of life. His evident social status is emphasized by the close proximity of the physician; contemporaries recounted medical personnel kept a distance from the sick unless they were affluent.

From the representation of the bodies of diseased individuals, the final section will return to the theme of the visualization of the physical suffering of holy bodies, through wounds and torture, as a metaphor for infirmity.

Physical suffering and infirmity

The first attempted martyrdom of Sebastian has been compared with the popular medieval image of the Man of Sorrows, where viewers were invited to share in the bodily sufferings to encourage them to do penance.[47] As we have seen for other parts of Italy, in Florence an emphasis came also to be placed more generally on the wounded body of saints. The aim was also to underline the efficacy of healing by holy people, following the long tradition of the role of medieval saints and the new Catholic religious Orders. Within this context, it is not always clear whether the marks on the body were the result of wounds or sores, and therefore representing the result of torture or disease. For the original viewers this distinction may not be that significant, since the representation of a wound may have been transmuted into a sore to reflect more closely the patron's concern with sickness.

Jacopo Vignali specialized in the representation of this nexus between religion and medicine, as reflected clearly in *Christ Showing His Wounds to St Bernard of Clairvaux* (Figure 3.3). The painting was commissioned in 1623 by the Miniati family for the Florentine church of SS. Simone e Giuda. The only known representation of this subject in Florence from this period,[48] Bernard, accompanied by two angels, is shown throwing up his hands in dismay and looking at Christ with deep compassion. Christ himself kneels with his back horizontal to the ground and points with his left forefinger to the bloody wounds or sores, presumably inflicted during the flagellation. Bernard was closely associated with healing miracles, providing spiritual medicine to treat the wounds. Christ's wounds were intended to lead viewers to participate in His sufferings and were an invitation to do penance for individual and general sin which causes sickness. Furthermore, as Christus Medicus, He was seen as curing the spiritual and physical sicknesses of the population.[49] Giovanni Pagliarulo has suggested that these sores or wounds in Vignali's painting may refer to the effects of typhus, which had afflicted Florence in these

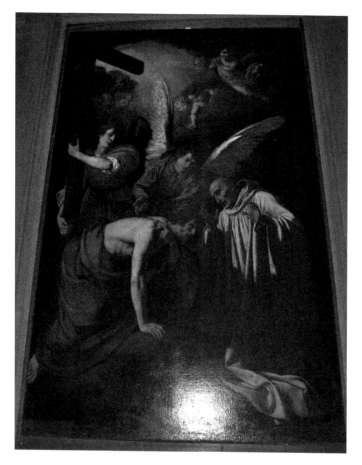

FIGURE 3.3 Jacopo Vignali, *Christ Showing His Wounds to St. Bernard of Clairvaux* (SS. Simone e Guida, Florence, 1623)

Source: Sailko, Wikimedia Commons: Creative Commons Attribution 3.0 Unported license

years (1620–23), killing over 3,000 people in the city.[50] Apart from the congruence of the dates of the commission and of the epidemic, Pagliarulo has suggested that Christ's wounds reflect a rash, one of the main symptoms of this disease. A clear contemporary description of the symptoms of lenticular fever, associated with exanthematic typhus, was provided by the well-known Veronese physician Girolamo Fracastoro in his book *De contagione et contagionis morbis* (1546): 'About the fourth or seventh day, red, or often purplish-red spots broke out on the arms, back and chest, and looked like flea-bites (punctiform), though they were often larger and in the shape of lentils, whence rose the name of the fever'.[51] Though it could be argued that there were large spots on Christ's back, some of which were purplish-red, these could also be read as the effect of a severe beating. Whether or not Vignali was directly representing lenticular fever, the wounds could equally well be a symbolic representation of general physical suffering from endemic and epidemic diseases present in the city in these years.

This altarpiece is important for the depiction of the lacerations on Christ's back and the reference to Bernard's miraculous healing powers. Similar themes were also explored at the time in secular painting, such as the works by Giovanni Battista Vanni and Ottavio Vannini depicting a scene of curing from Torquato Tasso's *Gerusalemme liberata*. Here, Erminia helps her beloved, the crusader knight Tancredi, by cutting off her hair, which has miraculous healing properties.[52]

Jacopo Vignali at San Marco

The final section of this chapter will explore further the joint themes of physical suffering and the curative role of saints in relation to one of Vignali's most important commissions between 1623 and 1630: four paintings for the pharmacy of the Observant Dominican convent of San Marco, which had been redesigned in the early seventeenth century.[53] These canvases are no longer on the premises of the pharmacy, but are nearby in a corridor off the cloister of Sant'Antonino. While the subjects of these four substantial canvases reflect iconographic themes current in seventeenth-century Italy, their combination in the same place gives special strength to their underlining message, the Christian endorsement of the combined power of physical and spiritual medicine. The panels, in chronological order, are *Tobias and the Angel* (1623), *The Baptism of Constantine* (1623–24), *St Peter Treats St Agatha* (1623–24), and *The Good Samaritan* (1630).

Miraculous healing is the central theme which unites these four images, especially relevant to their location within the pharmacy of a religious Order. The first picture to be commissioned was set in a rural landscape and shows Tobias, accompanied by his faithful dog, gazing at an enormous fish (Figure 3.4). The other main figure is the Archangel Raphael, dressed as an affluent young man, who was the patron saint of travellers and renowned for his miraculous powers as a healer. Tobias is shown holding a knife in his right hand, and, under the guidance of Raphael, making an incision in the fish's side in order to extract the fish's gall, which was to be used as a medicine to anoint the blind eye of Tobit, his father, to restore his sight.[54] To the left of the fish's head lies a small white-and-gold medicinal jar, or albarello, with the lid beside it, into which the gall would be placed and which he carried to his father (Figure 3.5).

Many fifteenth-century Florentine paintings of Tobias and the angel show them walking side by side, with Tobias carrying the fish (usually much smaller) on their way to administer the gall to Tobit.[55] Although this traditional iconography did not disappear, by the later sixteenth century, more painters placed greater emphasis on treatment, be it the action of extracting the gall or administering it to Tobit.

Vignali's San Marco *Tobias and the Angel* thus clearly reflects the strength of both spiritual and physical medicine, based, on the one hand, on Raphael's reputation for miraculous healing and, on the other, on the surgical knife being employed

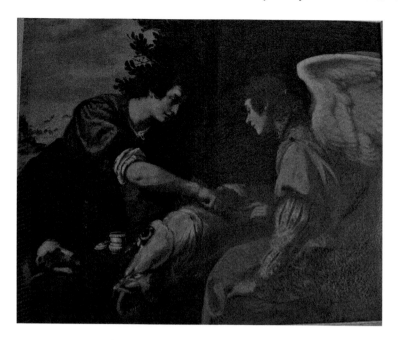

FIGURE 3.4 Jacopo Vignali, *Tobias and the Angel* (1623)

Source: Maggie Bell with the concession of the Museo di S. Marco, Ministero per i beni e le attività culturali, Polo museale della Toscana

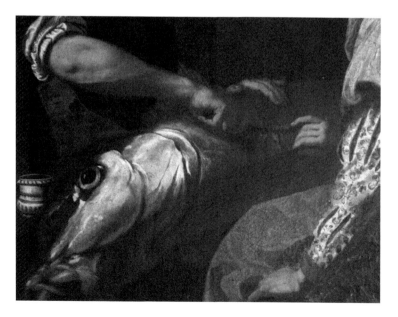

FIGURE 3.5 Jacopo Vignali, *Tobias and the Angel* (detail showing the fish's head and the white-and-gold albarello)

Source: Maggie Bell with the concession of the Museo di S. Marco, Ministero per i beni e le attività culturali, Polo museale della Toscana

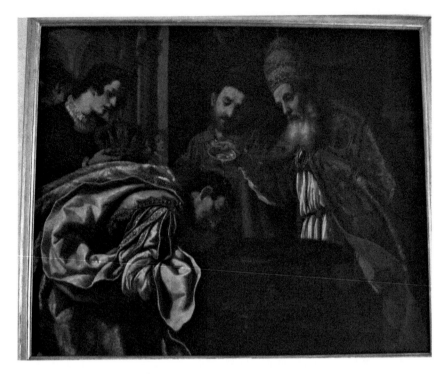

FIGURE 3.6 Jacopo Vignali, *Baptism of Constantine* (1623–24)

Source: Maggie Bell with the concession of the Museo di S. Marco, Ministero per i beni e le attività culturali, Polo museale della Toscana

by Tobias and the representation of the albarello, a type of container which would have been found in abundance within the pharmacy itself. The second picture in the series, *The Baptism of Constantine*, painted a year later, also contains a clear reference to the miraculous effect of spiritual medicine (Figure 3.6). Pope Silvester 1, who is shown baptising Constantine, is elaborately dressed in a crimson-lined cope faced with elaborately woven images of saints, fastened with a clasp containing a large precious stone, underlining his status as the head of the Roman Catholic Church. The Emperor is also richly dressed in clothes encrusted with pearls to denote his status, although the white of his garments would also have been understood as reflecting penitence and humility. This scene thus reflects the power of the unguent of spiritual medicine, as the Pope freed Constantine from original sin, washing away its impurities. However, there was also a subtext appropriate for the context of a Dominican pharmacy. It was believed that through the act of baptism, Silvester also had cured the Emperor of the physical sickness of leprosy. Although Vignali does not show Constantine with the sores associated with this terrible sickness, the holy baptismal water had evidently already cured him, just as medicinal unguents and salves wash and cleanse physical wounds and sores on a patient's body.[56]

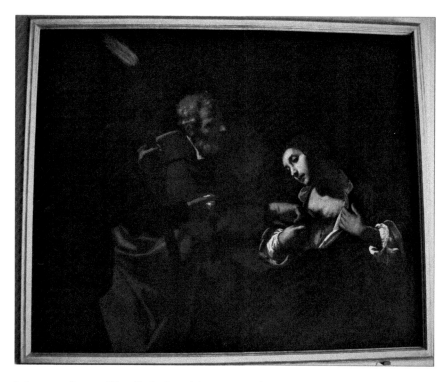

FIGURE 3.7 Jacopo Vignali, *St. Peter Treats St. Agatha* (1623–24)

Source: Maggie Bell with the concession of the Museo di S. Marco, Ministero per i beni e le attività culturali, Polo museale della Toscana

The third canvas is a shocking and very unusual scene of St Agatha exposing her bloody chest to St Peter, after she had had her breasts removed through torture (Figure 3.7). Her patient martyred expression is matched by St Peter's compassionate glance as he spreads unguent on the wounds, taken from a small phial, which he holds in his right hand. It is a curiously intimate scene and is certainly a challenging picture. This image is particularly violent when compared with a contemporary painting by Lorenzo Lippi (1632–34), who shows a much softer and more sensual view of St Agatha, who simply points to her bared, right-hand breast, with little indication of the torture she will suffer, except to the *conoscenti*.[57] Within ten years, Lippi painted another picture of the same subject. Again, he presents a sensuous, well-dressed young lady, who engages the viewer with her direct gaze. Here too her body is presented as unmutilated, but she provides a graphic reminder of her martyrdom, since two breasts are shown in a dish in front of her, while she holds a sharp knife in her left hand.[58]

The fourth picture was painted in 1630 during the plague epidemic. Vignali shows the Good Samaritan pouring ointment on the wounds of the sickly young man, who, like plague victims in that year, had collapsed at the side of the road

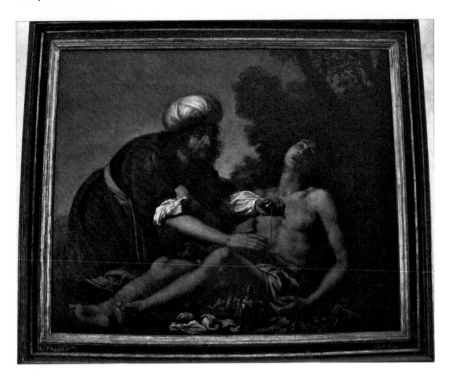

FIGURE 3.8 Jacopo Vignali, *The Good Samaritan* (1630)

Source: Maggie Bell with the concession of the Museo di S. Marco, Ministero per i beni e le attività culturali, Polo museale della Toscana

(Figure 3.8). He is shown with a number of abrasions on his body, the worst at the level of his waist. He had evidently already received treatment, because there is a bandage on his right-hand leg above his ankle. Giovanni Pagliarulo in his description of the picture argues that this body covered with sores may very well have been a reference to the body of the plague victim. This may be true in a metaphorical sense, although in terms of more accurate representation, it is difficult when looking at the picture to determine whether he is suffering from cuts resulting from a beating or the sores of disease.[59]

The role of these four paintings was to advertise the power of these saints and at the same time the healing role of the newly refurbished friars' pharmacy. The central medical message of each picture was underlined by the use of liquids or unguents. In the case of Constantine, it was baptismal water which cured him of original sin. While holy water was kept within the church, the other medicines would have been made up and stored in the pharmacy in the types of storage jars represented in some of pictures. This underlines the importance of the process of treatment within the friars' pharmacy and explains Vignali's emphasis on the curative properties of medicines.

Conclusion

In the canvases by Vignali at San Marco, as with the other images discussed in this chapter, spiritual and physical medicine were invoked to work in combination to treat and cure the sick and wounded. While Christ was seen as the divine physician, he also administered punishment for the sins of mankind, hence the necessity to invoke the help of saintly intercessors, such as Sebastian and Rocco, together with local cults, such as that of Sant'Antonino. However, the Virgin Mary remained the most important intercessor and she was represented at the apex of the hierarchy in many altarpieces, as well as being the subject of miraculous images, at the shrines of Santissima Annunziata and Santa Maria Impruneta. Other imperatives behind the visualization of infirmity included the desire to advertise the role of religious Orders in the care of the sick or the role of cities in successfully defending themselves against plague.

This range of contexts, then, has helped to determine how sickness and infirmity were represented. In the vast majority of cases, the main motivation was religious rather than medical, which helps to explain why it was less rather than more common to show specific physical symptoms when a generic picture of a pale, languishing body would serve the purpose. It should also not be forgotten that as Galenic humoral medicine conceived disease as an imbalance of humours and a collection of symptoms, infirmity was not easy to represent in visual terms. The exceptions were major epidemics, such as leprosy, plague, and the Great Pox. While it has been shown by historians that there was a general tendency in early modern Italy to reveal fewer and less marked specific symptoms among saints and individual plague victims, it has been argued here that this pattern was not always reflected at the local levels, as seen in the case of Florence and its hinterland. However, where the iconography of infirmity in Florence does follow more general trends is the greater emphasis placed on the vivid depiction of wounds. Indeed, as has been pointed out in relation to Vignali's oeuvre in the 1620s and 1630s, the wounds themselves may have acted as a metaphor for epidemic disease.[60] Thus, given this variety of motivations and styles of representation, an overly emphatic distinction between sickness, infirmity, and wounds risks returning us to the traditional filter of retrospective diagnosis. After all, the aim in depicting physical suffering was to induce penitence within the viewer, which provided hope for individuals and communities to recover from sickness.[61]

Notes

1 Cohn, *The Black Death Transformed*; Green, *Pandemic Disease in the Medieval World*.
2 Boeckl, *Images of Leprosy*.
3 See Lynteris, *Ethnographic Plague*, chapter 1.
4 For an image, see https://en.wikipedia.org/wiki/Giovanni_del_Biondo.
5 Barker, 'The making of a plague saint', 90–131, and on Del Biondo, 100–02. See also Marshall, 'Reading the Body of a Plague Saint', 237–72.
6 For an image, see https://en.wikipedia.org/wiki/Palla_della_Peste_(Guido_Reni).
7 Puglisi, 'Guido Reni's *Pallione del Voto*', 403–06.

8 Puglisi, 'Guido Reni's *Pallione del Voto*', 404.

9 For an image, see https://en.wikipedia.org/wiki/Domenico_Gargiulo, cf. Clifton, 'Art and Plague at Naples', 97–152.

10 Cipolla, *Fighting the Plague*, 101.

11 Jones, 'San Carlo Borromeo', 65–74; Barker, 'Plague art', 45–64; Clifton, 'Art and plague at Naples', 97–152.

12 Pellicini, *Discorso sopra de' mali contagiosi pestilenziali*, 6–7.

13 For a more detailed consideration of this image, see Henderson, *Florence under Siege*, 156–58.

14 Pellicini, *Discorso sopra de' mali contagiosi pestilenziali*, 6–7.

15 Borea, 'Pietro Dandini'.

16 On the representation of Borromeo during the Milanese plague, see Jones, 'San Carlo Borromeo', 65–96. Images of Borromeo in Venice, for example, from the earlier seventeenth century include Pietro Damini, *San Carlo Borromeo e gli appestati*, and Camillo Procaccini, *San Carlo Borromeo in gloria*: see Comune di Venezia, *Venezia e la peste*, 255–56, a.29 and a.30.

17 Boeckl, *Images of Plague*, 1–9, 113–14; Barker, 'Plague art', 48–49.

18 For an image, see https://commons.wikimedia.org/wiki/File:Giovan_battista_vanni,_deposizione_di_san_sebastiano,_1626,_01.jpg; cf. Barker, 'Plague art', 47–48; Guidi and Marcucci, *Il Seicento Fiorentino*, I, 292–93.

19 Boeckl, *Images of Plague*, 108–18. On this theme for an earlier period, see the chapter in this volume by Diana Bullen Presciutti, and on the Camilliani's nursing role at the Incurabili hospital of San Giacomo in Rome: Arrizabalaga, Henderson and French, *The Great Pox*, 171–73.

20 On the important role of nursing staff in Florence, see Henderson, *The Renaissance Hospital*, chapter 6.

21 Barker, 'Plague art', 47–49.

22 Guidi and Marcucci, *Il Seicento Fiorentino*, vol. 1, 124–25.

23 Boeckl, *Images of Plague*, 108–18; Barker, 'Plague art', 47–49.

24 See Mason Rinaldi, 'Le immagini della peste', 209–24, 225–86.

25 Marshall, 'A plague saint for Venice', 153–88; Marshall, 'A new plague saint', 543–49.

26 For an image, see https://it.m.wikipedia.org/wiki/File:Peste_del_1630_a_Venezia,_Bozzetto_-_Zanchi.jpg. Cf. Riccorboni, 'Antonio Zanchi', 57–58.

27 On plague in Florence in the 1520s, see Henderson, 'Plague in Renaissance Florence', 165–86; and on the 1570s, see Preto, *Peste e società*, and Cohn, *Cultures of Plague*.

28 Cipolla, *Fighting the Plague*, 100–01, tables A.1 and A.2.

29 Henderson, *Florence under Siege*, 164–67.

30 See Henderson, *Florence under Siege*, chapter 6, for a detailed discussion of these events during the epidemic.

31 Henderson, *Florence under Siege*, chapter 6.

32 Barker, 'Plague art', 47–48. On Florence, see Pagliarulo, 'Jacopo Vignali' (1994), 144; Pagliarulo, 'Jacopo Vignali', in *Il Seicento Fiorentino*, vol. 3, 183–87.

33 Pagliarulo (1994), 184, 186; Iarocci, 'The Santissima Annunziata', 210.

34 Pagliarulo, 'Jacopo Vignali' (1994), 185–86.

35 Bellesi, *Vincenzo Dandini*, 83, cat. no. 8.

36 Bellesi and Bisceglia, *Carlo Dolci*, 182–83, cat. no. 11; Baldassari, *Carlo Dolci*, 158–59, cat. no. 62.

37 Pagliarulo, 'Jacopo Vignali' (1994), 140.

38 Pagliarulo, 'Jacopo Vignali' (1994), 158.

39 Pagliarulo, 'Jacopo Vignali' (1994), 153–55.

40 Guidi and Marcucci, *Il Seicento Fiorentino. Pittura*, 298–99, cat. no. 1.150.

41 D'Afflitto, *Lorenzo Lippi*, 196: *Madonna col Bambino e i santi Rocco, Sebastiano, Antonio da Padova, Michele e Donato* (Ronta, chiesa di San Michele, 1634).

42 On Dandini, see Guidi and Marcucci, *Il Seicento Fiorentino*, vol. 3, 69–73, and for a more detailed consideration of this image, see Henderson, *Florence under Siege*, 156–58.

43 On this cycle, see Jenni Kuuliala's chapter in this volume.
44 Papi, *Andrea Commodi*, 101, cat. no. 32; see the earlier examples: Papi, *Andrea Commodi*, 90, cat. no. 20; 97, cat. no. 26. Another image of Borromeo appears in Vignali's *Pietà*, in which he meditates on the Passion and Christ's wounds: Pagliarulo, 'Jacopo Vignali' (1994), 142.
45 Papi and Petrioli Tofani, *Andrea Commodi*, 34–35, plate 17; 212, cat. no. 62; registro cronologico, 221–23. Cf. Guidi and Marcucci, *Il Seicento Fiorentino*, vol. 2, 144–45.
46 On Baccio, see *Il Seicento Fiorentino*, vol. 3, 76–78.
47 Boeckl, *Images of Plague*, 55–56; Barker, 'The making of a plague saint'; Marshall, 'A new plague saint'.
48 Guidi and Marcucci, *Il Seicento Fiorentino*, vol. 2, 249–50.
49 Henderson, *The Renaissance Hospital*, chapter 4.1.
50 Cipolla, *I pidocchi e il granduca*, 95.
51 Fracastorii, *De contagione*, 103.
52 For these paintings, see Baldassari, *La collezione Piero ed Elena Bigongiari*, 18 (Pl. 7, Giovanni Battista Vanni), 19 (Pl. 8, Giovanni Battista Vanni, painted in Rome after 1629).
53 The most detailed discussion of these paintings is in Pagliarulo, 'Jacopo Vignali' (1994). See most recently, Pagliarulo, 'Jacopo Vignali, *San Pietro cura Sant'Agata*, 314–15.
54 See also, Giovanni Battista Vanni (1600–60), *Tobiolo e l'angelo* painted in the late 1620s-early 1630s, *Il Seicento*, vol. 2, 294–96.
55 For example, Antonio and Piero del Pollaiuolo, *Tobias and the Angel* of 1460 (Galleria Sabauda, Turin), and Andrea del Verrocchio, *Tobias and the Angel* of 1470–75 (National Gallery London).
56 Boeckl, *Images of Leprosy*, 81–82, 110–13. See also the discussion in this volume by Diana Bullen Presciutti of the lepers illustrated in 'La Franceschina'.
57 D'Afflitto, *Lorenzo Lippi*, 195, cat. no. 25.
58 D'Afflitto, *Lorenzo Lippi*, 240, cat. no. 67.
59 Pagliarulo, 'Jacopo Vignali' (1994), 146.
60 See, Pagliarulo, 'Jacopo Vignali' (1994), 144.
61 I am very grateful to Giovanni Pagliarulo for his help and advice while writing this chapter, especially his expertise on Jacopo Vignali, and to Maggie Bell for taking many of the photographs used here.

Bibliography

Primary sources

Fracastorii, Hieronymi, *De contagione et contagionis morbis et eorum curatione, libri III*, trans. and ed. Wilmer Cave Wright (New York and London: Putnams, 1930).
Pellicini, Antonio, *Discorso sopra de mali contagiosi pestilenziali. Raccolto dall'Eccellentissimo Sig. Antonio Pellicini D'ordine del Colegio de Medici Fiorentini. Per comandamento del sereniss. Gran Duca di Toscana* (Florence: Zanobi Pignoni, 1630).

Secondary sources

Arrizabalaga, Jon, John Henderson, and Roger French, *The Great Pox. The French Disease in Renaissance Europe* (New Haven and London: Yale University Press, 1997).
Bailey, Gauvin Alexander, Pamela M. Jones, Franco Mormando, and Thomas W. Worcester (eds), *Hope and Healing: Painting in Italy in a Time of Plague, 1500–1880* (Chicago: Chicago University Press, 2005).
Baldassari, Francesca, *Carlo Dolci. Complete Catalogue of the Paintings* (Florence: Centro Di, 2015).

Baldassari, Francesca, *La collezione Piero ed Elena Bigongiari: Il Seicento Fiorentino tra 'favola' e dramma* (Pistoia: Editore Cassa di Risparmio di Pistoia e Pescia, 2004).

Barker, Sheila, 'Art, Architecture and the Roman Plague of 1656–1657', in Irene Fosi (ed.), *La Peste a Roma (1656–1657), Roma Moderna e contemporanea*, 14 (Rome: Università degli Studi di Roma Tre, 2006), 243–62.

Barker, Sheila, 'The making of a plague saint. Saint Sebastian's imagery and cult before the Counter-Reformation', in Franco Mormando and Thomas W. Worcester (eds), *Piety and Plague from Byzantium to the Baroque* (Kirksville, MO: Truman State University Press, 2007), 90–131.

Barker, Sheila, 'Plague art in early modern Rome: Divine directives and temporal remedies', in Bailey, Jones, Mormando and Worcester (eds), *Hope and Healing*, 45–64.

Bellesi, Sandro, *Vincenzo Dandini e la pittura a Firenze alla metà del Seicento* (Pisa: Editore Felici, 2003).

Bellesi, Sandro and Anna Bisceglia, eds, *Carlo Dolci, 1616–1687* (Città di Castello: Sillabe, 2015).

Boeckl, Christine M., *Images of Leprosy: Disease, Religion and Politics in European Art* (Kirksville, MO: Truman State University Press, 2011).

Boeckl, Christine M., *Images of Plague and Pestilence. Iconography and Iconology* (Kirksville, MO: Truman State University Press, 2001).

Borea, Evelina, 'Pietro Dandini', in *Dizionario biografico degli Italiani* (Rome: Istituto dell' Enciclopedia italiana, 1986), vol. 32.

Cipolla, Carlo M., *Fighting the Plague in Seventeenth-Century Italy* (Madison: University of Wisconsin Press, 1981).

Cipolla, Carlo M., *I pidocchi e il granduca. Crisi economica e problem sanitari nella Firenze del '600* (Bologna: Il Mulino, 1979).

Clifton, James, 'Art and Plague at Naples', in Bailey, Jones, Mormando and Worcester (eds), *Hope and Healing*, 97–152.

Cohn, Samuel Kline, Jr., *The Black Death Transformed: Disease and Culture in Early Renaissance Europe* (London: Hodder Arnold, 2002).

Cohn, Samuel Kline, Jr., *Cultures of Plague: Medical Thinking at the End of the Renaissance* (Oxford: Oxford University Press, 2010).

Comune di Venezia, *Venezia e la peste, 1348–1797* (Venice: Marsilio Editore, 1979).

D'Afflitto, Chiara, *Lorenzo Lippi* (Florence: Edifir, 2002).

Green, Monica H., ed., 'Pandemic disease in the medieval world: Rethinking the Black Death', *The Medieval Globe*, 1.1 (Kalamazoo, MI: Arc Medieval Press, 2014).

Guidi, Giuliana, and Daniele Marcucci (eds), *Il Seicento Fiorentino* (Florence: Cantini Edizioni d'Arte, 1986–87), 3 vols.

Henderson, John, *Florence Under Siege: Surviving Plague in an Early Modern City* (New Haven and London: Yale University Press, 2019).

Henderson, John, 'Plague in Renaissance Florence: Medical theory and government response', in Neithard Bulst and Robert Delort (eds), *Maladies et société (xii—xviiie siècles)* (Paris: CNRS Editions, 1989), 165–86.

Henderson, John, *The Renaissance Hospital: Healing the Body and Healing the Soul* (New Haven and London: Yale University Press, 2006).

Iarocci, Bernice Ida Maria, *The Santissima Annunziata of Florence, Medici Portraits, and the Counter Reformation in Italy* (unpublished PhD Dissertation, University of Toronto, 2015).

Jones, Pamela M., 'San Carlo Borromeo and plague imagery in Milan and Rome', in Bailey, Jones, Mormando and Worcester (eds), *Hope and Healing*, 65–74.

Lynteris, Christos, *Ethnographic Plague: Configuring Disease on the Chinese-Russian Frontier* (London: Palgrave Macmillan, 2016).

Marshall, Louise, 'A new plague saint for Renaissance Italy: Suffering and sanctity in narrative cycles of Saint Roch', in Janie Anderson, ed., *Crossing Cultures: Conflict, Migration and Convergence: The Proceedings of the 32nd International Congress of the History of Art* (Melbourne: The Miegunyah Press, 2009), 543–49.

Marshall, Louise, 'A plague saint for Venice: Tintoretto at the Chiesa di San Rocco', *Artibus et historiae*, 66 (XXXIII) (2012), 153–88.

Marshall, Louise, 'Reading the body of a plague saint: Narrative altarpieces and devotional images of St. Sebastian in Renaissance Art', in Bernard J. Muir (ed.), *Reading Texts and Images* (Exeter: Exeter University Press, 2002), 237–72.

Mason Rinaldi, Stefania, 'Le immagini della peste nella cultura figurative veneziana', in Comune di Venezia, *Venezia e la peste, 1348–1797* (Venice: Marsilio Editore, 1979), 209–24, 225–86.

Pagliarulo, Giovanni, 'Jacopo Vignali', in Giuliana Guidi and Daniele Marcucci (eds), *Il Seicento Fiorentino* (Florence: Cantini Edizioni d'Arte, 1986–87), vol. 3, 183–87.

Pagliarulo, Giovanni, 'Jacopo Vignali e gli anni della peste', *Artista. Critica dell'Arte in Toscana*, 6 (1994), 138–98.

Pagliarulo, Giovanni, 'Jacopo Vignali, *San Pietro cura Sant'Agata*, 1623–1624', in Gianni Papi (ed.), *Caravaggio e caravaggesci a Firenze* (Florence: Gruppo Editoriale Giunti, 2010), 314–15.

Papi, Gianni, *Andrea Commodi* (Florence: Edifi, 1994).

Papi, Gianni and Annamaria Petrioli Tofani, *Andrea Commodi dall'attrazione per Michelangelo all'ansia del nuovo* (Florence: Edizioni Polistampa, 2012).

Preto, Paolo, *Peste e società a Venezia* (Vicenza: Neri Pozza, 1992).

Puglisi, Catherine R., 'Guido Reni's *Pallione del Voto* and the Plague of 1630', *Burlington Magazine*, 130, 8 (1995), 402–12.

Riccorboni, Alberto, 'Antonio Zanchi e la pittura veneziana del seicento', *Saggi e memorie di storia dell'arte*, 6 (1966), 57–58.

PART II

Institutions and visualizing illness

4

ON DISPLAY

Poverty as infirmity and its visual representation at the hospital of Santa Maria della Scala in Siena

Maggie Bell

Beginning in the eleventh century, the hospital of Santa Maria della Scala in Siena provided medical care and assistance to the local and foreign poor. The hospital grew organically over the centuries, absorbing almost half of the buildings around the piazza it shares with the cathedral of Siena. By the mid-fifteenth century, similar to other massive civic hospitals at the time, the Scala was a sprawling complex allowing for varying types of care that included treating the sick, housing foundling children, distributing alms, and sheltering pilgrims and travellers, all of whom had no grounding in the community or were unable to seek aid at home.

This chapter investigates how the social condition of poverty shaped depictions of infirmity, taking as a case study the fifteenth-century frescoes painted in the *pellegrinaio*, or central male ward, of the hospital of Santa Maria della Scala (Figure 4.1).[1] The cycle, painted between 1440 and 1444, is composed of eight monumental frescoes representing the history and good works of the hospital and offers numerous and varied depictions of the infirm. At the time, the ward opened on to the Piazza del Duomo, and given the location and permeability of the *pellegrinaio*, the frescoes would have been seen by a wide audience, including staff, hospital inmates, and outside visitors. This highly visible cycle was probably designed by the rector Giovanni di Francesco Buzzichelli and his predecessor Carlo d'Agnolino di Bartoli, then bishop of Siena, who together created a complex system of iconography that spoke to the identity of the hospital as a civic and religious institution that served the needs of the poor and infirm.[2]

A shared characteristic of all hospital beneficiaries was their vulnerability, typically exacerbated by poverty, which was understood in the period as having a causal relationship with ill health.[3] Fifteenth-century documents from the hospital of the Misericordia in Prato frequently use the words *povari* (poor) and *infermi* (infirm) interchangeably when describing reason for admittance. Though the Scala's inmate records from this period do not survive, studies of similar documents from the Prato

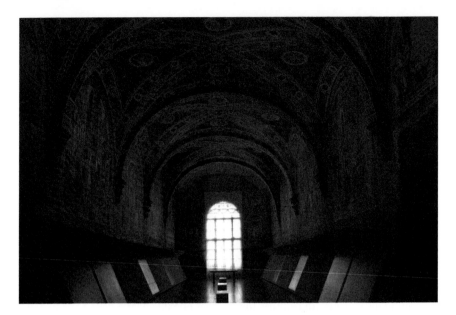

FIGURE 4.1 View of *Pellegrinaio*, Hospital of Santa Maria della Scala, Siena

Source: Photo by author

institution reveal that a majority of people who came to the hospital were economically disadvantaged or outside their networks of care and were often admitted for ailments caused by their poverty.[4] Period documents from Santa Maria della Scala confirm that at the time the *pellegrinaio* frescoes were painted, the primary concern of the hospital was providing services for the poor. The most commonly used word to refer to those taken in by the hospital was 'povari', which appears frequently in the generic language of the Libro Vitale chronicling donations made to 'Spedale Santa Maria e i suoi povari' (the hospital of Santa Maria and its poor). On the rare occasions when inmates are mentioned in the financial accounts, it is often in association with the adjective 'povero', as in 'povari pellegrini' ('poor pilgrims') or 'venti soldi si dero a tre huomini povari' ('twenty soldi [given] to three poor men').[5] In the original hospital statutes from 1305, the primary recipients of care are the poor or the poor and infirm—language that is reused in the later editions of the hospital statutes in 1454.[6]

To represent the infirmity of the poor was to depict both physical ailment and social position, which were intertwined conditions. On the wall containing four scenes of the hospital's history, those who are both indigent and ailing are shown according to typical representational tropes. They occupy marginal compositional and architectural spaces, in some cases displaying their infirmities, such as an injured limb, to verify their need and attract the generosity of others. A consequence of being poor in the period often meant that one's infirmity was experienced in a public or semi-public environment. As a result, the poor sick were depicted as being more visually present in daily urban life than their affluent counterparts, who were cared for in their homes.

On the opposite side of the hall, the compositional marginalization of the poor sick changes completely in the four frescoes representing the curative and charitable works inside the hospital. In these images, the bodies of the infirm are centrally located and are observed by doctors, hospital staff, visitors, and inmates. These central positions expose the depicted poor sick to scrutiny while also identifying them as individuals worthy of attention. This dual aspect was rooted in broader societal attitudes towards the poor, who were simultaneously recipients of judgemental evaluation and acts of charity. At the Scala, where poverty and infirmity were essentially synonymous, the *pellegrinaio* frescoes reveal the highly visible condition of being sick while poor in a large civic hospital. Caring for infirmity began with seeing it, and the artistic strategies employed in the *pellegrinaio* frescoes modelled the sorts of looking (ideal and practised) that occurred in the hospital space, which will be addressed in three overlapping categories: assessment, spectacle, and contemplation.

Infirmity of the poor in public spaces

The *pellegrinaio* frescoes are dominated by architectural settings that have the same complexity as the narratives unfolding within them. While imaginative, aspects of the architecture are meant to evoke specific places in the hospital and in its surrounding urban environment, allowing viewers to readily draw connections between the frescoes and the hospital itself. The scenes suggestively render the vivacity of daily hospital life by depicting varied crowds of staff, inmates, and visitors moving within spaces dedicated to particular kinds of care, such as medical wards, chapels in which alms were distributed, and the living quarters for foundling children. The frescoed architecture of the Scala is not merely illustrative; rather, it represents the structured relationships between figures that shape social and aesthetic definitions of the poor sick.

In the frescoes recounting the hospital's history, the poor sick are situated in relationship to the built environment in ways that are consistent with contemporary pictorial traditions. Fifteenth-century paintings often locate such figures in marginal places like loggias or city gates, notably in scenes set around the Temple of Solomon, such as the Presentation of the Virgin and the Presentation of Christ.[7] These poor and infirm figures, who are usually found on the stairs of the Temple or in the peripheral urban surroundings, have varying significance, including 'ornaments' for principal scenes, reminders of the virtue of poverty and charity, or as foils for wealthy bystanders.[8] The *pellegrinaio* frescoes repeat this convention in two scenes: *The Expansion of the Hospital* and *The Investiture of the Rector* (Figure 4.2 and Figure 4.3), both of which depict the piazza between the Scala and the cathedral. The *Expansion* scene, painted by Domenico di Bartolo in 1443, shows the hospital as an active construction site covered in scaffolding. In the centre, above a builder carrying bricks and a mason holding a divider, the rector lifts his hat as he accepts a donation from a bishop's

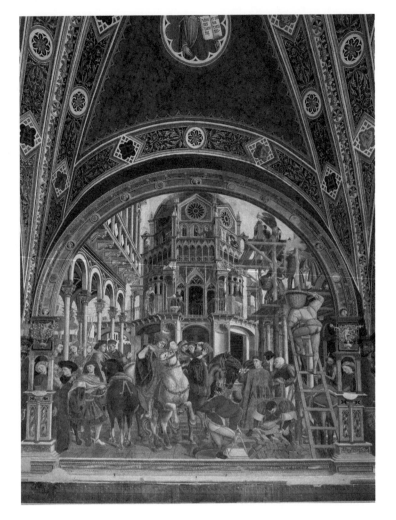

FIGURE 4.2 Domenico di Bartolo, *The Expansion of the Hospital*

Source: Comune di Siena, photo by Bruno Bruchi, 2013

messenger.[9] Immediately behind the rector is the builder's ladder, a clear reference to the hospital's emblem of a *scala*, or ladder, crowned with a cross. On the other side, a bearded figure emerges from the doorway of the hospital, leaning heavily on a walking stick, dressed in a ragged tunic that exposes his arms and chest. The man is removed from the central narrative and serves rather as an attribute of the hospital behind him, indicating the Scala's status as a charitable institution.[10]

The Investiture of the Rector, painted by Priamo della Quercia in 1442, depicts another foundational moment in 1305, when the Beato Agostino Novello changed

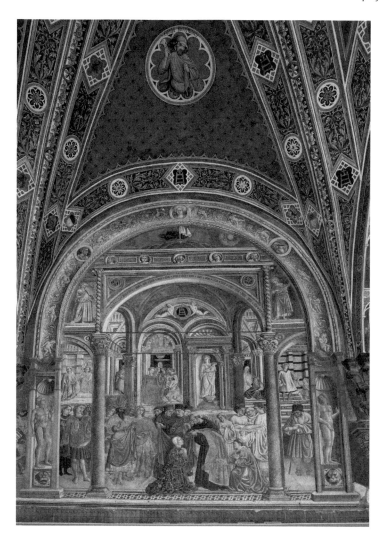

FIGURE 4.3 Priamo della Quercia, *The Investiture of the Rector by Beato Agostino Novello*

Source: Comune di Siena, photo by Bruno Bruchi, 2013

the administrative structure of the Scala to follow that of the Augustinian Order (Figure 4.3). In the foreground, the rector of the hospital receives a cloak from Beato Agostino, indicating his acceptance of the Augustinian Rule. The ceremony is observed by an elderly man whose ill-fitting tunic and dependency on his walking stick suggests bodily discomfort and sets him in contrast with the well-dressed visitors on the left side of the fresco. The scene takes place in a baldachin-like

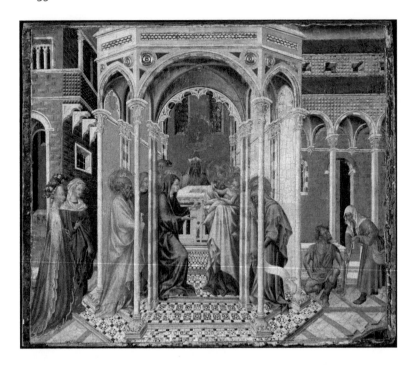

FIGURE 4.4 Giovanni di Paolo, *The Presentation of Christ in the Temple*

Source: The Metropolitan Museum of Art, public domain

structure reminiscent of Giovanni di Paolo's 1435 predella panel depicting the presentation of Christ at the Temple (Figure 4.4). This panel also shows a contrast between the elegant observers to the left, who stand in front of a residential palace, and the beggar couple to the right in front of a loggia, who display signs of physical malady. The disintegrated pavement establishes a further contrast between the left and right sides of the image and enhances the symbolic weight of the beggars, connecting poverty and illness to civic instability.[11]

On the opposite side of the *pellegrinaio*, the frescoed scenes of care reinforce the public vulnerability of the individuals whom the hospital served. In *The Distribution of Alms* (Figure 4.5), a crowd of people, including beggars, pilgrims, and mothers with children, enters a chapel of the Scala from the piazza through a large door.[12] After receiving alms, they re-enter the city through the door to the left. The figures appear in a frieze-like arrangement close to the picture plane, so viewers can clearly see their infirmities, some wrapped in bloodied bandages and others relying on walking sticks or other devices for mobility. Visible through the large portals are buildings surrounding the piazza outside. Indicating the proximity of the poor sick to the urban environment, these views implicitly reinforce the fact that these individuals needed to travel through the city in order to find remedy and sustenance at the hospital.

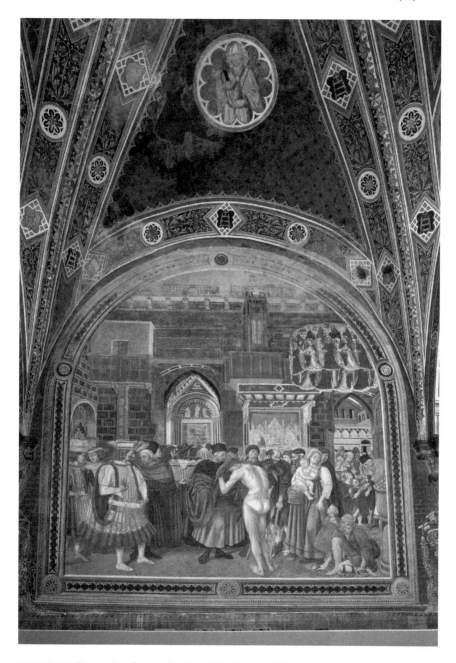

FIGURE 4.5 Domenico di Bartolo, *The Distribution of Alms*

Source: Comune di Siena, photo by Bruno Bruchi, 2013

The Distribution of Alms adheres to period conventions of representing gatherings of the poor and sick in urban spaces. Visual representations of crowds of urban poor tended to be associated with charitable scenes, such as Andrea di Bartolo's panel painting *Joachim and Anna Giving Food to the Poor and Offerings to the Temple* (1400–05) at the Washington National Gallery of Art. Here the Virgin's parents stand in open porches and distribute food to a group with physical ailments similar to those in the *Distribution* scene in the *pellegrinaio*. In these examples, the alms-seekers approach the alms-givers and receive temporary shelter from the urban environment in the permeable spaces of the loggia or open chapel.[13] These scenes show charity as a public act serving not only the needs of the individual but also that of the city.

Although the other three frescoes representing the Scala's daily good works take place within the hospital itself, they reinforce the public experience of the poor sick. Each fresco depicts spaces dedicated to a particular type of care: a ward (Figure 4.6), the women and children's living quarters (Figure 4.7), and a refectory for feeding large numbers of hospital inmates and the city's hungry (Figure 4.8). While less obviously enmeshed with the urban environment than the chapel in the *Distribution of Alms*, these spaces appear permeable, with figures entering and exiting the boundaries of the scenes, diminishing any sense of a hermetically sealed clinical environment.[14] Though modern viewers might expect single-occupancy hospital beds, the Scala provided care in large open wards, in which two, and sometimes up to four, people would share a bed.[15] Writing in 1400, a papal jubilee year, the chronicler Tommaso Montauri described such a scene, saying that 'so full were the hospitals of the infirm, both foreigners and countrymen, that it was a mercy [*pietà*] to behold.'[16] The image Montauri evokes suggests an intimacy between infirm individuals placed into very close contact that made privacy in the modern sense impossible. Additionally, the very fact that the chronicler claims to have observed the inmates in their beds reveals the accessibility of the ward to outsiders.

Poverty added a dimension of visibility to the condition of infirmity that was not diminished when one had recourse to a hospital but rather was part of institutional practices of observing inmates. For the purposes of this chapter, I use 'observation' to mean any act of concerted looking, which took various forms in an early modern hospital setting. The *pellegrinaio* frescoes not only represent the wounds and maladies of inmates with excruciating detail but also depict the specific ways in which such conditions could be observed in the real ward. While not analogous to the medicalizing clinical gaze as has been discussed in an eighteenth-century context, the *pellegrinaio* frescoes suggest an *institutional* gaze, or gazes, facilitated by the unique aspects of life in an early modern civic hospital.[17]

Assessment

Different types of institutional gazes appear with particular clarity in the four frescoes representing the curative and charitable activities of the Scala. At the far end of the *pellegrinaio*, on the north wall, *The Care of the Sick* (Figure 4.6) shows a busy ward, whose activities focus on the assessment and treatment of the wounded and

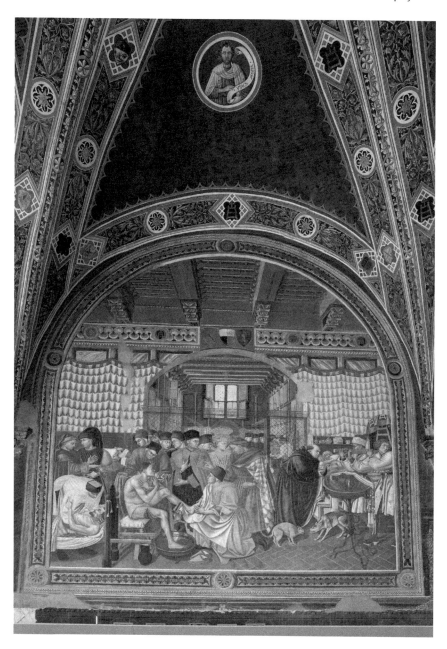

FIGURE 4.6 Domenico di Bartolo, *The Care of the Sick*

Source: Comune di Siena, photo by Bruno Bruchi, 2013

sick. A nude man sits in the foreground of the image just to the left of centre, a bloody laceration sliced violently across his right thigh. A surgeon dressed in a fur cape and red turban, holding an instrument in his right hand and a vial of ointment in his left, looks fixedly at the injured man.[18] Kneeling in the centre of the image, a *pellegriniere*—the official responsible for the daily operations of the wards—also looks intently at his charge, washing his feet in hot water; this is both a symbolic gesture of mercy and a reference to actual medical practice.[19] The rector stands between the surgeon and his subject, his left hand touching his distinctive cloak, as if indicating his authority to compel the surgeon to intervene.

An attentive gaze also appears in the scene to the left, where a hospital brother embraces an emaciated man in a cot, whose lower body extends beyond the frame of the image. Above, two physicians attempt a diagnosis, discussing the appearance of the infirm man's urine. The physician holding a vial, or *matula*, of urine studies it closely in order to discern the imbalance of humours causing the man's suffering. This illustrates a practice recommended as a means of diagnosis by Hippocrates and Galen, who describe visible clues, such as discolouration, that indicate particular maladies.[20]

These vignettes in *The Care of the Sick* are arranged close to the picture plane for the sake of visual clarity in order to demonstrate the various ways that the hospital served the bodily needs of inmates. The effect is similar to Santi Buglioni's terracotta frieze (1526) on the façade of Il Ceppo, Pistoia's civic hospital, which represents aspects of hospital care.[21] As in *The Care of the Sick*, the central panel of the Ceppo frieze shows the staff and physicians performing examinations and caring for inmates. These scenes are framed by a blank background, which isolates the actions of the figures, making them more visible from below. This is unlike the scenes of assessment and care depicted in *The Care of the Sick*, which are given a spatial context, situated at the end of an expansive ward that extends beyond a wrought-iron gate, similar to what would have separated the *pellegrinaio* from the entrance to the hospital.[22] The proximity of these scenes to the picture plane not only increases their legibility but also sets them apart from the background activity beyond the gate, suggesting that they occur in an antechamber of the ward.

Creating a compositionally distinct space may be a visual interpretation of a practice described in the statutes of 1305 regarding the assessment of incoming individuals prior to their placement in the hospital. The fifteenth statute dictates that 'we order and desire that one of the brothers of the aforementioned hospital—one who is benign and pious—or the *pellegriniere*, to receive and to tend to and assign to a bed all the infirm [*li infermi*] that come or are brought or carried to said hospital, so that they will be put in bed according to what appears worthy and convenient to the rector and said *pellegriniere* given their infirmity and need'.[23] Santa Maria Nuova, Florence's large civic hospital, processed inmates in a similar way, evaluating their need in the entrance hall before assigning them a bed.[24] These statutes reveal the exposing nature of the assessment of new arrivals, which involved not only official scrutiny but also the probability of being seen by other inmates and staff. They also indicate that assessment procedures were typically not assigned to physicians, who were rarely on staff. In this period, there would have been only two designated hospital physicians, who would have significantly limited their time with individual inmates.[25] Rather, as the statutes suggest, hospital brethren or officials who managed the wards, like the *pellegriniere* or the *infermiere*, would be the first to examine new arrivals. In this vein, *The Care of the Sick* shows the institutional gaze of the Scala as being shared across a range of caregivers, operating in their various capacities to assess and place inmates. *The Care of the Sick* reinforces the institutional imperative for observation of infirm bodies—a first step in incorporating inmates into the hospital. The fact that the scene takes place in a ward very similar to the *pellegrinaio* implicates the viewer, who participates in the visual assessment of the depicted inmates. Their infirm bodies are not relegated to the margins of the composition but are almost life-size and are readily visible in the foreground of the image.

Spectacle

The observation of the poor sick also had a spectacular dimension at the Scala, one bound up in the creation of the institution's public-facing self-image. While today most tourists overlook the unadorned facade of the Scala, it made quite an impression in the fifteenth century. Decorated with now-lost frescoes of the life of the Virgin painted by Simone Martini, and Ambrogio and Pietro Lorenzetti in 1335, and located on the spiritual acropolis of Siena across from the cathedral, the hospital regularly participated in civic and religious ceremonies and processions.[26] The Scala was both a charitable institution and a showcase for Siena, and the civic government as well as St Bernardino, Siena's prolific and beloved preacher, urged citizens to donate to the hospital not only for the sake of the poor but to inspire a favourable impression of the city. In the face of the hospital's financial difficulties in the 1420s, Bernardino lamented the lack of beds for pilgrims and expressed his desire that the hospital return to the 'fame it once had.'[27] Bernardino's anxieties were grounded in the fact that in the fifteenth century the Scala was a standard destination for travellers to Siena. The 1495 chronicles of the German pilgrim Arnold von Harff, for example, list the hospital as one of the important sights to visit in Siena, and it enjoyed this status through the eighteenth century.[28]

In addition to caring for pilgrims, hospital administrators felt the need to impress high-profile visitors, such as Pope Eugenius IV and Sigismund, the emperor-elect of the Holy Roman Empire.[29] Representations of elite visitors appear throughout the *pellegrinaio* frescoes, a pictorial strategy that accentuates social and bodily difference through visual contrast.[30] Importantly, the elite visitors function not only as foils for the poor sick but also as observers. In *The Distribution of Alms* (Figure 4.5), adjacent to *The Care of the Sick*, a hectic crowd presses into the chapel. Mothers and children, the poor, elderly and infirm appear in the foreground, displaying the array of needs the hospital met through regular almsgiving. In the centre foreground, a nude man receives clothing from a hospital brother.[31] This charitable interaction is regarded from the opposite side of the space by an extravagantly dressed visitor; he has been convincingly identified as Emperor Sigismund based on his distinctive profile and headdress.[32] The rector stands by the onlooker's side, lifting his cap and directing the Emperor's attention with a gesture of his hand, which binds the Emperor and the alms-seeker as a conceptual pair. The alms-seeker's nudity conveys his physical vulnerability, his naked back covered in loose flesh with skin stretched across protruding vertebrae. His exposure suggests that his condition was likely caused by deprivation. Similarly, the meagre garments of two bearded men huddled in the right foreground reveal bloodied and bandaged legs—maladies preventing them from working and thus signalling their dependence on alms. Such unobstructed access to these disabled bodies is in direct contrast to the figure of the Emperor; his upright, presumably healthy body obscured by elaborate clothing that creates an imposing profile at the left edge of the fresco. The peripheral location of the Emperor and his retinue demarcate the scene and direct the viewer's attention towards the nude alms-seeker. This figure's central position close to the picture plane and at the centre of semicircle of figures further focuses the viewer's attention on him—aligning the viewer's gaze with that of the wealthy observer.

The adjacent scene of *The Care and Marriage of Foundling Children* (Figure 4.7) is similarly composed so that the gaze of wealthy outsiders is turned towards the vulnerable charges of the Scala. The scene emphasizes the exposure of foundlings indicated by the *pila*, or stone basin in which infants could be placed anonymously outside of the hospital.[33] The *pila* is located in the centre of the fresco, marking the divide between the space outside of the safety of the hospital and the enclosed space of the foundling's quarters. Immediately behind the *pila*, the rector places a swaddled infant in the arms of a nurse, inducting the foundling child into the care of the hospital, which culminates in her marriage depicted to the right. In the foreground, two women in fine clothing observe the scene, redirecting the viewer's eye from the edge of the image towards the vignettes of foundling care.

While the few travellers' descriptions of the Scala that remain do not mention inmates, their authors must have encountered the infirm served by the hospital. The revised statutes of 1454, which recommend that children 'sing for alms at the altar of the church, as is customary', indicate the expectation that visitors would be moved by seeing the poor and needy in the hospital.[34] The foundling children would have been difficult to overlook, becoming objects of special attention, whose plight was sanctified by their proximity to the altar. Similarly, the fresco known as *The Banquet for the Poor* (Figure 4.8), closest to the original entrance of the ward, likely refers to a practice described in the hospital statutes in which the rector would personally serve food to 'the infirm, the poor and the foundlings both male and female' of the hospital 'six times per year' on major feast days, including Easter, the feast of St John and the Assumption, 'and that of these things there should be made a public notice'.[35] In the scene, the rector embraces a semi-nude man, whose physical weakness is indicated by his reliance on a crutch. Again, the depleted body of the stooped figure occupies the centre foreground of the image.

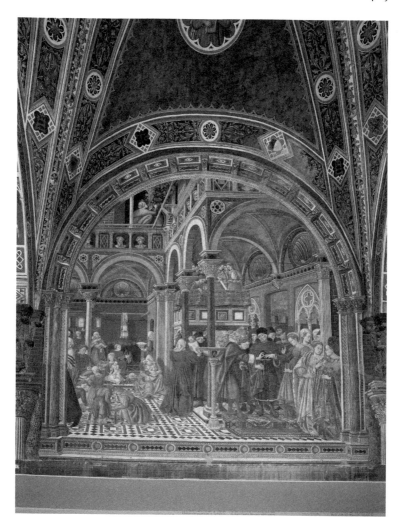

FIGURE 4.7 Domenico di Bartolo, *Care and Marriage of Foundling Children*

Source: Comune di Siena, photo by Bruno Bruchi, 2013

As the rector looks into the man's face, his right hand points behind his exposed back towards the young servant entering the hall with a bowl of food, who is in turn directed with a pointing gesture by a staff member, possibly the *pellegriniere*, who urges the servant in the direction of the emaciated man. To the far right, wealthy onlookers observe the exchange, their gazes directed toward the rector and his charge. That this practice took place on high-profile feast days and required public notice suggest that this was a public or semi-public event, as suggested by

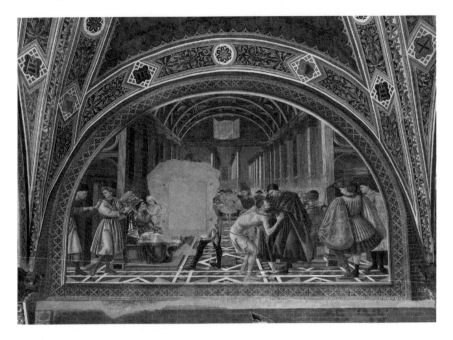

FIGURE 4.8 Domenico di Bartolo, *Banquet for the Poor*

Source: Comune di Siena, photo by Bruno Bruchi, 2013

the well-dressed observers, in which the infirm participated in the spectacle as ceremonial and actual recipients of the hospital's beneficence performed by the rector.

Like the ritualized distribution of food by the hospital rector, or the performances of foundling children for alms, the *pellegrinaio* cycle as a whole elevated and monumentalized charity and caregiving, showing hospital staff and wealthy visitors directing physical and visual attention to inmates. Jonathan Smith identifies one of the central functions of ritual practice as creating scenarios of 'paying attention' to everyday things through their emplacement within ritual environments.[36] Describing temples, for instance, Smith argues:

> The temple serves as a focusing lens, establishing the possibility of significance by directing attention, by requiring the perception of difference. Within the temple, the ordinary (which to any outside eye or ear remains wholly ordinary) becomes significant, becomes "sacred," simply by being there.[37]

Building on the public and ceremonial status of the Scala, the *pellegrinaio* frescoes, like rituals, marked as significant the everyday process of care and healing, turning mundane activities into noteworthy acts. In identifying the poor and sick inmates of the hospital as worthy of attention, the *pellegrinaio* frescoes asserted the power of the Scala as a society-shaping institution. Rather than displaying wounds and maladies in the doorways and loggias of the city in hopes of acquiring donations, the cycle emphasized the hospital's mercy, inviting in and caring for those who were simultaneously feared and overlooked in the wider urban environment. In inverting the compositional position of the poor sick depicted within the walls of the hospital from peripheral to central, the frescoes remind the viewer of the Scala's capacity to direct attention to those in most need.

Contemplation

The *pellegrinaio* frescoes, like many similar images in charitable houses, are versions of the Works of Mercy. Christ describes these seven acts as means through which the faithful can aid their 'least brethren' and, in doing so, demonstrate their devotion to Christ.[38] Christ was both the model recipient and enactor of mercy. This was at the fore in the minds of viewers looking at images such as the *pellegrinaio* frescoes, some of which refer directly to merciful acts in the New Testament. For instance, *The Care of the Sick* depicts feet washing, a both hygienic and highly symbolic practice that alludes to the story of Christ washing the feet of his Apostles.[39] The frescoes were not merely illustrative of the hospital's intake and treatment routines but also, in the context of period devotional practice, guided the viewer's emotional and spiritual engagement with the recipients of hospital care, and ultimately with the human suffering and divine mercy of Christ.[40]

Activating the viewer's emotions was also an important concept in fifteenth-century art theory—Leon Battista Alberti, in his 1427 treatise on painting, recommends that the viewer be guided through the image by a figure gesturing or looking towards the main action. He states: 'It seems opportune then that in the scene [*historia*] there is someone who informs the spectators of the things that unfold . . . or invites you with his own gestures to laugh together or cry in company'.[41] In each of the four scenes of care, hospital staff and elaborately dressed visitors fill the role of observer. Located close to the picture plane, but removed from the action, these peripheral figures serve as stand-ins for the viewer in the ward observing both the frescoes and the real acts of care. Although this was a conventional strategy in fifteenth-century painting, in the context of the hospital, the artistic device of directing the viewer's engagement with the image has particular social and spiritual significance. The act of looking in these cases is not modelled for the poor sick individuals who would have been in the beds below the frescoes but rather for their caretakers and for visitors and donors, who may in turn have been motivated to observe and contemplate the actual inmates in the *pellegrinaio*.

Contemplative observation fits within the hypothesis that the infirm bodies of the poor sick were more accessible than other bodies in the early modern period and that in this accessibility they carried a certain symbolic weight.[42] Christian devotional practices suggest that proximity to the poor and sick was a means of approaching God or enhancing one's chance of salvation. In Siena, St Catherine legendarily slept in the bowels of the Scala—her simple bed marked today by an effigy of the saint in the Oratorio di Santa Caterina—and drank the pus of a sick man to emulate Christ-like suffering.[43] In a less visceral example, throughout his

1425 sermons in the Campo of Siena, St Bernardino urges his listeners to practise appropriate giving to the poor, which includes caring for those who are ill.[44] He also stated that young men should exert themselves in caring for the poor to avoid idleness.[45] The *pellegrinaio* frescoes demonstrate the virtuous exercise of charity by representing the caregiving works of the hospital—the physical engagement on the part of the rector and his staff with the vulnerable bodies of the poor sick.

This institutionalized care placed expectations on the poor and infirm in terms of how they were supposed to receive assistance. Gerald Guest has argued that in French medieval visual culture, 'beggars' who sought alms in the streets were treated with less sympathy than 'paupers' who 'passively, humbly and shamefully receive alms'.[46] Bernardino's sermons similarly describe the appropriate way for the needy to ask for and accept charity, always with humility. He asks: 'you give a piece of bread to a poor man: who is more worthy, you who gave it freely or he who received it? It will be he who receives rather than he who gives by these measures: first the humility with which he asks, and second, the [level of] poverty he has, and his contemplation'.[47]

The *pellegrinaio* frescoes model the appropriate acceptance of charity on the part of the inmates. In the *Care of the Sick*, the man being prepared for surgery crosses his arms in a gesture that can be read as humble gratitude, which he performs with a Christ-like tranquillity that overrides the pain the deep gash in his thigh would undoubtedly produce. The same gesture appears on the opposite wall in the fresco depicting the investiture ceremony, in which, like the Virgin Mary in scenes of the Annunciation, the rector solemnly and obediently accepts his responsibilities. The similarity between the gesture of the wounded man and the kneeling rector in the *Investiture* scene underscores a public and ceremonial aspect to the receipt of care on the part of the hospital inmates, more overtly represented in scenes like *The Banquet for the Poor*, in which the rector serves a meal to hospital inmates on certain feast days. The gesture of humility also reinforces the power dynamics already established through the system of gazes in the scenes of caregiving, in which the poor sick are both recipients of charity and subject to observation. The *pellegrinaio* frescoes depict the hospital as an institution imbued with civic and spiritual virtue, under whose scrutiny infirmity is verified, and care is deservedly received.

Conclusion

At Santa Maria della Scala, where poverty was treated alongside infirmity, the *pellegrinaio* frescoes offer insight into how the social category of the poor sick was represented and viewed in the context of a large civic hospital. On one side of the ward, the poor and infirm are shown in marginal urban spaces that are clear references to recognizable locations around the hospital. These frescoes, particularly *The Expansion of the Hospital* and *The Investiture of the Rector*, establish the communal need for the Scala by depicting the poor sick in marginal architectural spaces in the Sienese urban environment. The frescoes across the hall showing scenes of caregiving taking place within the hospital suggest that the hospital remedies the problem of exposure and vulnerability, giving a place to those typically relegated to the margins of the city. The specificity of the rooms indicates that the structure is especially dedicated to the particular needs of the inmates, providing medical attention, alms, and shelter. However, these scenes also reinforce the accessibility of poor and sick bodies, particularly through pointed depiction of staff and wealthy visitors observing hospital inmates.

The poor and infirm invariably occupy central positions in the frescoes. This transforms their bodies into discursive sites, or meeting places for the different subject positions of the real viewers in the ward, identifying the inmates as 'attended-to' or deserving of societal attention.[48] For wealthy visitors, whose depicted counterparts occupy marginal positions in the frescoes gazing inwardly towards the beneficiaries of the hospital, their role is a supporting one, ideally in the form of financial contributions. For hospital staff, the *pellegrinaio* frescoes have a similar function to other images of caregiving in charitable houses, visualizing the implementation of the Works of Mercy in a familiar contemporary setting—a daily reminder of their role in caring for the poor of Christ for the benefit of the social whole.[49] These staff members are also depicted as attention-givers, if more immediately involved in the processes of care than the wealthy visitors. Through gesture and gaze, these figures direct the viewers' own gaze towards the infirm and suffering. For the living inmates in the ward, they saw themselves represented as the epicentres of institutional and communal attention, their bodies in need, and worthy of, interpretation and treatment in both Galenic and Christian medical and spiritual practices that shaped systems of care at the Scala.[50]

Notes

1 Van Os, *Vecchietta and the Sacristy of the Siena Hospital Church*; Gallavotti Cavallero, *Lo Spedale di Santa Maria della Scala*, 157; Christiansen, Kanter and Strehlke, *Painting in Renaissance Siena 1420*, 6–12; Scharf, *Der freskenzyklus des pellegrinaios in S. Maria della Scala zu Siena*; Costa and Ponticelli, 'L' iconografia del pellegrinaio'; Sordini, *Dentro l'antico ospedale*, 314–21.

2 Costa and Ponticelli, 'L' iconografia del pellegrinaio', 111–14.

3 Carmichael, *Plague and the Poor*, 109; Pullan, *Poverty and Charity*, 28; Whitley, 'Concepts of ill health and pestilence in fifteenth-century Siena', 157; Henderson, *The Renaissance Hospital*, 71; Nichols, 'Secular charity, sacred poverty',148.

4 Paolucci and Pinto, 'Gli "infermi" della Misericordia di Prato', 118, 120; Henderson, *The Renaissance Hospital*, 11.

5 Archivio di Stato di Siena, Ospedale 519 f.174v; Ospedale 519 f.182r. (All translations in this chapter are my own, unless otherwise noted.)

6 For instance in the fourth statute, which states: 'In which each conventual brother who finds himself in the city of Siena in these times must and should be present personally and actually every Sunday morning, and all the others that the rector gives food to the *poor sick . . .*'. [In che ogni frate conventuale el quale si ritrovarra nela citta di Siena in quelli tempi sia tenuto et debbi essare e intervenire personalmente et actualmente ogni domenicha en mattina et in tutti glaltri dì che maestro [rettore] da magiare [mangiare] agli *povari infermi* al desinare dessi dietro a maestro [rettore] o suo vicario et da loro non partirsi senza licentia dessi maestro [rettore] o suo vicario ad la pena di soldi venti per ciaschuna volta]. Archivio di Stato di Siena, Ospedale 24, f.44r.

7 On the beggars represented at 'interstices of urban space', see Nichols, *The Art of Poverty*, 17. On scenes from the Temple of Solomon, see Helas, 'Die Bettler vor dem Temple', 62–99.

8 Argenziano, 'La santità della malattia, la malattia della santità: le raffigurazioni dei malati e delle loro infermità nell'iconografia senese tra la fine del XII e la seconda metà del XV secolo', 192.

9 Costa and Ponticelli have identified the donor, mounted on a mule in the centre of the fresco, as a bishop because he wears a similar head covering to the carved effigies of entombed Sienese bishops in the cathedral. Costa and Ponticelli, 'L' iconografia del Pellegrinaio', 121.

10 On the use of beggars as 'attributes' of saints, see Helas, 'Der Körper des Bettlers', 372.

11 Helas, 'Ricchezza e povertà', 28. Leon Battista Alberti expressed anxiety about the destabilizing effect of too many poor in public urban spaces. In his treatise on architecture, published in 1482, Alberti prescribes a time limit of three days in which the poor can remain in a city without working so as to prevent them from publically begging and to spare the city 'from their loathsome presence'. Alberti, *On the Art of Building in Ten Books*, 130.

12 This last space was the Capella delle Reliquie, whose function is identified by the rear view of the balcony from which the hospital's relics were displayed. The chapel became the Cappella del Manto in 1441. Loseries, 'Der Dom im städtebaulichen Zusammenhang vom mittleren 14', 691–92; Sordini, *Dentro l'antico ospedale*, 92–95; Gallavotti, *Lo Spedale di Santa Maria della Scala in Siena*, 106, 418; Scharf, *Der freskenzyklus des pellegrinaios*, 253; Pertici, *The Fabric of History: Power, Prestige and Piety in Siena*, 51.

13 On loggias as sites of urban charity, see Henderson, *The Renaissance Hospital*, 77.

14 There is evidence for the flexible boundaries of the hospital, which required regulation on the part of the administration. The forty-fifth regulation of the hospital statutes states that while visitors to the hospital may eat with family members who are inmates, they may not sleep overnight in the wards, suggesting this was a problem that occurred with some regularity. *Statuti volgari de lo spedale di Santa Maria Vergine di Siena*, section XLV.

15 Henderson, *The Renaissance Hospital*, 254.

16 'Erano pieni li spedali d'infermi forestieri e paesani, che era una piatà [pietà] a vedere' Montauri *Cronaca*, 761, quoted in Travaini and Piccinni, *Il libro del pellegrino*, 44.

17 For critiques of the 'clinical gaze' in the early modern period, see Colin Jones, 'The construction of the hospital patient in early modern France'; Flora, 'Representing women and poverty in medieval art'.

18 On the attire of surgeons, see Strehlke, 'Domenico di Bartolo', 119; Park, *Doctors and Medicine*, 64.

19 Scharf, *Der freskenzyklus des pellegrinaios in S. Maria della Scala zu Siena*, 189; Henderson, *The Renaissance Hospital*, 162.

20 'Now the diseases as well as the seasons, and the extent of the periods, whether occurring daily, on alternative days, or at longer intervals, will indicate the paroxysms and their constitutions. Similar information is derived from the supervening occurrences: as the sputum in pleuritics, when it appears at the approach of the disease, shortens it: but of afterwards prolongs it. In the same manner the urine, stools and sweat announce when they appear, the facility or difficulty of the crisis; the length or shortness of the disease'. Hippocrates *Aphorisms*, 10. See also Galen, *On the Structure of the Art of Medicine*, 373.

21 The Ceppo was under the direction of Leonardo Buonafede, the rector of the hospital Santa Maria Nuova in Florence, which had already employed the Buglioni for lunettes and medallions between 1511 and 1515, though nothing as ambitious as this frieze, which spans the entire length of the Ceppo's facade. Giancarlo Gentilini, *I della Robbia*, 439–40. See also Boyd, 'Narrating Charity at the Ospedale del Ceppo', in press.

22 Sordini, *Dentro l'antico ospedale*, 121.

23 *Statuti volgari*, section XV.

24 Translation in Henderson, *The Renaissance Hospital*, 163.

25 Whitley, 'Concepts of ill health', 129. Jones also discusses the limited contact between inmates and physicians in early modern French hospitals. Jones, 'The construction of the hospital patient in early modern France', 58.

26 Beatrice Sordini, *Dento l'antico ospedale*, 94.

27 Quoted in Piccinni and Travaini, *Il libro del pellegrino*, 20.

28 Harff, Arnold von, *The Pilgrimage of Arnold von Harff*, 14.

29 Strehlke, 'Domenico di Bartolo', 40–45.

30 Examples of this are vast—for specific discussions in relationship to class, see Bettella, 'The marked body as otherness in Renaissance Italian culture', 149–81; Healy, 'Fashioning civil bodies and others', 205–26; Mellinkoff, 'Outcasts: signs of otherness in Northern European art of the Late Middle Ages'; Tom Nichols, *Others and Outcasts in Early Modern Europe: Picturing the Social Margins*.

31 For more on the significance of depictions of clothing in scenes of almsgiving, see Cordelia Warr, 'Clothing, charity, salvation and visionary experience in fifteenth-century Siena', 187–211.

32 Strehlke, 'Domenico di Bartolo', 138.

33 Presciutti, *Visual Cultures of Foundling Care in Renaissance Italy*, 54.

34 'Item che fanciulli dello spedale predecto vadino per la Hra [main altar] chiegiendo e achattando limonsine come sempre per lo passato si costumo.' Archivio di Stato di Siena, Ospedale 24 f.2v.

35 Banchi, *Statuti volgari*, LVII: 'Che lo Rettore del Spedale sei volte ne l'anno serva a li povari, infermi e gittati; e che di ciò se faccia piubica scrittura.' (My translation.) This ritualized serving of the poor is also the subject of a monochrome fresco painted in an adjacent ward by Carlo di Giovanni in 1445–58, in which the rector is shown holding a tray of food in a ward lined with beds.

36 Smith, *To Take Place*, 103.

37 Smith, *To Take Place*, 104.

38 Botana, *Works of Mercy*, 3.

39 The standard hygienic practice of washing the feet of inmates at the Hospital of Santo Spirito in Rome was given spiritual significance through the weekly re-enactment of the *mandatum pauperum*, or the story of Christ washing his disciples' feet. Botana, *Works of Mercy*, 132.

40 Depictions of the *Man of Sorrows*, for instance, inspired pangs of suffering akin to what Christ felt, and in scholarly and monastic traditions images served as mnemonic devices to guide meditation. Foundational texts on the affective role of images in early modern devotional practice include David Freedberg, *The Power of Images*; Hans Belting, *Likeness and Presence*; Mary Carruthers, *The Craft of Thought*; Nina Bolzoni, *The Web of Images*.

41 Alberti, *On Painting*, 212.

42 On the symbolism of beggars in sixteenth-century Venice, see Nichols, 'Secular charity, sacred poverty', 163.

43 Bynum, *Holy Feast and Holy Fast*, 172.

44 Bernardino, *Le prediche volgari inedite*, 263.

45 'And how should the life of a young man be conducted? In mercantile affairs, giving oneself to morality, study, letters the good of the poor, aiding justice: if a man can exert himself in these things, he will not be idle.' In che debba essere esercitata la vita dell'uomo giovane? In fare mercanzia, a darti alle moralità, allo studio, alle lettere, ne' beni de' poveri, agiutare [aiutare] la giustizia: che l'uomo si può esercitare in qualche cosa, per non stare ozioso.' Bernardino, *Le prediche volgari inedite*, 271.

46 Flora, 'Representing Women and Poverty in Medieval Art', 70.

47 'Tu dai uno pezzo di pane al povero: chi merita più, o tu che 'l dai liberamente, o colui che 'l riceve? Potrà meritare più colui che 'l riceve, che colui che 'l dà, per le cagioni: prima per la umiltà del chiedere, per la povertà che tiene, e per la contemplazione.' Bernardino, *Le prediche volgari inedite*, 263.

48 Perkins, *The Suffering Self*, 7.

49 Botana, *Works of Mercy*, 166, 191–92.
50 On the relationship between Early Christian and Galenic modes of interpreting and caring for the body, see Perkins, *The Suffering Self*, 142–72.

Bibliography

Primary sources

Unpublished

Archivio di Stato di Siena, Ospedale 24, 2v, f. 44r.
Archivio di Stato di Siena, Ospedale 519, 174v, f. 182r.

Published

Alberti, Leon Battista, *On the Art of Building in Ten Books*, ed. and trans., Joseph Rykwert (Cambridge, MA: MIT Press, 1988).

Alberti, Leon Battista, *On Painting: A New Translation and Critical Edition*, ed. and trans., Rocco Sinisgalli (Cambridge: Cambridge University Press, 2011).

Bernardino, *Le prediche volgari inedite: Firenze 1424–1425 Siena 1425*, ed., Dionisio Pacatti (Siena: Ezio Cantagalli, 1935).

Galen, *On the Structure of the Art of Medicine; The Art of Medicine; On the Practice of Medicine to Glaucon*, trans., Ian Johnston, The Loeb Classical Library, 523 (Cambridge MA: Harvard University Press, 2016).

Harff, Arnold von, *The Pilgrimage of Arnold von Harff, Knight, from Cologne, Throughout Italy, Syria, Egypt, Arabia, Ethiopia, Nubia, Palestine, Turkey, France and Spain, Which He Accomplished in the Years 1496 to 1499*, trans., Malcolm Letts (London: Hakluyt Society, 1946).

Hippocrates *Aphorisms*, trans., Thomas Coar (New York: The Classics of Surgery Library, 1994).

Statuti volgari de lo spedale di Santa Maria Vergine di Siena scriti l'Anno MCCV: e ora per la prima volta pubblicati, ed., Luciano Banchi (Siena: I. Gati Editore, 1864).

Secondary sources

Beatrice Sordini, *Dentro l'antico ospedale: Santa Maria della Scala, uomini, cose e spazi di vita nella Siena medievale* (Siena: Protagon, 2010).

Belting, Hans, *Likeness and Presence: A History of the Image before the Era of Art*, trans., Edmund Jephcott (Chicago: University of Chicago Press, 1990).

Bettella, Patrizia, 'The marked body as otherness in Renaissance Italian culture', in Linda Kalof and William Bynum (eds), *A Cultural History of the Human Body in the Renaissance*, vol. 3 (Oxford and New York: Berg, 2010), 149–81.

Bolzoni, Lina, *The Web of Images: Vernacular Preaching from Its Origins to St Bernardino da Siena* (Aldershot: Ashgate, 2003).

Botana, Federico, *The Works of Mercy in Italian Medieval Art (c. 1050–c. 1400)* (Turnhout: Brepols, 2012).

Boyd, Rachel, 'Narrating charity at the Ospedale del Ceppo', in Jack Hartnell (ed.), *Continuous Page: Scrolls and Scrolling from Papyrus to Hypertext* (Courtauld Books Online). https://doi.org/10.33999/2019.10.

Bynum, Caroline Walker, *Holy Feast and Holy Fast: The Religious Significance of Food to Medieval Women* (Berkeley: University of California Press, 1986).

Carmichael, Ann, *Plague and the Poor in Renaissance Florence* (Cambridge: Cambridge University Press, 1986).

Carruthers, Mary, *The Craft of Thought: Mediation, Rhetoric, and the Making of Images 400–1200* (Cambridge: Cambridge University Press, 1998).

Christiansen, Keith, Laurence B. Kanter, and Carl Brandon Strehlke, *Painting in Renaissance Siena 1420–1500* (New York: Harry N. Abrams, 1988).

Cordelia Warr, 'Clothing, charity, salvation and visionary experience in Fifteenth-century Siena', *Art History*, 27, 2 (2004): 187–211.

Costa, Elda and Laura Ponticelli, 'L' iconografia del pellegrinaio nello spedale di Santa Maria della Scala di Siena', *Iconografia*, 3 (2004): 111–14.

Flora, Holly, 'Representing women and poverty in medieval art', in Carlee A Bradbury and Michelle Moseley-Christian (eds), *Gender, Otherness and Culture in Medieval and Early Modern Art* (Cham: Palgrave Macmillan, 2017), 67–89.

Freedberg, David, *The Power of Images: Studies in the History and Theory of Response* (Chicago: University of Chicago Press, 2007).

Gallavotti Cavallero, Daniela and Duccio Balestracci, *Lo Spedale di Santa Maria della Scala in Siena: vicenda di una committenza artistica* (Pisa: Pacini, 1985).

Gentilini, Giancarlo, *I della Robbia: La scultura invetriata nel Rinascimento* (Florence: Cantini, 1992) vol. 2.

Giulio Paolucci and Giuliano Pinto, 'Gli "infermi" della Misericordia di Prato (1401–1491)', in Giuliano Pinto (ed.), *La Società del bisogno: povertà e assistenza nella Toscana medievale* (Florence: Salimbeni, 1989), 101–29.

Healy, Margaret, 'Fashioning civil bodies and others: Cultural representations', in Linda Kalof and William Bynum (eds), *A Cultural History of the Human Body in the Renaissance*, vol. 3 (Oxford and New York: Berg, 2010), 205–26.

Helas, Philine, 'Die Bettler vor dem Temple: zur "invensione" und Transformation eines Bildmotivs in der Italienischen Malerei der Renaissance (1423–1552)', *Iconographica*, 3 (2004): 62–99.

Helas, Philine, 'Der Körper des Bettlers: zur Darstellung und Ausblendung von körperlicher Versehrtheit in der Italienischen Kunst zwischen dem 14. und frühen 16. Jahrhundert', in Cordula Nolte (ed.), *Homo debilis. Behinderte—kranke—versehrte in der gesellschaft des mittelalters* (Korb: Didymos-Verlag, 2009).

Helas, Philine, 'Ricchezza e povertà: la Presentazione al Tempio della pala Strozzi', in Andrea de Marchi (ed.), *Nuovi studi sulla pittura tardogotica: intorno a Gentile da Fabriano* (Leghorn: Sillabe, 2007), 19–32.

Henderson, John, *The Renaissance Hospital: Healing the Body and Healing the Soul* (New Haven: Yale University Press, 2006).

Jones, Colin, 'The construction of the hospital patient in Early Modern France', in Norbert Finzsch and Robert Jütte (eds), *Institutions of Confinement: Hospitals, Asylums and Prisons in Western Europe and North America, 1500–1950* (Cambridge: Cambridge University Press, 1996), 55–74.

Loseries, Wolfgang, 'Der Dom im städtebaulichen Zusammenhang vom mittleren 14. Bis zum 20. Jahrhundert', in *Kirchen von Siena*, 3.1, 1.2 (Munich: Bruckman, 2006), 691–722.

Mellinkoff, Ruth, *Outcasts: Signs of Otherness in Northern European Art of the Late Middle Ages*, California Studies in the History of Art, vol. 1 (Berkeley: University of California Press, 1993).

Nichols, Tom, *The Art of Poverty: Irony and Ideal in Sixteenth-Century Beggar Imagery* (Manchester: Manchester University Press, 2007).

Nichols, Tom, *Others and Outcasts in Early Modern Europe: Picturing the Social Margins* (Aldershot: Ashgate, 2007).

Nichols, Tom, 'Secular charity, sacred poverty: picturing the poor in Renaissance Venice', *Art History*, 30 (2007), 138–69.

Perkins, Judith, *The Suffering Self: Pain and Narrative Representation in the Early Christian Era* (Abingdon: Taylor & Francis, 1995).

Pertici, Petra, *The Fabric of History: Power, Prestige and Piety in Siena in the Pellegrinaio of Santa Maria della Scala* (Siena: Betti, 2015).

Piccinni, Gabriella and Lucia Travaini, *Il libro del pellegrino: Siena, 1382–1446: affari, uomini, monete nell'Ospedale di Santa Maria della Scala* (Naples: Liguori, 2003).

Presciutti, Diana Bullen, *Visual Cultures of Foundling Care in Renaissance Italy* (London: Routledge, 2018).

Pullan, Brian, *Poverty and Charity: Europe, Italy, Venice, 1400–1700* (Aldershot: Variorum, 1994).

Scharf, Friedhelm, *Der Freskenzyklus des Pellegrinaios in S. Maria della Scala zu Siena: Historienmalerei und Wirklichkeit in einem Hospital der Frührenaissance* (Hildesheim: Georg Olms Verlag, 2001).

Smith, Jonathan Z., *To Take Place: Toward Theory in Ritual* (Chicago: University of Chicago Press, 1987).

Strehlke, Carl Brandon, *Domenico di Bartolo* (unpublished PhD dissertation, Columbia University, 1986).

van Os, Hendrick W., *Vecchietta and the Sacristy of the Siena Hospital Church: A Study in Renaissance Religious Symbolism* ('s-Gravenhage: Staatsuitgeverij, 1974).

Whitley, Antonia, *Concepts of Ill Health and Pestilence in Fifteenth-Century Siena* (unpublished PhD dissertation, Warburg Institute, University of London, 2004).

5

THE FRIAR AS *MEDICO*

Picturing leprosy, institutional care, and Franciscan virtues in *La Franceschina*

Diana Bullen Presciutti

The best-known illustration from *La Franceschina*, a late-fifteenth-century collection of Franciscan *vitae*, depicts St Francis of Assisi and three of his brethren caring for victims of leprosy in an institutional environment (Figure 5.1).[1] In the watercolour image Francis appears at the top left, offering alms in the form of coins to one leprous man. To the right, a pair of friars tend to the sores of a patient, using sponge and ointment. Below them, another man receives bread in his left hand, while in his right, he holds a clapper, a noisemaker carried by lepers to alert others to their presence. Two additional patients appear in the lower-left corner, one clasping his hands in prayer, the other seated beside two rolls of bread, also wielding a clapper.

This illustration combines a hagiographic episode from the life of Francis with the newly popular iconography of the hospital scene, an unusual combination that positioned Francis and his companions as effective medical practitioners. While lepers were featured in a number of thirteenth-century St Francis altarpieces, these mostly posthumous miracle scenes are economic in composition, with minimal detail, and emphasize the healing power of relics rather than the close description of individual maladies.[2] Franciscan narrative cycles from the fourteenth and fifteenth centuries, heavily influenced by the Assisi Upper Church fresco cycle, rarely include lepers or leprosy imagery; when lepers do appear, the symptoms of their disease are rendered schematically.[3] We see a very different pictorial strategy at work in the *La Franceschina* miniature. This illustration, which places a strong emphasis on the disfiguring symptoms of leprosy, shows the Franciscans offering sustenance and comfort to the sufferers of the disease; their grateful patients are, in turn, presented as pious and deserving. Care is depicted as taking place in an idealized hospital environment, and there is no indication of miraculous healing—it is instead humility, made manifest through hospital work, that is highlighted.

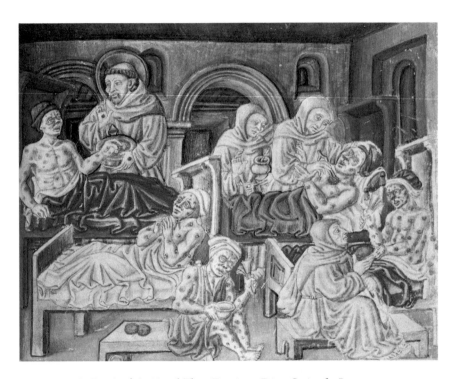

FIGURE 5.1 *St Francis of Assisi and Three Franciscan Friars Caring for Lepers*

Source: akg-images/De Agostini/A. Dagli Orti

Through a close examination of this illustration, along with related visual evidence from elsewhere in *La Franceschina* and other sources, I elucidate in this chapter the visual strategies through which the early Franciscans were constructed in the manuscript as both efficient medical practitioners and models of humility for a fifteenth-century Observant audience. I will also show how the leprosarium image registers tensions in the representation of both ideal Observant behaviour and the institutional care of the afflicted, particularly the challenge of balancing the unrestrained embrace of bodily subjugation with the more circumspect requirements of appropriate medical care. While leprosy has been the subject of considerable attention in the scholarly literature, the focus has largely been on the late medieval period;[4] by the fifteenth century, plague and other social problems had displaced leprosy in discourses on charity, a shift reflected in the scholarship.[5] Among the few who have considered the illustrations of *La Franceschina* in relation to leprosy are Roberto Cobianchi, who has identified a link between the rise of the Observant movement within the Franciscan order and a new interest in representations of leprosy,[6] and Angelita Marques Visalli, who has explored the value of images as historical evidence by using the illustrations of *La Franceschina* as a case study.[7] Building on these contributions through a more sustained consideration of the leprosarium scene, I demonstrate here how illustrations could work on their own terms—in conversation with, but independent of, accompanying text—to negotiate the relationship between leprous bodies and ideal Observant Franciscan behaviour in late-fifteenth-century Italy.

While I am mindful of the derogatory connotations of the word 'leper' when applied today to sufferers of Hansen's disease, I use the term to be faithful to my sources.[8] To be diagnosed with leprosy in late medieval and Renaissance Italy was to be a leper—the disease was inextricably linked with social identity, in a way quite distinct from other afflictions. In this chapter, the term 'leprosy' does not refer specifically to Hansen's disease.[9] Nor can we speak of a monolithic notion of 'leprosy' in the late medieval and early modern period; in fact, the terms 'lebbra' and 'lebbrosi' could be applied to sufferers of a host of different maladies characterized by a broad range of symptoms. Recent interventions by François-Olivier Touati and Carole Rawcliffe have convincingly established that leprosaria, institutions founded largely in the twelfth and thirteenth centuries, were more akin to monastic communities than sites of forced quarantine; lepers, in turn, were viewed in both positive and negative lights, as Luke Demaitre and others have shown.[10] Leprosy could be both a punishment for sinful actions and a sign of predetermined salvation, with miseries in this world counting against suffering in the next. While this contradictory and ambivalent attitude towards leprosy endured in the late fifteenth century, my interest here is not in how 'leprosy' or related diseases were diagnosed or treated at the time.[11] For the Observant readers of *La Franceschina*, leprosy is instead an *idea*, a social construct—one associated with certain symptoms, such as skin lesions, disfigurement, and a generic 'unclean' status, as well as with broader concerns about contamination, contagion, and sin.[12]

The mirror of the Observants

The stated goal of *Lo Specchio dell'Ordine Minore*—the official title of *La Franceschina*—is to operate as a mirror for, or model of, ideal Franciscan behaviour.[13] The treatise is written in a Tuscan-Umbrian dialect, rather than scholarly Latin, and was aimed at Observant friars of all levels of education. The author, the Perugian Observant Giacomo Oddi,[14] organized the text into thirteen chapters. The first eleven address principal Franciscan virtues, such as poverty and humility; the remaining two consider the punishment of bad *frati* and the celebration of their good counterparts.[15] Each chapter begins with examples from the life of Francis that demonstrate the virtue under consideration, followed by the lives of other Franciscan saints, *beati*, and friars. Several virtues are explicitly associated with specific activities: charity, for example, is identified with preaching; patience is linked with martyrdom; and, most significant for this chapter, humility is exemplified by the care of lepers.

La Franceschina participated in a well-established tradition of Franciscan hagiographical writing, one that traced its origins to the lives of Francis written by Thomas of Celano and Bonaventure in the thirteenth century.[16] In compiling his text, Oddi drew extensively upon earlier *vitae*, especially Bartolomeo da Pisa's *De conformitate vitae beati Francisci* (1385–90). Through his engagement with Bartolomeo, Oddi also accessed Bonaventure's *Legenda maior* (1260–66), the *Speculum perfectionis* (*c.* 1318), and the *Actus beati Francisci* (*c.* 1322), among other texts.[17] As was typical of such treatises, Oddi incorporated large sections of previous texts almost word-for-word, thereby buttressing his claims through the words of his predecessors. Even the format of the treatise had precedents: by organizing the lives around virtues, Oddi followed the model of the *Vita Rigaldina* (*c.* 1300).

While *La Franceschina* was completed in 1474, it is believed to have been gestating for at least two decades. Four manuscript versions survive, all from Umbria: the earliest, dated 1474, originates from the Observant Franciscan Convent of Monteripido in Perugia.[18] This version, identified by Nicola Cavanna as the prototype,[19] includes forty-five illustrations painted by three different hands, among them the image discussed earlier (Figure 5.1).[20] A second manuscript, dated to 1482–84, is from the Convent of the Porziuncola, or Santa Maria degli Angeli, outside Assisi; this version, which is the most heavily illustrated of all four surviving manuscripts, comprises 152 miniatures, including the scene of Francis and his brethren in the leprosarium (Figure 5.7). The other fifteenth-century manuscript, from Norcia, does not contain leprosy imagery, probably because only eight of a projected forty-nine miniatures were executed. The final manuscript, also from Perugia, is from the late sixteenth century and thus falls outside the chronological limits of this study.[21] Plans to publish the treatise never came to fruition, but it was nevertheless widely influential in the Franciscan community.[22]

Picturing leprosy

While the various iterations of *La Franceschina* have received surprisingly little attention from art historians, the scene of the leprosarium from the Perugia manuscript is regularly reproduced as an illustration of late medieval medical care. *HistoryExtra*, the official website of the *BBC History Magazine*, for example, uses it to illustrate 'the hospital experience in Medieval England'.[23] The image has also been incorrectly identified with the bubonic plague, one among many such errors that Monica Green, Lori Jones, and others have worked tirelessly to correct.[24] The reasons for this frequent instrumentalization and misidentification are the same: the miniature stands out for its atypically detailed visual description of diseased bodies covered with cutaneous lesions. To create a naturalistic and detailed rendering of each skin lesion, the artist of the leprosarium scene used red and blue paint, with uneven patches of red signalling scabs, and blue circles of paint indicating bruising.[25]

In contrast to the naturalistic detail found in the *La Franceschina* illustration, conventional representations of leprosy, such as a fourteenth-century miniature from the *Omne Bonum* encyclopaedia (Figure 5.2), use only unmodified dots of reddish paint to symbolize leprotic sores.[26] In addition to the carefully described lesions, the Perugia illumination also departs from schematic depictions of leprosy by highlighting the ravages inflicted by the disease on the faces of the patients. All of the lepers exhibit damage to their noses, marked by visible nostrils that suggest decay, as well as missing teeth.[27] The *Omne Bonum* miniature, in common with other conventional depictions of leprosy, shows no such facial disfigurement.

Leprosy, as both a disease and a social identity, occupied a dual role in late medieval and early modern culture. Lepers were perceived to be sinful, their disease a punishment for their actions.[28] They were required to wear hats and gloves to cover the disfiguring signs of their ailment, and they had to use clappers or bells to alert passers-by to their presence.[29] Because the disease was understood to be at least selectively contagious, lepers were housed in leprosaria to separate them from the rest of the community.[30] And yet they were also loved by Christ, who demonstrated the depth of His compassion through His embrace of lepers. Leprosy could be a sign of divine punishment, in the tradition of Job, but it also allowed for the possibility of redemption.[31] By cleansing the leper with his touch, Christ forged a model for self-negating humility, a willingness to sacrifice His bodily health in the service of *amor proximi*. Unsurprisingly, it was Christ who provided the template for the representation of leprosy in visual hagiography. In this twelfth-century mosaic from Monreale cathedral (Figure 5.3), for example, we can see Christ holding out his hand to heal the afflicted man, whose leprotic state is readily identifiable from the red marks that cover his skin. This image, like most examples from visual hagiography, shows leprosy being miraculously healed by the grace of God.

Leprosy in Franciscan hagiography

Leprosy played an important role in the hagiography of St Francis of Assisi, imitator of Christ *par excellence*. In the text of *La Franceschina*, Oddi details several encounters between Francis and lepers, all sourced from thirteenth- and fourteenth-century Franciscan *vitae*, in order to illustrate the extent of the saint's humility. Among these is the tale of Francis's conversion from Bonaventure's *Legenda maior* (1260–66), which was itself an elaboration of accounts from Francis's own testament and

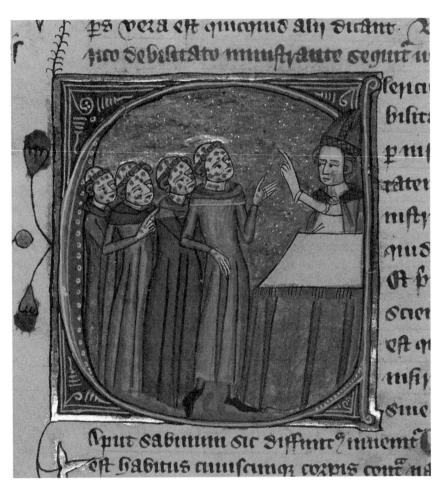

FIGURE 5.2 *A Bishop Instructing Clerics Suffering from Leprosy*

Source: © The British Library Board, MS Royal 6 E vi, vol. 2

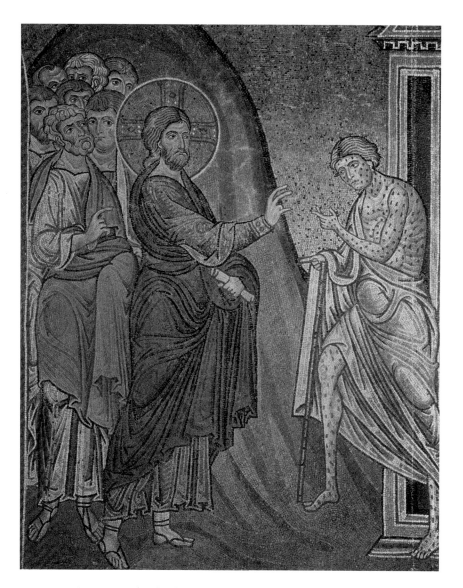

FIGURE 5.3 Byzantine school, *Christ Heals the Leper*

Source: Duomo, Monreale, Sicily, Italy/Bridgeman Images

Thomas of Celano's *Vita prima* of 1228.[32] The story, as recounted by Oddi in the chapter concerning the virtue of rejecting the world, tells of how a leper appeared before Francis as he rode on horseback, still in secular garb, over the plain of Assisi. Although he found the sight of lepers to be very unpleasant, Francis knew that his quest for perfection required him to conquer himself by embracing that which he found most repellent.[33] Despite his revulsion, Francis descended from his horse, gave the leper alms, and, taking him by the hand, kissed him. After the kiss, Francis remounted his horse and, from then on, through much self-abnegation, worked towards his eventual spiritual victory.[34]

Following this encounter, Oddi, this time quoting liberally from Bonaventure, tells of how a converted Francis took a purse of coins and went into the leprosarium, where he distributed the money and kissed the hands of all the lepers.[35] And thus, Oddi tells us, 'that which previously had been bitter for him, to see and speak with the lepers, was made sweet and most sweet'.[36] As a 'true lover of humility', Francis later diligently served the lepers, washed their feet, bandaged their lesions, cleansed away the putrefaction, and attended to their needs 'with a great excess of fervour'.[37]

While in his testament Francis had dwelt upon his time spent living amongst (and caring for) lepers, Celano's *vitae* shifted the focus away from what Pietro Maranesi calls the 'quotidian' aspect of work in the leprosarium in favour of the 'heroic act' of the meeting on horseback.[38] In his *Legenda minor* (1260–62), Bonaventure, in turn, had identified the miracle of the speaking crucifix of San Damiano as the true moment of Francis's conversion, displacing the encounter with the leper.[39] This shift in the hagiographical texts is reflected in the absence of the care of lepers from Bonaventure-inspired pictorial cycles, most notably the one in the Basilica di San Francesco in Assisi (and its many imitators). While he eagerly borrows from both Celano and Bonaventure, Oddi reinstates the primacy of the care of lepers in discursive constructions of ideal Franciscan identity; in *La Franceschina*, Francis's imitation of Christ is concomitant with his humble, quotidian charity towards lepers.

The most expansive discussion of leprosy in *La Franceschina* comes in the Humility chapter. Importantly, in the Perugia manuscript, the scene of Francis and the early Franciscans in the leprosarium is the only illustration found in the chapter on Humility; for its reader, therefore, the scene visually encapsulated the entirety of the multifaceted virtue. In the accompanying text, Oddi again recounts, using virtually the same language, the *Legenda maior*'s tale of Francis's conversion, as well as his later care and solicitude towards lepers.[40] What is new in the Humility chapter is Oddi's emphasis on the institutional environment. In addition to Bonaventure, Oddi cites the *Prima regola* in order to establish that Francis wanted his followers to labour in leprosaria and to beg for alms on behalf of lepers:

> After some time, when he began to have friars, he wanted them to stay in the hospitals for lepers, to serve them, and to make them the foundation for holy humility; and in the *Prima regola*, St. Francis allowed that the brothers

could beg for alms on behalf of the lepers, excepting for money, from which in every way they must guard against.[41]

The leprosarium scene, which appears on the facing folio (fol. 223r), surely refers to these activities. For Oddi, the leper hospital becomes the key site for the performance of humility—and, by extension, ideal Observant Franciscans become effective medical practitioners.

La Franceschina does not focus on *curing* the leprosy. Oddi does recount two instances when Francis healed lepers—one with his kiss, another through bathing—but the emphasis of these stories is not the miraculous nature of cleansing, and these scenes are not illustrated in the Perugia manuscript. Instead, Oddi presented the interaction with lepers as, first and foremost, a means to demonstrate humility: Francis and his followers overcame profound disgust at the symptoms of the malady, thereby 'conquering themselves'. The physical symptoms that engender the response of revulsion to the leprous body, emphasized in the Perugia miniature, are part and parcel of the display of holiness—the worse the lesions, the more disfigured the body, the more worthy the act of embracing, kissing, and tending. As Maranesi has elucidated, leprosy served for the early Franciscans as a 'paradigmatic event' that enabled both Francis and his followers to forge and perfect their devotional practice.[42] Oddi builds on this discursive tradition by presenting the care of lepers as concomitant with the ideal humility of the early Franciscans and, by extension, their Observant heirs.[43]

The friar as *medico*

Echoing the emphasis on the leprosarium context in Oddi's text, the Perugia miniature shows the care of lepers taking place in a hospital ward. Instead of miraculous healing, we see Francis and his brethren operating as hospital workers in an institutional environment. As previously mentioned, this innovation is a departure from conventional representations of the subject, including the few precedents in the visual hagiography of Francis.[44] The composition takes as its template the idealized depiction of hospital activities, a subject newly popular in the fifteenth century. As we can see in this fifteenth-century illustration from an illuminated edition of Avicenna's *Canon* (Figure 5.4), now in Florence's Biblioteca Laurenziana, such scenes construct the hospital ward as a salubrious environment where competent medical practitioners tend to patients.[45] Emphasis is placed on the variety of treatments on offer: as in the *La Franceschina* illustration, the Laurenziana miniature shows patients receiving both medical care and sustenance. In light of the close relationship between care and cure in medical discourses of the time, the efforts of the friars in the leprosarium scene to regulate the 'non-naturals' through the provision of food and drink can be understood as complementary to that of medical doctors.[46] Although bed-sharing seems to have been common practice in late medieval and Renaissance hospitals, idealized representations of ward life, including the *La Franceschina* miniature, often show beds occupied by single patients.

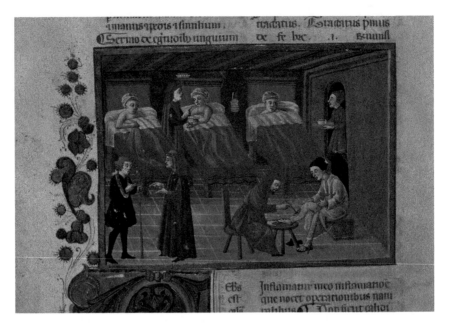

FIGURE 5.4 *Doctors Treating Patients in a Hospital Ward*

Source: Tarker/Bridgeman Images

In contrast to the more capacious ambit on view in the Florentine example, the Perugian illustration presents a compressed compositional space populated with outsized figures, allowing observers maximum access to the bodies of the afflicted. These visual strategies draw the attention of the intended viewer—probably an Observant, perhaps a novice—both to the symptoms of the disease and to the solicitous care offered by Francis and his followers. Importantly, that care aligns with the behaviour displayed by the medical practitioners in the Florentine illustration: while Francis and his fellow friars exhibit no sign of revulsion or unwillingness to be in contact with the bodies of the lepers, neither do they embrace the lepers as Francis himself did on the plain of Assisi and elsewhere—the friars are represented here as hospital workers, not as saints.

The friars in the Perugian miniature, confronted with the grisly symptoms of leprosy, respond not with kisses nor with revulsion; instead, they work, in tandem with the idealized ward environment, to respond to the medical and nutritional needs of the patients. Francis offers alms to a leper, who is appropriately ensconced in his own bed beneath a blanket.[47] His head, like that of the other lepers in the miniature, is covered with a hat; this was prescribed both for the health of the lepers and to conceal from view the disfiguring impact of the disease.[48] While Francis's hands lie close to that of the leper, he does not make physical contact with him. The two Franciscans at the top right, in turn, attend to the lesions of the leprous patient as solicitous and competent nursing staff. One friar holds a jar of ointment, and the other applies a soaked sponge to the lesions on the man's chest. The use of red for the sponge and silver for the tongs makes it clear—through sharp chromatic contrast with pale, rose-tinged skin—that the friar is not in direct contact with the lesions of the patient. In these vignettes, we see the miniature deftly balancing the demands of self-abnegating humility with that of ideal Renaissance hospital practice.

This tension between touch and revulsion, between contact and separation, is further explored in the text of *La Franceschina*. An additional tale told by Oddi—sourced from two early-fourteenth-century sources, the *Speculum perfectionis* and the *Assisi compilation* (also known as the *Legenda Perusina*)—elaborates further on the relationship between the bitter and the sweet, and between *imitatio Christi* and normative institutional care.[49] This story, which also appears on the folio facing the leprosarium scene, tells of the aptly named Iacomo Semplice, a man of great holiness and simplicity. Iacomo 'was like a doctor' ('era como medico'), and he 'had great grace from God to govern the sick, and he willingly took care of all the needs of those lepers'.[50] One day, Iacomo led a leper covered with lesions to the convent of Santa Maria degli Angeli, and, seeing him, Francis rebuked him for bringing the leper amongst the healthy brothers:

> 'You must not, brother Iacomo, lead these lepers so lesioned among the healthy brothers; in as much as it is not beneficial nor for you, nor for them'. It follows that while St. Francis wanted his friars to serve the lepers, he did not want them to lead them out of their hospitals, when they were so lesioned, considering that the human mind typically is greatly disgusted by it.[51]

Thus the text presents Francis as devoted to the care of lepers but also mindful of the need for their separation from the rest of society in a properly administrated leprosarium.

Seeing Iacomo's humility, however, Francis soon reverses course and reproaches himself for his actions.[52] In penitence, Francis eats from the same dish as a leper, an act described in excruciating detail by Oddi, who elaborates here on his textual sources.[53] The leper, described as a 'Christian friar', was 'all lacerated and abominable to look at'.[54] His fingers were consumed, chewed up, and bloody.[55] Most graphically, Oddi states, '[the leper] could not dip his fingers into the bowl to take a morsel, without some bloody discharge first falling into it'.[56] The sight of Francis eating from this contaminated bowl filled the friars who witnessed it with both fear and reverence. We can imagine Observant novices responding similarly to both the text and the leprosarium illustration in *La Franceschina*.[57]

Stigmata, lesion, wound, emblem

It is in the figure of Francis that we see most fully realized the tension I have identified in the image between intimate contact with lepers as an expression of humility and the more restrained engagement prescribed by idealized representations of fifteenth-century hospital practice. Despite Francis's placement at the rear of the compositional space, the gold of his halo and the red of the blanket draw the eye back to his oversized figure. The positioning of Francis's oddly foreshortened right arm ensures that the viewer notes the relationship between the stigmata marks and the red lesions that cover the skin of the leper.[58] And yet the naturalistic rendering of the scabby, bruised lesions, with their uneven contours, clearly differentiates them from the saturated red colour and crisp borders of the stigmata. The Observants were meant to ponder the relationship between the two marks without, however, confusing one for the other.

The unusual emphasis in the illumination on the physical impact of leprosy on the body, along with the filiation between skin lesions and the stigmata, also places in conversation three types of wounded bodies: stigmatic, leprotic, and martyred. This is underscored in *La Franceschina*, in both text and image, by the exceptional stress placed on martyrdom, associated in the text with the virtue of Patience. Twenty-nine of the forty-five illustrations in the Perugia manuscript come from the single chapter on Patience, whereas most of the other chapters, including the one on Humility, feature a single illustration.[59] The Patience chapter also follows the one on Humility, encouraging the reader to consider the synergies between the text and images presented in both. The Patience chapter begins with the Crucifixion, followed a few folios later by Francis receiving the stigmata. Both miniatures emphasize the perforation of the body, with copious amounts of blood pouring from the wounds of Christ, and the body of Francis again awkwardly foreshortened so that every wound is clearly visible to the viewer. In particular, the side wound of Christ, and its echo in the stigmata of Francis, draws the viewer's eye to the brutal penetration and sanguineous fissuring of flesh.

Most of the martyrdom scenes in the Patience chapter depict the deaths of early Franciscan martyrs in Morocco; the subject was timely, as their cult would be officially recognized by the Franciscan pope Sixtus IV in 1481.[60] Isabelle Heullant-Donat has identified a shift in Franciscan discourse on martyrdom between the thirteenth and fourteenth centuries, arguing that after a period of ambivalence about voluntary martyrdom, 'in the mind of Francis of Assisi—as imagined in the second half of the fourteenth century—martyrdom was the very essence of the Franciscan vocation'.[61] The wounds of martyrdom were explicitly linked to Francis's stigmata by Thomas of Celano, who, in the *Vita prima*, wrote that Francis greatly desired martyrdom and received the stigmata instead as a kind of consolation prize; his second *vita* and Bonaventure's *Legenda maior* took a different tack, moving away from the celebration of voluntary martyrdom.[62] Representations of the bloody deaths of the Franciscans in Morocco enjoyed a brief revival in the first half of the fourteenth century, with frescoes in Franciscan friaries in Verona (San Fermo Maggiore), Siena (San Francesco), and the chapter house of the Santo in Padua. The visual emphasis on martyrdom imagery in *La Franceschina* constitutes a return to these earlier themes, and the sheer number of such scenes must have made a forceful impact on the Observant reader—equating the patient suffering of the early Franciscans with that of Christ's crucifixion and Francis's stigmatization.

The martyrdom scenes in the Perugia manuscript of *La Franceschina* are exceptionally graphic, with bodies subjected to all manner of violence. Some of the miniatures use a limited chromatic range, creating a contrast between brown robes and muted backgrounds and bright-red blood, as we see in a scene of mass beheading (Figure 5.5).[63] In other examples, Franciscan bodies are stabbed, crucified, burned, mauled, dragged, cleaved, flayed, sawn apart, and more. This emphasis on the graphic rendering of violent martyrdoms would have complemented the detailed description of lesions and disfigurement in the leprosarium scene, as well as the accompanying textual descriptions of lepers with lacerated faces and bloody fingers. This pictorial strategy elides the leprous body with that of the martyred saint, a connection reinforced by the inclusion, in the hospital scene, of the leper who holds his hands together in pious gratitude. The virtue of Patience, the images tell us, necessitates the willing sacrifice of bodily integrity, resulting in broken skin and gushing wounds. The suffering of martyrs, described between the adjacent Humility and Patience chapters, is equated with the suffering of lepers, both constructed on the model of Christ's suffering. If Francis and his brethren are the humble caregivers in the leprosarium, then the lepers are patient martyrs, their flesh sacrificed for divine will. To be humble is to be patient—both virtues are centred on the sweet reward on offer for those willing to embrace the comparatively unimportant sacrifice of the body.

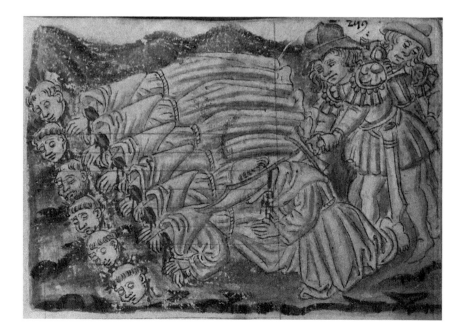

FIGURE 5.5 *Martyrdom of Early Franciscans*

Source: Author, with the concession of the Biblioteca Comunale Augusta

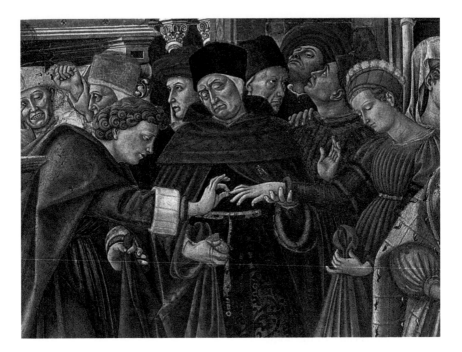

FIGURE 5.6 Domenico di Bartolo, *Care and Marriage of Foundlings*, detail

Source: Ospedale di Santa Maria della Scala, Siena, Italy © F. Lensini, Siena/ Bridgeman Images

The institutional context gives yet another signification to Francis's stigmata, working to mitigate the emphasis on self-abnegation and bodily sacrifice. Whereas the wound in Francis's torso is usually depicted in his side, as is that of Christ, the artist of the Perugia illustration represented it in his chest, giving priority to visibility over tradition and naturalism. In addition to serving as a mark of his sanctity, as a form of martyrdom, and as a kind of holy skin lesion, the wound also reads as an institutional insignia. It appears as something affixed to the habit, rather than as something seen through a hole in it. In combination with the habit itself, the chest wound thus operates as a hospital *stemma*, or emblem, in much the same way as the ladder symbol on the uniform of the rector in a mid-fifteenth-century fresco depicting hospital activities in the *pellegrinaio* ward of Siena's Ospedale di Santa Maria della Scala (Figure 5.6).[64] This pictorial strategy calls attention to Francis's status as a hospital worker and reinforces the immediacy of this institutional environment for a fifteenth-century viewer. Francis and his brethren, the illustration tells us, make their humility manifest not just by caring for lepers but by doing so in an institutional environment administered according to fifteenth-century notions of appropriate governance. Instead of the more affective acts of kissing and embracing, with their high risk of contagion, Francis's humility in the *La Franceschina* illustration operates within the bounds of institutional medical practice—and the 'emblem' serves to make this official.

Observant values

Presenting Francis as a hospital worker, complete with *stemma*, would have linked the founder of the Franciscan order to the most important Observant saint, Bernardino da Siena. Bernardino's work with plague victims in Siena's Scala hospital formed an important part of the *vita* of the saint, who was canonized in 1450, around the same time Oddi began work on *La Franceschina*.[65] Bernardino was also venerated as a plague saint in Umbria, where he appears with St Sebastian on numerous plague banners, such as that painted by Benedetto Bonfigli, now housed in the Oratorio di San Bernardino in Perugia. Further afield, in Lombardy, Bernardino was constructed as a solicitous and effective hospital worker in the fresco cycle in the chapel of San Bernardino in San Francesco, Lodi, executed at roughly the same time as the Perugia manuscript.[66]

The Observant movement within the Franciscan Order had, over the first half of the fifteenth century, shifted from a more ascetic ideal, emphasizing absolute poverty, isolation, and prayer, towards one focused more on dynamic preaching and community engagement.[67] In this vein, *imitatio Francisci* took a back seat to obeying the Observant leadership. This new iteration followed the more radical Spirituals of the late thirteenth and early fourteenth centuries, their heirs, the militantly eschatological Fraticelli, and the more moderate but still less socially engaged late-fourteenth- and early-fifteenth-century Observance of Paoluccio de' Trinci.[68] This shift towards an active pastoral life and an emphasis on obedience over poverty was exemplified in the person of Bernardino. Yet Oddi's treatise, with its stress on martyrdom, poverty, and the imitation of Francis, harkens back to the early Observant ideal of asceticism and rejection of the world.[69] While the text highlights these more severe values in its discussion of humility and the care of lepers, the Perugia illustration shifts the balance back towards the Bernardinian *via media*. The graphic description of symptoms evokes martyrdom and the negation of the body, but the avoidance of intimate contact and the use of the hospital scene template signals the importance of community engagement and obedience to institutional norms.

In the illustrations in the Assisi manuscript of *La Franceschina*, produced 1482–84, we see a move away from the Bernardine model and towards a more militant, Spiritual-influenced Observantism. While the surrounding text remains much the same, the illustration of the leprosarium scene in the Assisi manuscript (Figure 5.7) differs from its Perugian precedent in significant ways.[70] The Assisi miniature, in common with the other illustrations in the manuscript, is more economic than the Perugia version, excluding much of the earlier image's precise detail and colouristic variation. Gone is the careful rendering of the ward itself; while the beds with their wood headboards remain, the architectural details found in the Perugia image, like the ribbed arches and coffered ceiling, have been replaced with the void of the parchment folio. These pictorial strategies have the effect of blending together blankets and pillows with the robes of the Franciscan friars, decreasing the separation between the caretakers and the institutional furnishings.

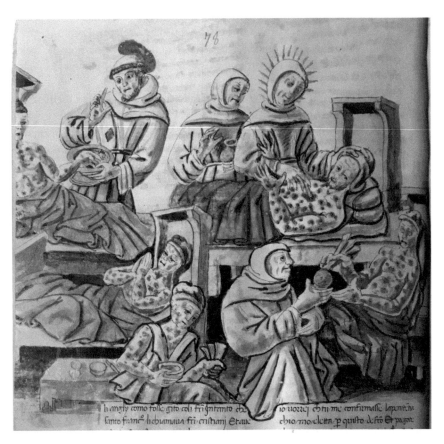

FIGURE 5.7 *St Francis of Assisi and Three Franciscan Friars Caring for Lepers*

Source: Author, with the concession of the Biblioteca Porziuncola

Interestingly, the Assisi image also departs from the Perugian model in the visual description of the symptoms of leprosy. The red lesions are less detailed, reading more as blotches than bruised, scabby sores. And yet the more muted, almost monochrome palette of the Assisi miniature makes the lesions stand out dramatically. The red marks are more numerous and more intense, threatening to overwhelm the bodies they cover. The faces of the lepers do not show clear signs of disfigurement; while this more schematic approach perhaps reflects the Assisi artist's less sophisticated technique, it also suggests that such descriptive detail was not considered necessary to communicate the essential messages of the illustration. Unlike the Perugia miniature, in which none of the lepers acknowledge the viewer, in the Assisi illustration, one of the patients is shown gazing directly out of the compositional space, soliciting both attention and sympathy. The effect of these visual strategies is that the viewer feels more connected to the lepers as people, as they appear less disfigured and more solicitous of the viewer's attention.

Another passage in the Assisi miniature underscores the virtuous humility of the Franciscans, highlighting the central theme of the chapter. The Franciscan friar, here distinguished as a *beato* by the gold rays emanating from his head, repeats the action of the Perugia manuscript by pressing the sponge to the flesh of the leper with tongs or an implement of some kind. And yet the looser, more schematic brushwork and reduced palette of the Assisi manuscript produces a strange effect here: at first glance it appears that the friar is sticking his finger directly into one of the lesions.[71] Unlike the Perugia miniature, where the tongs are clearly distinguished by their crisp contours and silver hue, here the implement is painted in the same flesh tone as the hands of the friar, which are in turn sketched in so loosely that they cannot be readily distinguished. The sponge itself is also less clearly articulated, blending as it does into the pattern of skin lesions. In tandem with the outward gaze of the patient, which pulls the eye to this area of the miniature, this visual confusion serves to underscore the intimate level of physical contact between the two figures.

The Assisi manuscript version of the scene of Francis and his brethren in the leprosarium highlights the challenges leprosy, or any contagious disease, posed as a mechanism for demonstrating ideal humility. The ravages leprosy visited on the body, especially on the skin, produced responses of revulsion and a desire to create physical separation between the healthy and the sick. Yet Francis himself identified the need to conquer this revulsion as central to the imitation of Christ and the attainment of holiness. While the text of *La Franceschina* describes the full-throated embrace of leprous bodies, risk of contagion and all, the Perugia leprosarium scene, with its depiction of orderly hospital activities, signals an ambivalence about unfettered physical contact, one that can be read in light of broader tensions between the Bernardine and more militant factions within the Observant movement. These tensions are on full view in the two leprosarium miniatures for *La Franceschina*, despite the virtually identical texts that accompany them. In the Perugia illustration, the symptoms of leprosy are highlighted, but physical contact is mediated through institutional norms. In the Assisi version, in contrast, the lesions are more schematic, yet the loose brushwork and limited colour palette blur the boundaries between the Franciscan bodies and their leprous counterparts. By comparing these closely related images, we can see how visual representations of a disease, in this case leprosy, could work in very different ways to negotiate what it meant to be an ideal Observant Franciscan in fifteenth-century Italy.

Notes

1 Illustration from Giacomo Oddi, *Lo Specchio dell'Ordine Minore* (known as *La France-schina*), 1474, Perugia, Biblioteca Comunale Augusta, MS 1238, fol. 223r.
2 On these altarpieces, see, among others, Ahlquist and Cook, 'Posthumous Miracles', 211–56.
3 On leprosy in fourteenth- and fifteenth-century Franciscan imagery, largely limited to manuscript illumination, see Cobianchi, '". . . Come vero amante"', esp. 59–60. On the Assisi cycle, see, most recently, Cooper and Robson, *The Making of Assisi*.
4 See Touati, *Maladie et société*; Demaitre, *Leprosy in Premodern Medicine*; Rawcliffe, *Leprosy in Medieval England*.
5 Although he overstated the case by suggesting that the disease, as a specific malady, had been eradicated, Michel Foucault identified this shift in the discourse on institutional charity; see Foucault, *Madness and Civilization*, 3–7.
6 Cobianchi, '". . . Come vero amante"'.
7 Visalli, 'Os caminhos da perfeição'.
8 In so doing I come to the same conclusion as Carole Rawcliffe, who uses the term: Rawcliffe, *Leprosy in Medieval England*, 10. Luke Demaitre, in contrast, chose to avoid it: Demaitre, *Leprosy in Premodern Medicine*, xii. On this debate, see also Elma Brenner, 'Recent perspectives', 389; Brenner also opts to use 'leper'. On Hansen's identification of the *Mycobacterium leprae*, see Demaitre, *Leprosy in Premodern Medicine*, vii.
9 For a very different approach, one that sees Hansen's disease and medieval leprosy as essentially one and the same, see Boeckl, *Images of Leprosy*.
10 Rawcliffe, *Leprosy in Medieval England*; Touati, *Maladie et société*; Demaitre, *Leprosy in Premodern Medicine*. See also the bibliography in Brenner, 'Recent Perspectives', 396–99.
11 On institutional responses to leprosy in the Umbrian region, see Sensi, 'Per la storia dei lebbrosi', 291–342.
12 As part of his broader analysis of the iconography of leprosy in biblical imagery, William Ober, a physician, addresses the slippery nature of terminology: Ober, 'The Iconography of Leprosy. Part I', 48. Ober's methodology, however, is firmly rooted in retrospective diagnosis. A more comprehensive and historically sensitive discussion is found in Demaitre, *Leprosy in Premodern Medicine*, 75–102. See also Brenner, 'Recent Perspectives', 389–91.
13 On the gestation of the manuscript, see Oddi, *La Franceschina* [hereafter cited as Oddi-Cavanna]. Cavanna decided to refer to the text as 'La Francheschina' to avoid confusion with other *Specchi* and also to lend greater significance to the work. For his justification of this choice, see Oddi-Cavanna, 1: x–xii. On the issue of the title, see also Pasqualin Traversa, *La 'minoritas' francescana*, 6–7. For the didactic function of 'literary mirrors' in the Observant context, see Lappin, *Mirror of the Observance*, 8.
14 Oddi's authorship is broadly but not universally accepted. On this issue, see Pasqualin Traversa, *La 'minoritas' francescana*, 16–19.
15 The number thirteen refers to Francis and his twelve companions: Pasqualin Traversa, *La 'minoritas' francescana*, 8.
16 Celano's *Vita prima* was written in 1228–29, just after Francis's death; he later followed with the *Vita secunda* (1244–47) and the *Tractatus de miraculis* (1250–52). In 1260, Bonaventure was commissioned to write a new life of Francis; this text, the *Legenda maior*, was established in 1266 as the official version, a status formalized with the destruc-

tion, on the orders of the General Chapter, of all previous lives: Ahlquist and Cook, 'Posthumous miracles', 211.

17 On the 'indirect' nature of Oddi's engagement with the early biographies, see Pasqualin Traversa, *La 'minoritas' francescana*, 2–3; 9–10; Lappin, *Mirror of the Observance*, 180.

18 On the four manuscripts, see Oddi-Cavanna, 1: LX–LXXX.

19 Oddi-Cavanna, 1: LXVI. Nevertheless, Cavanna uses the Assisi version as the basis for his edition, rather than the Perugia manuscript. On this issue, see Pasqualin Traversa, *La 'minoritas' francescana*, 15–16. As the focus of this chapter is the Perugia leprosarium scene, I have chosen to use the Perugia text as the basis for quotations, with reference also to Cavanna's edition of the Assisi manuscript.

20 On the illustrations, see Oddi-Cavanna, 1: L–LIX; Scarpellini, 'I tre illustratori', 701–18.

21 On the illustrations of the late-sixteenth-century version, which comes from the Monteluce convent in Perugia, see Mancini, *Miniatura a Perugia*, 86–97. The Monteluce manuscript also includes the leprosarium scene. While clearly modelled on the fifteenth-century illustration, the later iteration does not feature the same level of descriptive detail in the rendering of leprotic symptoms.

22 On the unrealized plans for publication, see Pasqualin Traversa, *La 'minoritas' francescana*, 5, note 3. On the influence of the text, see Oddi-Cavanna, 1: XXXII–L; Pasqualin Traversa, *La 'minoritas' francescana*, 11–14; Lappin, *The Mirror of the Observance*, 182.

23 For the *HistoryExtra* website, see Sweetinburgh, 'The hospital experience'.

24 See Green, Walker-Meikle, and Müller, 'Diagnosis of a "plague" image'; Jones and Nevell, 'Plagued by doubt'.

25 Scarpellini believes that this illumination, along with several others in the Perugia manuscript, was 'reinforced' with more saturated colours at some point in its history: Scarpellini, 'I tre illustratori', 707. While some of the illuminations feature more opacity and saturation than others, distinguishing earlier from later interventions is difficult. Scarpellini does not specify any 'reinforced' areas of the leprosarium scene. Based on my examination of it, I believe these to be limited to the blankets on the beds and the background architecture.

26 On the iconography of leprosy, see Ober, 'The iconography of leprosy. Part I'; Ober, 'The iconography of leprosy. Part II'; Boeckl, *Images of Leprosy*. The illustration is a detail from James le Palmer, *Omne Bonum*, British Library, London, MS Royal 6 E VI, vol. 2, fol. 301r.

27 For the collapsed nose as a recognized symptom of leprosy, see Demaitre, *Leprosy in Premodern Medicine*, 61 and 92.

28 Sensi, 'La lebbra e i lebbrosi', 35.

29 On the shifting status of the clapper—used to call for aid within the leprosarium, to appeal for alms, to warn others of imminent danger—see Touati, *Maladie et société*, esp. 417–20; Demaitre, *Leprosy in Premodern Medicine*, 57–59. Demaitre's current research concerns the discursive multivalence of the clapper.

30 This attitude shifted over the course of the late medieval period, as Touati has demonstrated. While in the twelfth and thirteenth centuries, leprosy was not explicitly identified as contagious, a greater belief in its infectiousness developed in the fourteenth century. On these shifts, see Touati, *Maladie et société*; Touati, 'Contagion and leprosy'.

31 Argenziano, 'Giobbe e Lazzaro', 76.

32 On the role of leprosy in Francis's conversion, with specific reference to these textual sources, see, among others, Cobianchi, '". . . Come vero amante"', 55–57; Maranesi, 'Il servizio ai lebbrosi'. For Francis's testament, see Menestò and Brufani, *Fontes Franciscani*, 227; for an English translation, see Armstrong, Hellmann, and Short, *The Saint*, 124–27. For the Latin texts of Celano's *Vita prima* and Bonaventure's *Legenda maior*, see Thomas of Celano, 'Vita prima S. Francisci' and Bonaventure, 'Legenda maior S. Francisci'; for English translations, see Armstrong, Hellmann, and Short, *The Saint*, 180–308 (Celano) and Armstrong, Hellmann, and Short, *The Founder*, 525–683 (Bonaventure).

33 Biblioteca Augusta Perugia (hereafter BAP), MS 1238, fol. 35r: 'Unde essendo tedioso molto a sancto francesco de vedere li leprosi et orribile. Uno di cavalcando esso [patre], essendo [anche] nello habito seculare, sescontro cum uno leproso. Et facendose violentia ad semedesimo . . .'. See also Oddi-Cavanna, 1:76. Here I am translating 'facendose

violentia ad semedesimo'—literally 'making violence against himself'—as 'conquer himself'; this seems to hew closer to the meaning of Oddi's source material (Bonaventure) and the theme of the chapter (self-abnegation as a means of rejecting the world). Unless otherwise noted, all translations are my own.

34 BAP, MS 1238, fol. 35r: '. . . descese subito del cavallo, et dielli certi denare et pigliandolo per lamano gli li bascio. Et receuto el bascio dalleproso, remonto acavallo, et da quillo in puoy se comenzo a fare per tale modo violentia ad se medesimo, che in breve pervenne mediante la gratia de dio ala vittoria'.

35 BAP, MS 1238, fol. 35r: 'In tanto che li a pochi de lui tolse una borscia de denare, et andosse alospedale delli leprosi, et radunatilj tutti insieme, tutti quilli denarj distribuj intra loro et atutti lo basciava lamano'.

36 BAP, MS 1238, fol. 35r: 'Et cosi quillo che prima gli era amaro de vedere, et conversare co li leprosi, li fo da poy dolce, et dolcissimo'.

37 BAP, MS 1238, fol. 35r: 'Et puoy che ebbe renuntiato al mondo nelle mane delo episcopo dassese, si como dice la seconda parte de la legenda maiure, senando alli leprosi como vero amatore dela humilita, et stando conessi diligentemente li serviva, lavando loro li piedi, legava le piaghe, et nettavale dala insania et curavali da omne loro neccessita, cum grande excesso de fervore'. By using 'insania' in this transcription, I diverge from Cavanna, who followed the Assisi manuscript and opted for 'sania'. In the Perugia manuscript, there is a gap in the text and an abbreviation mark that suggests that there was a *y*, which is no longer visible. Cavanna acknowledges in a footnote that both the Norcia and Monteluce manuscripts use 'insania'. See Oddi-Cavanna, 1:77. On Oddi's use of the term 'insania' elsewhere in the text to denote a bloody discharge or pus, see note 56.

38 Maranesi, 'Il servizio ai lebbrosi', 36.

39 Maranesi, 'Il servizio ai lebbrosi', 37–38.

40 The description of the encounter on horseback is very similar to that in the 'desprezo del mondo' chapter, though here Oddi includes the detail that the leper is later revealed to be Christ in disguise: 'Et remontando acavallo resguardando per lo leproso, nollo vidde in nulla parte. Impero che quillo fo Christo in spetie deleproso' (BAP, MS 1238, fol. 222r).

41 BAP, MS 1238, fol. 222v: 'Depo alquanto tempo, quando comenzò ad avere deli frati, volse che essi frati staessero per li hospitalj de li leprosi ad servire ad essi. Et li facessero lo fondamento dela santa humilita. Et nella prima regula sancto francesco concessi alli frati che per li leprosi podessero gire ad cercare la limosina. Salvo la pecunia, da la quale in ogne modo se devessero guardare'. See also Oddi-Cavanna, 2:62.

42 Maranesi, 'Il servizio ai lebbrosi', 34–35.

43 Interestingly, Oddi's vision of perfect Franciscan self-abasement excludes St Elizabeth of Hungary, famed for her institutional care of lepers. Elizabeth appears only in passing in *La Franceschina*—the text largely ignores female followers of Francis—and no mention is made of her hospital work. For Oddi, the early Franciscans operate as models for his Observant readership, a role that excluded female tertiaries like Elizabeth. On the visual hagiography of Elizabeth of Hungary as hospital worker, see Boeckl, *Images of Leprosy*, 60–61; 122–29.

44 On this earlier iconography, see Cobianchi, '". . . Come vero amante"', 58–59.

45 The illustration is from Avicenna, *Canon*, Biblioteca Medicea Laurenziana, Florence, MS Gaddi 24, fol. 247v. Additional examples of hospital scenes include the frescoes in the *pellegrinaio* of the Ospedale di Santa Maria della Scala, Siena (1441–43) (see Bell, in this volume); the detached frescoes of the Works of Mercy from the Consorzio dei Vivi e Morti, Parma (c.1450, Galleria Nazionale di Parma); the glazed terracotta frieze on the loggia of the Ospedale del Ceppo, Pistoia (c.1515).

46 On this relationship, and the importance to medical practice of regulating Galen's 'non-naturals' (food and drink, rest and exercise, etc.), see Henderson, *The Renaissance Hospital*, xxix–xxx.

47 Lesioned bodies raised special concerns about bed-sharing, as we see from the c.1500 prescriptive statutes of the Ospedale di Santa Maria Nuova in Florence: '[The infirmarer] assigns the feverish and those with skin lesions or wounds to empty beds . . .', as quoted in Park and Henderson, '"The first hospital among Christians"', 181.

48 See Demaitre, *Leprosy in Premodern Medicine*, 49; Boeckl, *Images of Leprosy*, 69.

49 For the story and its textual sources, see Manselli, *Nos qui cum eo fuimus*, 215.

50 BAP, MS 1238, fol. 222v: 'Iacomo era como medico. Et avea grande gratia da dio, de governare linfirmj. Et volontiere curava de ogne loro bisogno quilli leprosi'. See also Oddi-Cavanna, 2:62–63.

51 BAP, MS 1238, fol. 222v: 'Unde che uno giorno frate Iacomo meno quillo leproso ad santa maria de li angeli. Et vedendolo santo francesco, disse ad frate Iacomo quasi reprehendolo. *Tu non deverete frate Iacomo menare quisti leprosi cosi piegati in tra li frati sani. Impero che non e, honesto ne per te, ne per loro.* Advenga che santo francesco volesse che li suoy frati servissero a li leprosi, non volea pero che li menasso fuore deli loro hospitalj, quando erano cosi piegati. Considerando che la mente humana ne sole prendere molta schifeza' [my italics]. See also Oddi-Cavanna, 2: 63.

52 BAP, MS 1238, fol. 222v: 'Et avendo santo francesco represo frate Iacomo, subito se represe se medesimo'.

53 BAP, MS 1238, fol. 222v: 'Allora dixe santo Francesco: questa sia la mia penitentia, che io magne in una medesima scutella insieme con frate cristiano'.

54 BAP, MS 1238, fol. 222v: 'Era quisto leproso tutto lacerato et habominevole ad vedere'.

55 BAP, MS 1238, fol. 222v: 'Li deti avea tucti consumati, rosi et sanguinolenti'.

56 BAP, MS 1238, fol. 222v: 'Non ponea may li deti nella scutella, che prima non cascasse de quilla insania nella scutella'. It is difficult to translate Oddi's phrase 'quilla insania' precisely. Oddi uses 'insania' to describe, in generic terms, the contamination or rot of leprosy (see note 37). The *Legenda Perusina*, one of his sources for this story, characterizes this event with the words 'cum mitteret ipsos in scutellam, deflueret in eam sanguis', specifying a bloody flow: Menestò and Brufani, *Fontes Franciscani*, 1561. While John Florio, in his 1611 dictionary, defines 'insania' as 'madnesse', he lists 'sanie' as meaning 'bloudy matter squized out of sores. Also putrefaction or poison': Florio, *Queen Anna's New World*, 258 and 463. In light of this, I have rendered 'insania' here as 'bloody discharge'.

57 This story was not illustrated in any of the extant manuscripts. On this omission, see Visalli, 'Miniaturas franciscanas', 123.

58 On the discursive filiation between leprotic sores and stigmata wounds, see Maranesi, 'Il servizio ai lebbrosi', 33. Cobianchi also observed the similarities between the two forms in the Perugia leprosarium scene: Cobianchi, '". . . Come vero amante"', 63.

59 On the disproportionate emphasis on martyrdom in the illustrations, see also Scarpellini, 'I tre illustratori', 708; Visalli, 'Miniaturas franciscanas', 117–18.

60 Heullant-Donat, 'Martyrdom and identity', 430.

61 Heullant-Donat, 'Martyrdom and identity', 433.

62 Heullant-Donat, 'Martyrdom and identity', 433.

63 The illustration is from Giacomo Oddi, *Lo Specchio dell'Ordine Minore* (known as *La Franceschina*), 1474, Perugia, Biblioteca Comunale Augusta, MS 1238, fol. 259r.

64 On the institutional *stemma* as a visual form, see Lincoln and Rihouet, 'Brands of Piety'.

65 On the canonization of Bernardino, see Pellegrini, *Il processo di canonizzazione*.

66 On the visual hagiography of Bernardino, see Pavone and Pacelli, *Iconografia*. The iconography of Bernardino as an idealized hospital worker also features in a sixteenth-century fresco cycle in the church of San Bernardino in Lallio.

67 On this shift and broader tensions within the Franciscan Order in the fifteenth century, see Moorman, *A History of the Franciscan Order*, 368–83; Nimmo, *Reform and Division*; the essays collected in *Il rinnovamento del Francescanesimo*; Merlo, 'Dal deserto alla folla'; Lappin, *The Mirror of the Observance*, 12.

68 Lappin, *The Mirror of the Observance*, 14–20. On Paoluccio de' Trinci and the early Observance, see Sensi, *Dal movimento eremitico*.

69 Lappin, *The Mirror of the Observance*, 33. On the Perugian context for the Observant movement in relation to *La Franceschina*, see Pasqualin Traversa, *La 'minoritas' francescana*, 37–41.

70 The illustration is from Giacomo Oddi, *Lo Specchio dell'Ordine Minore* (known as *La Franceschina*), *c.* 1482–84, Biblioteca Porziuncola, Santa Maria degli Angeli (Assisi), MS 3, fol. 233v.

71 This gesture has an obvious parallel with the act of the sceptical knight Jerome, who stuck his hand into the stigmatic side wound of the dead St Francis to verify its authenticity; this moment often appears in depictions of Francis's death, such as the version frescoed *c.* 1300 in the Upper Church of the Basilica di San Francesco in Assisi. Jerome's act, in turn, echoed that of St Thomas examining the side wound of Christ. Observant readers of the Assisi version of *La Franceschina* would have been well prepared to identify both references.

Bibliography

Primary sources

Armstrong, Regis J., J. A. Wayne Hellmann, and William J. Short, eds, *The Founder. Volume II of: Francis of Assisi: Early Documents* (Hyde Park, NY: New City Press, 2000).

Armstrong, Regis J., J. A. Wayne Hellmann, and William J. Short, eds, *The Saint. Volume I of: Francis of Assisi: Early Documents* (Hyde Park, NY: New City Press, 1999).

Bonaventure, 'Legenda maior S. Francisci', in PP. Collegii S. Bonaventurae (ed.), *Analecta Franciscana sive Chronica aliaque varia documenta ad historiam Fratrum Minorum spectantia*, vol. 10 (Florence: Quaracchi, 1941), 555–652.

Florio, John, *Queen Anna's New World of Words, or Dictionarie of the Italian and English tongues* (London: Melch. Bradwood, 1611).

Menestò, Enrico and Stefano Brufani, eds, *Fontes Franciscani* (Assisi: Edizioni Porziuncola, 1995).

Oddi, Giacomo, *La Franceschina. Testo volgare umbro del secolo XV*, ed. Nicola Cavanna, 2 vols (S. Maria degli Angeli: Tipografia Porziuncola, 1929, rpt. 1981) [cited as Oddi-Cavanna].

Oddi, Giacomo, *Lo Specchio dell'Ordine Minore* (La Franceschina), 1474, Biblioteca Comunale Augusta, Perugia, MS 1238 [cited as BAP, MS 1238].

Oddi, Giacomo, *Lo Specchio dell'Ordine Minore* (La Franceschina), 1482–84, Biblioteca Porziuncola, Assisi, MS 3.

Pellegrini, Letizia, ed., *Il processo di canonizzazione di Bernardino da Siena (1445–1450)* (Grottaferrata: Quaracchi, 2009).

Thomas of Celano, 'Vita prima S. Francisci', in PP. Collegii S. Bonaventurae (ed.), *Analecta Franciscana sive Chronica aliaque varia documenta ad historiam Fratrum Minorum spectantia*, vol. 10 (Florence: Quaracchi, 1941), 3–115.

Secondary sources

Ahlquist, Gregory W. and William R. Cook, 'The representation of the posthumous miracles of St Francis of Assisi in thirteenth-century Italian painting', in William R. Cook (ed.), *The Art of the Franciscan Order in Italy* (Leiden: Brill, 2005), 211–56.

Argenziano, Raffaele, 'Giobbe e Lazzaro: santi, malati e protettori. L'iconografia della lebbra a Siena e nel contado tra il XIII e il XV secolo', in Giuseppina De Sandre Gasparini and Maria Clara Rossi (eds), *Malsani. Lebbra e lebbrosi nel medioevo* (Caselle di Sommacampagna: Cierre, 2013), 73–117.

Boeckl, Christine M., *Images of Leprosy: Disease, Religion, and Politics in European Art* (Kirksville, MO: Truman State University Press, 2011).

Brenner, Elma, 'Recent perspectives on leprosy in Medieval Western Europe', *History Compass*, 8, 5 (2010), 388–406.

Cobianchi, Roberto, '". . . Come vero amante della umiltà perfetta . . .": assistenza ai lebbrosi nell'iconografia francescana (XIII—XV secolo)', in Philine Helas and Gerhard Wolf (eds), *Armut und Armenfürsorge in der italienischen Stadtkultur zwischen 13. und 16. Jahrhundert. Bilder, Texte und soziale Praktiken* (Frankfurt am Main: Peter Lang, 2006), 55–67.

Cooper, Donal and Janet Robson, *The Making of Assisi: The Pope, the Franciscans and the Painting of the Basilica* (New Haven and London: Yale University Press, 2013).

Demaitre, Luke, *Leprosy in Premodern Medicine: A Malady of the Whole Body* (Baltimore: The Johns Hopkins University Press, 2007).

Foucault, Michel, *Madness and Civilization: A History of Insanity in the Age of Reason*, trans. Richard Howard (New York: Vintage Books, 1988).

Green, Monica H., Kathleen Walker-Meikle, and Wolfgang P. Müller, 'Diagnosis of a "plague" image: a digital cautionary tale', *The Medieval Globe*, 1, 1 (2014), 309–26.

Henderson, John, *The Renaissance Hospital: Healing the Body and Healing the Soul* (New Haven and London: Yale University Press, 2006).

Heullant-Donat, Isabelle, 'Martyrdom and identity in the Franciscan Order (Thirteenth and Fourteenth Centuries)', *Franciscan Studies*, 70 (2012), 429–53.

Il rinnovamento del Francescanesimo: l'Osservanza. Atti dell'XI Convegno Internazionale, Assisi, 20–21–22 ottobre 1983, ed. Società Internazionale di Studi Francescani (Assisi: Università di Perugia, 1985).

Jones, Lori and Richard Nevell, 'Plagued by doubt and viral misinformation: the need for evidence-based use of historical disease images', *The Lancet Infectious Diseases*, 16, 10 (2016), 235–40.

Lappin, Clare, *The Mirror of the Observance: Image, Ideal and Identity in Observant Franciscan Literature, c. 1415–1528* (unpublished PhD dissertation, University of Edinburgh, 2000).

Lincoln, Evelyn and Pascale Rihouet, 'Brands of piety', *UC Davis Law Review*, 47 (2013), 679–703.

Mancini, Francesco Federico, *Miniatura a Perugia tra Cinquecento e Seicento* (Perugia: Electa, 1987).

Manselli, Raoul, *Nos qui cum eo fuimus: Contributo alla questione francescana* (Rome: Istituto storico dei cappuccini, 1980).

Maranesi, Pietro, 'Il servizio ai lebbrosi in san Francesco e nei francescani', *Franciscana*, 10 (2008), 19–81.

Merlo, Grado Giovanni, 'Dal deserto alla folla. Persistenti tensioni del francescanesimo', in Giorgio Cracco (ed.), *Predicazione francescana e società veneta nel Quattrocento: committenza, ascolto, ricezione. Atti del II Convegno internazionale di studi francescani, Padova, 26–27–28 marzo 1987*, 2. ed. riv. (Padua: Centro Studi Antoniani, 1995), 61–77.

Moorman, John R. H., *A History of the Franciscan Order from Its Origins to the Year 1517* (Oxford: Clarendon Press, 1968).

Nimmo, Duncan, *Reform and Division in the Medieval Franciscan Order, from Saint Francis to the Foundation of the Capuchins* (Rome: Capuchin Historical Institute, 1987).

Ober, William B., 'Can the leper change his spots? The iconography of leprosy. Part I', *The American Journal of Dermatopathology*, 5, 1 (1983), 43–58.

Ober, William B., 'Can the leper change his spots? The iconography of leprosy. Part II', *The American Journal of Dermatopathology*, 5, 2 (1983), 173–86.

Park, Katherine and John Henderson, '"The First Hospital Among Christians": The Ospedale di Santa Maria Nuova in Early Sixteenth-century Florence', *Medical History*, 35 (1991), 164–88.

Pasqualin Traversa, Giovanna, *La 'minoritas' francescana nell'interpretazione della 'Franceschina' (Testo volgare Umbro del secolo XV)* (Assisi: Edizioni Porziuncola, 1995).

Pavone, Mario Alberto and Vincenzo Pacelli (eds), *Iconografia* [*Enciclopedia Bernardiniana*, vol. 2] (Salerno: Arti grafiche Boccia, 1981).

Rawcliffe, Carole, *Leprosy in Medieval England* (Woodbridge, UK and Rochester, NY: Boydell Press, 2009).

Scarpellini, Pietro, 'I tre illustratori della Franceschina (MS 1238 della Biblioteca Augusta di Perugia)', in Emanuela Sesti (ed.), *La miniatura italiana tra Gotico e Rinascimento: Atti del*

II Congresso di Storia della Miniatura Italiana, Cortona 24–26 settembre 1982 (Florence: Leo S. Olschki, 1985), 701–18.

Sensi, Mario, *Dal movimento eremitico alla regolare osservanza francescana. L'opera di fra Paoluccio Trinci* (Assisi: Edizioni Porziuncola, 1992).

Sensi, Mario, 'La lebbra e i lebbrosi nel medioevo e ad Assisi', *Convivium Assisiense*, 11, 2 (2009), 31–52.

Sensi, Mario, 'Per la storia dei lebbrosi tra Umbria e Marche (secoli XII-XV)', in Giuseppina De Sandre Gasparini and Maria Clara Rossi (eds), *Malsani. Lebbra e lebbrosi nel medioevo* (Caselle di Sommacampagna: Cierre, 2013), 291–342.

Sweetinburgh, Sheila, 'The hospital experience in medieval England', *HistoryExtra* (24 June 2019), www.historyextra.com/period/medieval/the-hospital-experience-in-medieval-england/.

Touati, François-Olivier, 'Contagion and leprosy: Myth, ideas and evolution in Medieval minds and societies', in Lawrence I. Conrad and Dominik Wujastyk (eds), *Contagion: Perspectives from Pre-Modern Societies* (Aldershot: Ashgate, 2000), 179–201.

Touati, François-Olivier, *Maladie et société au Moyen âge: La lèpre, les lépreux et les léproseries dans la province ecclésiastique de Sens jusqu'au milieu du* XIVe *siècle* (Brussels: De Boeck Université, 1998).

Visalli, Angelita Marques, 'Miniaturas franciscanas: a construção da virtude da humildade entre observantes na *Franceschina* (1474)', *Territórios e fronteiras*, 9, 1 (2016), 112–30.

Visalli, Angelita Marques, 'Os caminhos da perfeição franciscana na *Franceschina* (1474)', *Domínios da Imagem*, 4, 7 (2010), 33–44.

PART III
Disease and treatment

6

THE DRAMA OF INFIRMITY

Cupping in sixteenth-century Italy

Evelyn Welch

With an emphasis on the idealized body, dramatic images of illness were unusual in Renaissance Italy. They appeared, if at all, in hospital cycles, or in narratives of charity, martyrdom, and miraculous interventions.[1] Depictions of medical treatment were rare unless they formed part of a larger story of instruction, salvation, or both. This makes it more surprising, therefore, that, in 1586, in the middle of a list of prints made after the works of the Mantuan artist Giulio Romano, the author and painter Giorgio Vasari recorded just such a picture of medical intervention:

> [A]nd of these there are engravings to be seen, executed by Giovan Battista Mantovano, who engraved a vast number of things drawn by Giulio, and in particular, besides three drawings of battles engraved by others, a doctor who is applying cupping-glasses to the shoulders of a woman and the Flight of Our Lady into Egypt, with Joseph holding the ass by the halter, and some Angels pulling down a date palm so that Christ could pluck the fruit.[2]

Little noticed by either art historians or historians of medicine, the reference is striking for its unusual subject matter.[3] From antiquity onwards, cupping—a treatment that involved heating bone, metal, or glass cups before placing them on the skin to create a seal—was undertaken with or without scarification and associated blood-letting.[4] However, images of cupping were usually provided for practical information rather than for visual pleasure. For example, illustrations of the surgical text of the fourteenth-century English surgeon, John of Arderne, carefully noted the sites where cups should be placed according to the relevant disorder.[5] In a late-fifteenth-century English version, red dots demonstrated the relevant points of

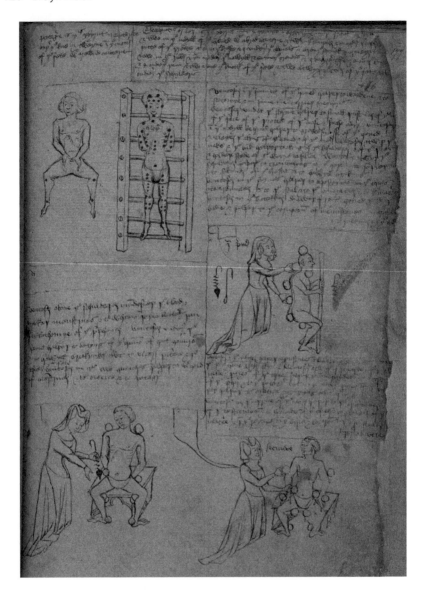

FIGURE 6.1 John of Arderne, surgical text

Source: © The British Library Board, Sloane 6, f.177

intervention, while a well-dressed, coifed woman placed the round cups, or *ventose*, on male and female bodies (Figure 6.1).

Similar pictures were included in manuscript and printed calendars such as the *regimina doudecim mensium*.[6] These texts informed readers of the right times of the year to take medicines, have sex, bathe, purge, or undertake sweat cures, enemas,

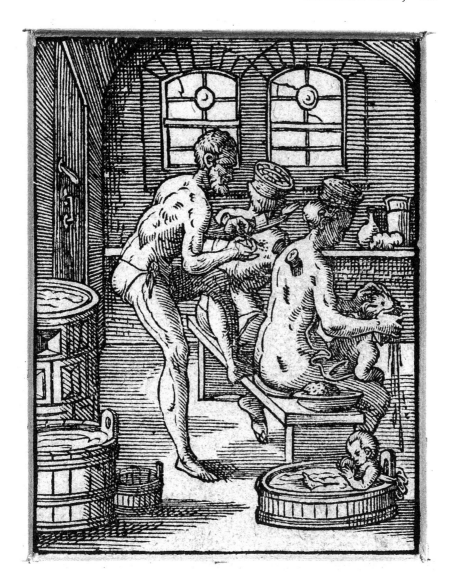

FIGURE 6.2 Joost Amman, *Eygentliche Beschreibung aller Stände auff Erden*
Source: Wellcome Collection

or bloodletting through cupping and venesection. In the sixteenth century, figures cupping their clients within bathhouses also appeared in 'Books of Trade', such as that of Joost Amman, in order to establish their professional standing (Figure 6.2). Very occasionally, as in the 1583 treatise on opthamology, *Ophthalmodouleia* by George Bartisch, the imagery combined the two, showing both the recommended treatment and celebrating its participants (Figure 6.3).

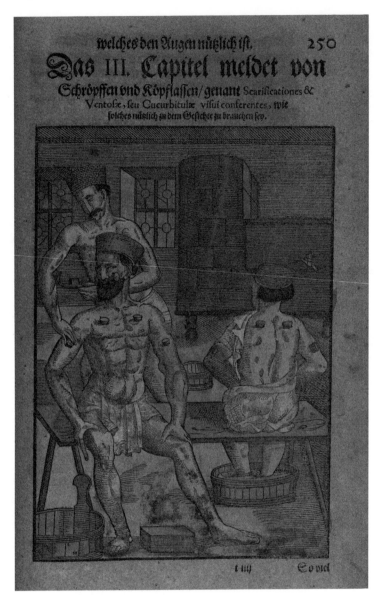

FIGURE 6.3 George Bartisch, *Ophthalmodouleia*

Source: Wellcome Collection

But the image that Vasari described earlier was very different in both purpose and format. It was neither a guide to nor an illustration of surgical practice. Instead, the engraving was a collectable item that demonstrated artistic and iconographic prowess; its fascination lay in the skill of its production and the drama of its narrative. Stemming from the visual legacy of Giulio Romano, these single sheets, often of considerable size, were designed for close observation and admiration. Why, then, would a sixteenth-century viewer want to purchase, study, or display an image of cupping?[7]

Tracing the image of 'a doctor who is applying cupping-glasses to the shoulders of a woman', its origins, and its multiple permutations allows insights into the way that medical interventions were reimagined using new forms of reproduction in the Renaissance. As importantly, exploring this imagery demands that in considering the development of new treatments for new diseases such as syphilis, or for the increasingly virulent versions of smallpox, we not only look at innovations in treatments but also consider how enduring and long-standing interventions such as cupping were asserted and promoted in the sixteenth century.

Imagining cupping: from paint to print

In his first edition of *The Lives of the Artists*, published in 1550, Giorgio Vasari rarely referred to prints and engravings, something he remedied in his second edition of 1568.[8] The image he listed was one of a series of engravings that he referenced in his life of Giulio Romano and, with a more extensive catalogue, in that of Marcantonio Raimondi, the prolific engraver associated with Raphael's designs. Remarkably, a version of the engraving showing 'a doctor who is applying cupping glasses to the shoulders of a woman' still survives today. It is not, however, by 'Giovanni Battista Mantovano', also known as 'Giovanni Battista scultori', but by a closely associated contemporary, the Mantuan engraver and damascene specialist Giorgio Ghisi (Figure 6.4).[9]

Unlike conventional surgical manuals of books of trades, this print does not show cupping taking place in a bathhouse. Instead, the action is set in a domestic environment, where a patient lies naked on an elegantly canopied bed. The gender of this figure is not obvious; but as we shall see, the nature of the treatment may provide the context for Vasari's assumption that the patient is female. A sheet is draped across the thighs, exposing the feet, buttocks, and the upper torso. Up-turned cups sit on each shoulder. The image captures the moment that the bearded, turbaned man is reversing the next cup, one that he will place on the figure's left buttock. Four female figures surround the bed. One sits below in mourning garb, another stands to the side in classicizing drapery, while two others, in indeterminate dress, hold the candle and plate used to create the hot air that will create the next cup's vacuum seal. A plate with poultry, the traditional food for the infirm, and a pair of sandals fill the floor space in front.

The print captures a moment of anticipation: the drama comes from the strong hatched lines on the walls, whose diagonals encourage the eye down to the bed. The curved space generated by the women who lean back and forth across the body creates a focal point, fixing the viewer's attention on the cupping that is about to take place. Nonetheless, as Vasari's note makes clear, this was not an original design. Its prestige came from its origins at the hands of Giulio Romano. The genealogy from paint to print, however, was a complex one. The Ghisi engraving

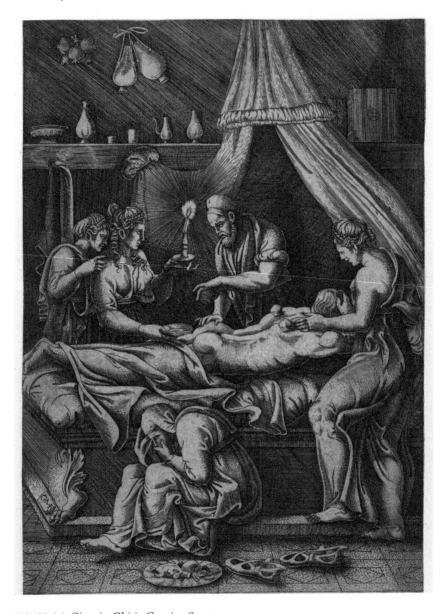

FIGURE 6.4 Giorgio Ghisi, *Cupping Scene*

Source: The Metropolitan Museum of Art, New York, public domain

took its iconography, in part, from a very private space originally designed for the Duke of Mantua, Federico II Gonzaga (1500–1540).[10] At some point in the early 1530s, Giulio Romano and his workshop designed and painted a set of frescoes in the *loggietta* of the so-called *giardino segreto*, a garden that led to a set of apartments reserved for the Duke himself.[11] The medical scene was not a separate, stand-alone

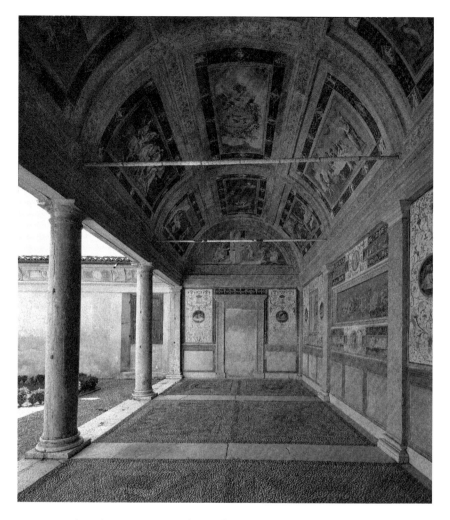

FIGURE 6.5 Agostino Mozzanego (after Giulio Romano), frescoed vault, Loggia Segreta

Source: Mantua, Palazzo Te

image. Instead, it was one of a series of nine narratives depicted on the barrel-vaulted ceiling of the *loggietta* (Figure 6.5).

The painted vault's precise iconography remains obscure. The imagery on the walls is strongly associated with wine, including scenes of Bacchus and Ariadne, as well as of Silenus. A sea scene fills the centre of the horizontal wall. At one end of the *loggietta*, figures make offerings to a pagan deity. At the other end, labourers and their animals lie asleep on the ground. The barrel vault itself has a row of central frescoes which show unidentified figures in apotheosis. The rectangular narratives on either side are more earth-bound, running from scenes of birth, labour (where men till the soil and a woman spins), love (as cupid draws his bow during a dance),

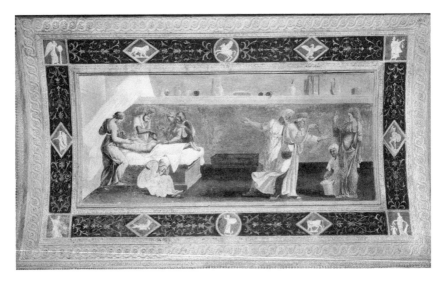

FIGURE 6.6 Agostino Mozzanego (after Giulio Romano), *Scene of Medical Treatment*

Source: Mantua, Palazzo Te

and a battle. The final rectangle (opposite the imagery of birth) shows the finality of life. It has two interconnected scenes: one where a physician peers at the patient's urine in a flask, the other where the bearded figure places a cupping glass on the figure extended across the bed.[12] In the frescoed version of the latter scene, the main focus is on the doctor, who faces a woman who gesticulates upwards, accompanied by a kneeling older woman holding a bucket; behind the doctor, a third male figure dramatically stretches out his arms as if in horror (Figure 6.6).

From the late nineteenth century onwards, this cycle has been described as an allegory of the human condition from birth to death.[13] Little, if any, attention has been paid to deciphering what is clearly a much more complex story. Given some of the specificity of the detail, it is likely that it does refer to an actual classical story, one perhaps related to Diana of Ephesus, who is shown in the birth scene.[14] Moreover, it is important to stress that while the actual meaning of the final panel depicting illness and, indeed, the full narrative itself might not be fully identifiable, the imagery did draw on a range of recognizable actors and actions. This meant that in looking upwards, the fresco's viewers were able to read the clear signs of a major illness, even if they could not identify its original classical source. The medical nature of the drama was signalled by the clothing and actions of the physician peering into a flask, work that would have been well understood as uroscopy, the identification of the internal state of the body through the reading of the colour and state of a patient's urine. There is a suggestion that the physician may then turn his attention to the patient's faeces in the bucket that is being held out by the woman below.[15] The seriousness of the eventual diagnosis is made clear by the dramatic gestures of the surrounding figures, who exclaim and gesticulate. Further down, another figure applies the cups to the recumbent patient, while a despondent woman sits at the foot of the bed, reminding the viewer of the seriousness of the situation.

Without the innovation of print, this scene of uroscopy, cupping, and patient care might have remained a minor episode in a small fresco hidden within the confines of Palazzo Te in Mantua. Instead it was translated and disseminated through two very different reproductions after the painting which survive today: the Ghisi print described earlier from about 1560, which only shows the cupping scene, and an earlier version dating from around 1542, which depicts the entire fresco in reverse (Figure 6.7). The latter was engraved, probably in France, by the Bolognese painter and engraver Antonio Fantuzzi, whose monogram appears on the bedframe.[16] Fantuzzi worked as Francesco Primaticcio's assistant on the frescoes of King François I's *Grande Gallerie* in Fontainebleau between 1541 and 1550 and the print has been dated to around 1542.[17] Primaticcio had trained with Giulio Romano and had worked at Palazzo Te himself. His Fontainebleau team clearly had access to Mantuan imagery, either through Giulio's original drawings or through copies after his works. This makes it difficult to be sure when a number of changes to the iconography were introduced, but the differences between the painting and the two prints were significant.

In the Fantuzzi engraving, the chest in the fresco has disappeared and the scene is highly condensed. There is greater emphasis on the wall hangings, whose sharp, swaying lines create a sense of energy, connecting the two sides of the drama. On the mantle above, an hourglass appears in both fresco and etching, suggesting the finite nature of time and the inevitability of death. But the engraving places greater

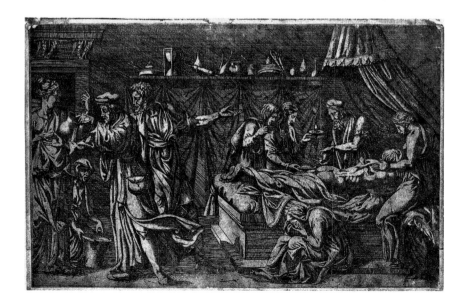

FIGURE 6.7 Antonio Fantuzzi, engraving

Source: Wellcome Collection

emphasis on treatments, with the very visible inclusion of an enema or a clyster on the shelf. At the same time as this very contemporary reference (clysters were often applied alongside cupping and venesection), the figures involved were given a more classicizing appearance. Nonetheless, despite their variations, the viewer of either the fresco or the Fantuzzi image would have been expected to recognize a set of shared responsibilities between the physician, who was undertaking the diagnosis through uroscopy and faecal analysis, and the barber-surgeon, who was applying the cupping remedy.

Studies on the Fontainebleau School of printing have noted the growing but still relatively small number of prints that were put into circulation.[18] In contrast, thirty years later, the marketplace for engravings had expanded considerably, offering new opportunities to represent older material. Again, it is not clear when and how Giorgio Ghisi, a Mantuan who might have seen the original Palazzo Te frescoes, obtained Giulio Romano's original designs. Ghisi himself was in France in the 1560s, where he may have seen either Fantuzzi's print or its original source such as a preparatory drawing for the fresco.[19] But whatever his inspiration, his own version is very different. It excludes the physician, focusing exclusively on the moment when the cup descends on the body. In Ghisi's hands, the engraving is no longer a sequential narrative from diagnosis to treatment but a moment of intense drama. All the attention is on the bearded figure, his sleeves rolled up, as he prepares to help his patient.

What prompted this shift? Certainly, Ghisi was thoughtful about how he attracted an audience for his works. Born in Mantua, he travelled widely, working in Rome, Antwerp, and at the French court. His plates were printed and sold in Rome by Antonio Lafreri, a Frenchman who made his reputation by commissioning and selling batches of engravings, such as the *Speculum Romanum*, which could be purchased as single images or as a complete set.[20] He also worked closely with the Antwerp publisher Hieronymus Cock, who had a similarly extensive distribution network for novel prints and engravings.[21]

The son of a merchant, Giorgio Ghisi was financially astute. The majority of his images reproduced or adapted works by Italy's most famous artists. These were figures who, thanks to Vasari and others, were gaining an international reputation. The largest number of his prints were after Giulio Romano, but he also copied works by Michelangelo, Raphael, Bronzino, Correggio, Primaticcio, and Luca Penni.[22] Part of his success was his willingness to rethink and re-present inaccessible frescoes and paintings, such as the Palazzo Te *loggietta*, to new audiences. But in these cases, he advertised them as new imagery rather than reproductions. For example, a second Ghisi print engaged with another of Giulio's designs for the *loggietta* vault: the narrative opposite the image of illness. This was a birth scene where a young woman is attended by a midwife, while Diana of Ephesus hands the new-born child to cherubs, as Aurora rises in her chariot and an old crone lights a fresh torch (Figure 6.8).

When Ghisi did a finely hatched engraving of this design by Giulio Romano in 1558, he was either confused by its meaning or believed that his audience would

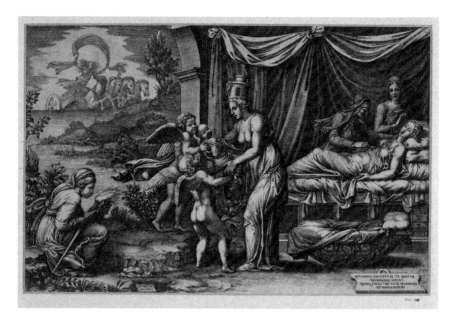

FIGURE 6.8 Giorgio Ghisi, *Birth of Memnon*

Source: © Victoria and Albert Museum, London

be. He deleted the characteristic but potentially troubling dangling breasts of Diana of Ephesus and added an inscription to suggest that this was the birth of Memnon, son of the goddess Aurora, who can be seen on her chariot in the background.[23] A drawing in the Minneapolis Institute of Art took this one stage further, removing the goddess's characteristic headdress and reducing the scene to a more conventional image of mythological birth.[24]

At some point around the same period in the 1560s, Ghisi took up the similar challenge of making the fresco of illness interpretable to an audience who would have never had access to the Palazzo del Te. Here, too, he tried to ensure that new viewers would be able to make sense of a scene whose original meaning had been lost. This time, however, Ghisi made no effort to introduce an Ovidian tale into the scene of attempted healing or to use explanatory inscriptions. Instead, he moved in the opposite direction. He reduced the classicizing elements, emphasizing the contemporary clothing of the setting through the bed-hangings, the implements on the shelves, and the domestic items in the foreground. Moreover, by removing the physician and the scene of diagnosis, Ghisi created a much calmer scene, one where the inherent drama lies in the tension of what is to come, not what had already happened. It is as much about what cannot be seen as it is about what can be observed. Thus, what is on the outside, the cup being placed on the body, will transform what cannot be seen, the impact within the body itself.

The sense of suspense was only possible if those with access to the print fully understood what it was they were seeing. Only close familiarity would have allowed sixteenth-century viewers to see the curved items on the shoulders as heated cups rather than, for example, stones or sponges. In the scene of Diana of Ephesus attending the birth scene, Ghisi thought it necessary to provide considerable amounts of additional information, such as inscriptions to make the iconography accessible. In the scene of illness, however, he made no such effort, presumably because he could safely assume they had a good knowledge of the practice of cupping. In the next section, therefore, we will explore the ways in which barbers, surgeons, and doctors competed, both in print and in practice, to bring humoral imbalances to the surface through cups and lancets. In doing so, we can attempt to bring a better understanding to what we might term 'the period body'. Like Michael Baxandall's 'period eye', thinking through the 'period body', or the intuitive, absorbed, and unquestioned understanding of how internal physiology worked in the Renaissance, changes our understanding of the original intentions of artist, engraver, and viewer.[25]

Cupping practices

In the shared classical and Arabic understanding of the body, four elements made up all living things: earth, air, fire, and water. These, in turn, created the four humours governing health: blood, which was hot and moist and associated with air; phlegm, which was characterized as cold and moist and connected to water; and black and yellow bile, which were regarded as cold and dry, and hot and dry, and associated respectively with earth and fire.[26] These gave rise to particular 'complexions' or types: sanguine, phlegmatic, melancholic, and choleric and their multiple variations. A healthy body had a harmonious balance between all four bodily fluids. Illness arose because of imbalance. This was often caused by interior circumstances, such as an excess of blood or the inability of the body to expel corrupt matter, or, as Michael Stolberg has shown, because of an inability to digest food properly, either in the stomach or in the liver.[27] The interior could also be disturbed by exterior forces, with a wide range of dangers arising from pathogenic air to the malevolent influence of the stars.

Attempts to manage a healthy internal balance by drawing blood, through venesection or scarification, or by raising blisters, date back to the earliest surviving medical writings, while lancets and cupping vessels used by Hippocratic practitioners from the fourth or fifth century BCE survive in forms that remained in use for millennia.[28] Recommended actions included various forms of phlebotomy, leeching, as well as wet and dry cupping. These were all used as regular prophylactics to maintain health as well as in emergencies. By the 1560s most printed calendars included symbols to indicate when cupping should be considered alongside bloodletting.[29] Thus, spring and autumn, when blood was regarded as plentiful due to moisture in the air, were propitious moments, while winter and summer, which were drier, were counter-indicated.[30]

In moments of crisis, cupping was particularly called for when corrupted matter was deep within the body. Plutarch, for example, used cupping as a metaphor in his aphorisms: 'For as cupping-glasses draw from the flesh what is worst in it, so the ears of busy-bodies attract the most evil stories.'[31] He also wrote, 'But, just as cupping-glasses draw the most virulent humour from the flesh, so you gather together against yourself the worst of your own condition.'[32] In their popular and much-adapted texts, the Roman physicians Galen and Celsus gave detailed information on bleeding and cupping, with an emphasis on what types of veins to approach, the cups to use, how and where to place them, and what conditions were appropriate for their use.[33] Thus, bleeding was primarily undertaken on the arm, usually from the median cubital vein at the elbow, but also from the temples and the ankle, and when necessary, even from the tongue. Cupping, which could be done with or without scarification, had a much broader range of sites to choose from, with fourteen separate potential locations depending on the disease. For example, German calendars, such as the popular *Teutsch Kalender*, which appeared in thirty-three editions between 1481 and 1522, recommended cupping on the forehead for eye complaints, headache, and dizziness. Cups were placed on the legs and buttocks 'to help reduce excessive sexual desire'.[34]

As this suggests, any sixteenth-century patient looking to ancient or contemporary sources would have found considerable written authority behind the practice of cupping.[35] However, despite the antiquity and the authorities associated with cupping, there were also numerous contradictions between the instructions and available advice. Should the treatment be undertaken close to the place of inflammation by placing, for example, the cup on a diseased area? Alternatively, should the cup be placed at a distance, encouraging the diseased matter to move away from the site?

Galen was clear that the latter course was correct, arguing:

> Likewise, the cupping glass is found to be an excellent remedy for the outward passage of those things in the depths and for the dislodgement, as it were, of those things that are already scirrhous. An exception is that the cupping glass must not be used on the inflamed part at the start, but only when you evacuate the body, and there is a need for you to evacuate and dislodge any of the things in the inflammation, or to drive them away to the outside.
>
> When affections are still evolving, do not apply the cupping glass to the actual structures that are beginning to suffer, but to those parts adjacent to them for the purpose of revulsion. And in this way, we place a cupping glass on the breasts when there is uterine bleeding, fixing the mouth of the cupping glass particularly to those vessels that are common to both the chest and the uterus. In the same way, when haemorrhage occurs through the nose, we place a very large cupping glass on the hypochondrium. The same also applies to every other haemorrhage: we draw it away to the opposite parts through the common veins, just as we also draw it back again should we need to do this. And if we wish to set in motion the menstrual flow, we place the cupping glass on the pubes and the inguinal glands. Also, a cupping glass placed over the inion (external occipital protuberance) is an excellent remedy

for a flux of the eyes. It is, however, necessary to evacuate the whole body beforehand, because, if it is plethoric, regardless of what part of the head you might place the cupping glass on, you will fill the whole head [with blood].[36]

Arabic instructions, such as Avicenna's *Liber canonis medicinae*, suggested a slightly different approach. In Book 4, chapter 21, 'On cupping glasses and their impact' ('De ventosis et earum affectibus'), Avicenna advised:

> Like bloodletting, cupping glasses can greatly heal a part of the skin/body [cutis], and take out much fine and thick blood. [. . .] Cupping glasses, which are placed on the legs, diminish [afflictions] nearby, and heal the blood and cause menstruation, and for this, which happens in pale women with a lack of thin blood, cupping glasses applied on the legs are better than bloodletting, for that which is hidden. [. . .] However, applying cupping glasses without scarification is therefore done so that the material is brought out by its own movement, and they are placed on the breasts to hold back the flow of menstrual blood. And when you wish to bring out a deep abscess to the exterior, so that the medicine can reach there [to the abscess], and when you require that the abscess is moved to another limb, because the vicinity is bad, and when it is needed that a limb is heated, so that blood flows back to its natural place, from where it has been flowing, as is the case of a rupture of blood (something missing here) [. . .] Cupping glasses applied to the buttocks drag out [afflictions] from the entire body, from the head to the intestines, and heal the corruption of menstrual blood, and in this way relieve the body.[37]

This passage makes it clear why Vasari identified the body as female: cups applied to the buttocks both helped reduce excessive sexual desire and, as importantly, 'heal the corruption of menstrual blood.' The sixteenth-century surgeon Ambroise Paré and his contemporary English translator also noted the importance of using cupping to encourage the flow of the menses:

> Of Cupping-glasses, or ventoses. Cupping-glasses are applyed especially when the matter conjunct and impact in any part is to be evacuated, and then chiefly there is place for scarification after the cupping-glasses: yet they are also applyed for revulsion and divertion; for when an humour continually flowes down into the eyes, they may be applyed to the shoulders with a great flame, for so they draw more strongly and effectually. They are also applyed under womens breasts, for to stop the courses flowing too immoderately, but to their thighes for to provoke them. They are also applyed to such as are bit by venemous beasts, as also to parts possessed by a pestiferous *Bubo* or Carbuncle, so to draw the poyson from within outwards. For (as *Celsus* saith) a Cupping-glasse where it is fastned on, if the skin be first scarified, drawes forth blood, but if it bee whole, then it draws spirit. Also they are applyed

to the belly, when any grosse or thick windinesse, shut up in the guts, or membraines of the muscles of the *Epigatrium*, or lower belly causing the Collick, is to bee discussed. Also they are fastned to the Hypocondry's, when as flatulency in the liver, or spleene, swels up the entraile lying thereunder, or in too great a bleeding at the nose. Also they are set against the Reines in the bottome of the belly, whereas the ureters run downe to draw downe the stone into the bladder, when as it stops in the middle or entrance of the ureter. You shall make choice of greater and lesser Cupping-glasses according to the condition of the part, and the conteined matter. But to those parts whereto these cannot by reason of their greatnesse be applyed, you may fit hornes for the same purpose.[38]

But while this might suggest a strongly gendered approach, cupping was recommended for many other conditions that afflicted both men and women. For example, as Paré noted, it was one of the treatments needed to shift tumours:

Matter contained in the part [where the tumour is located] . . . is against nature, [so] it requires to be evacuated by resolving things, as cataplasmes, ointments, formentations, cupping glasses or by evacuation, as by scarifying or by suppurating things as by ripening and opening the impostumes [abscesses].[39]

Paré also went to the trouble of illustrating the different sizes and scales of the cups that were required along with the lancets needed to pierce the skin before application.

In 1586, the Roman barber-surgeon Pietro Paolo Magni published his *Discorsi sopra il modo di sanguinare [. . .] & le ventose*, a treatise that focused exclusively on how different diseases and conditions should be treated using phlebotomy, leeches, and cups.[40] Magni explained that cupping glasses should be applied to the head, forehead, the nape of the neck, and under the beard and that they were suitable for everything from blows to the skull to nosebleeds. For women, they could be applied to her breasts, above the navel, on the shoulders, and on the buttocks.[41]

As this indicates, the classical treatises that validated cupping were numerous. Nonetheless, Vasari, who served the Medici court in Florence, would not have needed to have read these ancient sources or even reference the works of his contemporaries, Paré or Magni, in order to identify the print he saw as 'a doctor who is applying cupping-glasses to the shoulders of a woman.' Cupping was a long-standing, standard practice amongst his peers at the Medici court. For example, when the King of Spain Philip II's wife, Elizabeth of Valois, died in 1568, the Medici envoy to Madrid blamed her physicians: 'the doctors have expressly killed the Queen having, on the same morning, given her a medicine, and then having placed an infinite number of cups to try to save her life and having taken blood from her foot.'[42] The same sequence of cupping and bleeding from the foot (taking blood from this saphena vein, sometimes described as the *vena della madre*, was specifically indicated to encourage menstruation and the release of trapped fluids in the womb) was also prescribed by doctors in the early seventeenth century in a similarly unsuccessful attempt to cure the Duchess of Mantua, Eleanora.[43] In these cases, the physicians were responsible for the cupping, or at least for ordering it—something that may explain Vasari's identification of the figure in the print after Giulio Romano as a doctor rather than a surgeon.[44]

Who did the cupping in these different circumstances could often be contested. While both surgery and medicine were taught at university, the division of labour between the physician and the surgeon should have been clear. Barber-surgeons, barbers, and bath-house assistants who offered phlebotomy services were even further down the hierarchy.[45] In Venice and the Veneto, barbers sat an exam in the vernacular that only gave them licence to treat 'sores, grazes, injuries, wounds and other minor, non-life-threatening cases'.[46] In Bologna, the list of questions authorities posed before licensing barber-surgeons included inquiries such as the following:

> If they have ever let blood, applied cupping glasses or dressed broken or twisted bones?
> Who taught them such things?
> What kind of people they have treated and for what illness?
> How much do they pay per year to have the licence to let blood, apply cupping glasses dress fractures and practice as barbers?
> If they know what are the good and bad times to let blood?
> If they know about changes and effects of the moon and which ones are harmful when letting blood.[47]

Most important, however, was the final question: 'If, when they have let blood, they had done so when asked by physicians or simply by the patients' relatives or their friends?' This was because the practice was supposed to be supervised and controlled by doctors, not self-prescribed.

The Mantuan fresco and the closely associated Fantuzzi print both depicted this traditional relationship between the physician undertaking uroscopy and the figure doing the cupping. A Renaissance viewer would have recognized that the former had diagnosed a serious illness (hence the dramatic response of the immediate onlookers). They may well have assumed that the bearded figure by the bedside was simply following the doctor's orders in an attempt to shift the dangerous distempers within the body itself.[48] This conventional hierarchy was well understood. In his 1586 *Piazza universale di tutte le professioni del mondo*, for example, the Venetian writer and satirist Tomasso Garzoni wrote of barbers:

> Since their end and purpose is the cleansing of the body, which is brought about by shaving, the trimming of hair, the washing and buffing of those who have recourse to them. [. . .] Barbers are also used for blood-letting of the sick, and for applying cupping glasses, dressing wounds, giving enemas,

extracting rotten teeth and other such things, so that their art, as Bernardino de Bistis says in his Rosary, is thereby inferior to the science of medicine.[49]

In the Ghisi print, however, the doctor has disappeared. Instead, the figure doing the cupping has become the focal point. Does this suggest a subtle change in attitudes towards barber-surgeons or simply a shift in where and how the dramatic tension was signalled in the print? A sixteenth-century observer would have known that cupping took time to learn. In one study of how barber-surgeons were trained in the town of Feltre, albeit in the early seventeenth century, the scholar noted that it took three years to qualify and that the skills of bleeding and cupping were only taught in the second year.[50] The same study recorded how the Feltre notary Antonio Cadore recorded the wide range of services he had paid for or received free of charge from the barber-surgeon Zanvittore Capra, between August 1570 and 26 July 1571: 'for having washed my head [. . .] for four cupping treatments [. . .] for washing me and shaving me [. . .] for shaving my nephew Iacomo [. . .] for a bloodletting'.[51]

As this suggests, cupping was a quotidian practice that was as familiar as shaving. Nonetheless, understanding its operation required a basic understanding of the humoral system, one where even hair-washing carried dangers to a highly porous body.[52] Given the expense and status of print purchases, the original viewers of the Ghisi print may have been well educated, with an even more sophisticated understanding of humoral physiology than the norm. It may be no coincidence that at the same time as the fresco was being painted, and certainly by the time the prints were produced, many of the classical texts that emphasized and explained the practice of cupping were being re-translated and re-circulated in Italy and across Europe.

In his work on the rise of medical humanism, Vivian Nutton has noted that the period shortly before the creation of the *loggietta* in Mantua saw a remarkable surge in the publication of ancient works in newly edited formats.[53] The first edition of the complete surviving works of Galen in Greek and of the Hippocratic corpus in Latin were published in 1525.[54] In 1529, Teodoro Gaudano published a new version of Galen's key text on bloodletting and cupping.[55] By the 1520s, medicine and surgery at the University of Padua were being taught using both the medieval texts of Mondino de' Liuzzi and the newly modernized versions of Galen. In the new 'humanist' version of medical texts, these seemingly 'everyday' activities regained their classical origins and context. Thus, when the eminent Paduan physician Girolamo Mercurialis published his edition of Hippocrates in 1588, he illustrated cupping as a key therapy, using a very similar image to that deployed by Ghisi, on his frontispiece (Figure 6.8).

Conclusion

When Giorgio Ghisi adapted Giulio Romano's original designs for an image of infirmity, he was relying on his viewers' knowledge of the delicate and difficult task of creating a seal between bodily flesh and the heated cup. He expected his audience to see this as a dramatic moment in time. The kneeling, mourning woman, the dropped plate of poultry, and the fact that the intervention was taking place at home rather than in a barber-shop or bath-house, all indicated the severity of what was about to come.

This episode helps us understand the multiple ways in which the increasingly wide availability of printed material challenged perceptions of traditional practices at a time of considerable change in medical knowledge. Cupping may have been a long-standing way of managing the interior of the body using external means, but it now carried its classical heritage more overtly. At the same time, anyone—whether medically trained or not—could appreciate the drama of an illness that could lead to death if not instantly treated. In this sense, the engraving's impact was only made possible through the contemporary sixteenth-century viewers' innate understanding of their own body and that of others. Whoever purchased or looked at the print had to know enough about bodily interiors to appreciate the tensions involved. The way the cups shifted humours and moved blockages to the surface of the body had to be suggested rather than spelt out as a set of instructions. The internal changes that might save the patient's life could only be imagined. Appreciating the print was an understanding not only of the way in which the engraved lines created narrative but also of what was taking place below the surface of the skin.[56]

Notes

1 Lincoln, 'Curating the renaissance body', 42–61.
2 Vasari, *Lives of the Most Excellent Painters, Sculptors and Architects*, 302, 'disegni in istampa, stati intagliati da Giovan Batista Mantovano, il quale intaglio infinite cose disegnate da Giulio e particolarment, oltre a tre carte di battaglie intagliate da altri, un medico ch'apicca le coppette sopra le spalle a una femina, una Nostra Donna che va in Egitto, e Giuseppo ha a mano l'asino per la cavezza, et alcuni Angeli fanno piegare un dattero perché Christo ne colga de' frutti'. On this passage, see Ronen, 'Il Vasari e gli incisori del suo tempo', 92–104, and Letwin, '*Old in Substance and New in Manner*', 4.
3 Boorsch, Lewis and Lewis, eds, *The Engravings of Giorgio Ghisi*, 35.
4 Akhtar Qureshi, Ibrahim Ali, and Shaban Abu, 'History of cupping', 172–81.
5 London, British Library, Sloane 9, fols 176v–77 and fol. 177v. See Murray Jones, 'John of Arderne and the Mediterranean tradition of scholastic surgery', 289–321.
6 Brévart, 'The German Volkskalender of the Fifteenth century', 316; Lyon, *Wreaths of Time: Perceiving the Year in Early Modern Germany*, 96.
7 Bury, 'The taste for prints in Italy to c.1600', 12–26; for a specific example of print purchases, see Carrara and Gregory, 'Borghini's print purchases from Giunti', 3–17.
8 Witcombe, *Copyright in the Renaissance*, 3; and Gregory, *Vasari and the Renaissance Print*.
9 Boorsch, Lewis and Lewis, *The Engravings of Giorgio Ghisi*, 16.
10 Verheyen, *The Palazzo del Te in Mantua*, 129. See also Maurer, *Gender, Space and Experience at the Renaissance Court*.
11 Verheyen, *The Palazzo del Te in Mantua*, 33, 130.
12 Stolberg, *A Cultural History of Uroscopy*, see chapter 3.
13 Verheyen, *The Palazzo del Te in Mantua*, 129–30. See also the detailed illustrations of the *loggietta* in Beluzzi, *Palazzo Te a Manova*, 646–71.

14 Diana appears at multiple points throughout the Palazzo Te iconography and elsewhere in Mantuan imagery of the same period. See Nielsen, 'Diana Efesia Multimammia', 455–96.
15 Stolberg, *A Cultural History of Uroscopy*.
16 Zerner, *École de Fontainebleau. Gravures*, xlii; and Zorach, *Blood, Ink, Milk, Gold*, 145.
17 Zerner, *École de Fontainebleau. Gravures*, xlii.
18 Zerner, *École de Fontainebleau. Gravures*, xiii–xvi.
19 Boorsch, Lewis, and Lewis, *The Engravings of Giorgio Ghisi*, 18.
20 Boorsch, Lewis, and Lewis, *The Engravings of Giorgio Ghisi*, 18.
21 Riggs, *Hyeronymus Cock (1510–1570)*.
22 Boorsch, Lewis, and Lewis, *The Engravings of Giorgio Ghisi*, 25; and Letwin, '*Old in Substance and New in Manner*', 16.
23 Boorsch, Lewis, and Lewis, *The Engravings of Giorgio Ghisi*, 107.
24 See, Minneapolis Institute of Art, Circle of Giulio Romano, *Birth of Memnon*, drawing, Gift of Herschel Jones, 1926. Accession number P. 10,905.
25 Baxandall, *Painting and Experience in Fifteenth-Century Italy*, 29–57.
26 For a general overview of the humoral system, see, Arikha, *Passions and Tempers*.
27 Stolberg, 'You Have No Good Blood in Your Body', 63–82. See also Kuryama, 'Interpreting the History of Bloodletting', 11–46.
28 Lindemann, 'Disease and Medicine', 100–01 and Bliquez, *The Tools of Asclepius*, 6, 26.
29 Lyon, *Wreaths of Time*, 96.
30 Lyon, *Wreaths of Time*, 96.
31 Plutarch, *On Being a Busybody*, 488–89.
32 Plutarch, *On Tranquillity of Mind*, 192–93.
33 Davis, *Phlebotomy*, 2.
34 Brévart, *German Volkskalender*, 327, 338.
35 Nutton, 'Humanist Surgery', 75–99.
36 Galen, *Method of Medicine, Volume III*, 394–97.
37 Avicenna, *Liber canonis medicinae*, Lib. Fen 1 Ch. 21 (*De ventosis et earum affectibus*), (Hildesheim: G. Olms, 1964), fol. 62r-v (reprint of 1507 Venice edition).
38 Johnson, *The Workes of that Famous Chirurgion Ambrose Parey*, 694, chapter LXI. On *Paré* see Poirier, *Ambroise Paré*.
39 Johnson, *The Works of that Famous Chirurgion Ambrose Parey*, 198.
40 Magni, *Discorsi di Pietro Paolo Magni Piacentino sopra il modo di sanguinare*. See also Lincoln, 'Curating the Renaissance Body', 42–44.
41 Magni, *Discorsi di Pietro Paolo Magni*, 96.
42 Archivio di stato, Florence, Archivio Medici dopo il principato, v.4902, insert 1, fol. 85. Leonardo di Antonio de'Nobili to Cosimo de' Medici, 3 October 1568: '. . . Mi par a proposito che V.E. sappia, come li medici espressamente hanno ammazzato la Regina havendoli dato la mattina medesima una medicina, et appiccato infinite coppette per la vita, et cavato sangue per li piedi.'
43 Florence, Archivio di Stato, Archivio Medici dopo il principato, v.6113, fol. 25. Claudia d'Albon Coppoli to Caterina de'Medici Gonzaga, 27 November 1617: '. . . il giovedi se cavo sangue per li piedi, perche li erano cominciato le purghe et non continuavano se con un poco de segno . . . non riposo quasi niente la note pero il venerdi si chiamo il Giudo, et se li aplico le copette, et il sbato, una medicina, et si vede che niente ligiovera, non si doleno pero se non la testa et perse il sono afatto, se li aplico altre copette con tagliarle. . . .' On the *vena della madre*, see Christopoulos, 'Nonelite male perspectives on procured abortion, Rome circa 1600', 163–64.
44 Stolberg, 'A sixteenth-century physician and his patients', 239; Pomata, 'Practicing between Heaven and Earth', 123; Pelling, 'Appearance and reality', 82–112.
45 Savoia, *Cosmesi e chirurgia*; Cavallo, *Artisans of the Body in Early Modern Italy*; Pomata, *Contracting a Cure*; Gentilcore, *Healers and Healing in Early Modern Italy*; and Pastore, *Le regole dei corpi: medicina e disciplina nell'Italia moderna*.

46 Bartolini, 'On the borders', 88.
47 Bologna, Archivio di Stato, Studio, *Atti per processi vari del Collego e del Protomedicato 1588–1736*, busta no. 213. My thanks to Paolo Savoia for this reference.
48 Bartolini, 'On the borders', 89.
49 Cavallo, *Artisans of the Body*, 38.
50 Bartolini, 'On the borders', 89.
51 Bartolini, 'On the borders', 95.
52 Evelyn Welch, 'Art on the edge', 241–68.
53 Nutton, 'The rise of medical humanism', 2.
54 Nutton, 'The rise of medical humanism', 2.
55 Galen, *De curandi ratione per sanguinis missionem*. On this text, see Brain, *Galen on Bloodletting*.
56 The research for this chapter was undertaken with the support of the Wellcome Trust. My thanks to Dr Hannah Murphy, Dr Paolo Savoia, Dr Kathleen Miekle-Walker, and Dr Natasha Awais-Dean for their assistance with this research and, above all, to Dr Juliet Claxton for her invaluable help.

Bibliography

Primary sources

Unpublished

Archivio di Stato, Bologna, Studio, *Atti per processi vari del Collego e del Protomedicato 1588–1736*, busta no. 213.
Archivio di Stato, Florence, Archivio Medici dopo il principato, v. 4902, insert 1, f. 85.
British Library, Sloane 9, fols 176v–77 and fol. 177v.

Published

Avicenna, *Liber canonis medicinae*, Lib. Fen 1 Chapter. 21 (*De ventosis et earum affectibus*) (Hildesheim: G. Olms, 1964), fol. 62 recto-verso (reprint of 1507 Venice edition).
Galen, *Method of Medicine*, Volume III: Books 10–14, ed. and trans., Ian Johnston, G. H. R. Horsley, Loeb Classical Library 518 (Cambridge, MA: Harvard University Press, 2011).
Galeni De curandi ratione per sanguinis missionem, liber. Eiusdem, De sanguisugis: reuulsione: cucurbitula: & scarificatione: tractatulus. Theodorico Gaudano interprete (Paris: Christian Wechel, 1529).
Johnson, Thomas, *The Workes of That Famous Chirurgion Ambrose Parey Translated out of Latine and Compared with the French* (London: Cotes and Young, 1634).
Magni, Pier Paolo, *Discorsi di Pietro Paolo Magni Piacentino sopra il modo di sanguinare, attacare li sanguisughe & le ventose, far le fregagioni & vessicatori a corpi humani* (Rome: Bartolomeo Bonfadino, 1584).
Plutarch, *On Being a Busybody* in *Moralia, Volume VI: Can Virtue Be Taught? On Moral Virtue. On the Control of Anger. On Tranquility of Mind. On Brotherly Love. On Affection for Offspring. Whether Vice Be Sufficient to Cause Unhappiness. Whether the Affections of the Soul Are Worse Than Those of the Body. Concerning Talkativeness. On Being a Busybody*, ed. and trans., W. C. Helmbold, *Loeb Classical Library*, 337 (Cambridge, MA: Harvard University Press, 1939).
Vasari, Giorgio, *Lives of the Most Excellent Painters, Sculptors and Architects*, ed. and trans., Gaston de Vere, I (London: Macmillan & The Medici Society, 1912).

Secondary sources

Akhtar Qureshi, Naseem, Gazzaffi Ibrahim Ali, and Tamer Shaban Abu, 'History of cupping (Hijama): a narrative review of literature', *Journal of Integrative Medicine*, 15, 3 (2017), 172–81.

Arikha, Nora, *Passions and Tempers: A History of the Humours* (New York: Harper Collins, 2007).

Bartolini, Donatella, 'On the borders: surgeons and their activities in the Venetian State, 1540–1640', *Medical History*, 59 (2015), 83–100.

Baxandall, Michael, *Painting and Experience in Fifteenth-Century Italy: A Primer in the Social History of Pictorial Style* (Oxford: Oxford University Press, 1971).

Belluzzi, Amedeo, *Palazzo Tè a Mantova. The Palazzo Tè in Mantua* (Modena: Franco Cosimo Panini, 1998).

Bliquez, Lawrence, *The Tools of Asclepius: Surgical Instruments in Greek and Roman Times* (Leiden: Brill, 2015).

Boorsch, Suzanne, Michael Lewis, and R. E. Lewis, eds, *The Engravings of Giorgio Ghisi* (New York: Metropolitan Museum of Art, 1985).

Brain, Peter, *Galen on Bloodletting: A Study of the Origins, Development and Validity of His Opinions, with a Translation of the Three Works* (Cambridge: Cambridge University Press, 1986).

Brévart, Francis B., 'The German Volkskalender of the Fifteenth century', *Speculum*, 63 (1988), 312–42.

Bury, Michael, 'The taste for prints in Italy to c.1600', *Print Quarterly*, 2 (1995), 12–26.

Carrara, Eliana and Sharon Gregory, 'Borghini's print purchases from Giunti', *Print Quarterly*, 17 (2000), 3–17.

Cavallo, Sandra, *Artisans of the Body in Early Modern Italy: Identities, Families and Masculinities* (Manchester: Manchester University Press, 2007).

Christopoulos, John, 'Nonelite male perspectives on procured abortion, Rome circa 1600', *I Tatti Studies in the Italian Renaissance*, 17, 1 (2014), 163–64.

Davis, Bonnie Karen, *Phlebotomy: From Student to Professional* (Clifton Park: Delmar, 2010).

Gentilcore, David, *Healers and Healing in Early Modern Italy* (Manchester: Manchester University Press, 1998).

Gregory, Sharon, *Vasari and the Renaissance Print* (Farnham: Ashgate, 2012).

Kuriyama, Shigehisa, 'Interpreting the history of bloodletting', *Journal of the History of Medicine and Allied Sciences*, 50 (1995), 11–46.

Letwin, Hilary, '*Old in Substance and New in Manner': The Scultori and Ghisi Engraving Enterprise in Sixteenth Century Mantua and Beyond* (unpublished PhD dissertation, Johns Hopkins University, 2013).

Lincoln, Evelyn, 'Curating the Renaissance body', *Word & Image*, 17 (2001), 42–61.

Lindemann, Mary, 'Disease and Medicine', in Hamish Scott (ed.), *The Oxford Handbook of Early Modern European History, 1350–1750*, i: *Peoples and Place* (Oxford: Oxford University Press, 2015).

Lyon, Nicole M., *Wreaths of Time: Perceiving the Year in Early Modern Germany* (unpublished PhD dissertation, University of Cincinnati, 2015).

Maurer, Maria, *Gender, Space and Experience at the Renaissance Court: Performance and Practice at the Palazzo Tè* (Amsterdam: Amsterdam University Press, 2019).

Murray Jones, Peter, 'John of Arderne and the Mediterranean tradition of scholastic surgery', in Luis García-Ballester, Roger French, Jon Arrizabalaga, and Andrew Cunningham (eds), *Practical Medicine from Salerno to the Black Death* (Cambridge: Cambridge University Press, 1994), 289–321.

Nielsen, Marjatta, 'Diana Efesia Multimammia: The metamorphosus of a Pagan goddess from the Renaissance to the age of Neo-Classicism', in Tobias Fischer-Hansen and Birte Poulsen (eds), *From Artemis to Diana: The Goddess of Man and Beast* (Copenhagen: Museum Tusculanum, 2009), 455–96.

Nutton, Vivian, 'Humanist surgery', in A. Wear, R. K. French, and I. M. Lonie (eds), *The Medical Renaissance of the Sixteenth Century* (Cambridge: Cambridge University Press, 1985).

Nutton, Vivian, 'The rise of medical humanism: Ferrara, 1464–1555', *Renaissance Studies*, 11 (1997), 2–19.

Pastore, Alessandro, *Le regole dei corpi: medicina e disciplina nell'Italia moderna* (Bologna: Il Mulino, 2006).

Pelling, Margaret, 'Appearance and reality: barber-surgeons, the body, and disease', in A. L. Beier and Roger Finlay (eds), *London 1500–1700: The Making of the Metropolis* (London: Longmans, 1985).

Poirier, Jean-Pierre, *Ambroise Paré: un urgentiste au xv siècle* (Paris: Pygmalion, 2005).

Pomata, Gianna, *Contracting a Cure: Patients, Healers and the Law in Early Modern Italy* (Baltimore: Johns Hopkins University Press, 1998).

Pomata, Gianna, 'Practicing between Heaven and Earth: women healers in seventeenth-century Bologna', *Dynamis*, 19 (1999), 119–43.

Riggs, Timothy A., *Hyeronymus, Cock (1510–1570): Printmaker and Publisher in Antwerp at the Sign of the Four Winds* (New Haven: Yale University Press, 1971).

Ronen, Avraham, 'Il Vasari e gli incisori del suo tempo', *Commentari*, 28 (1977), 92–104.

Savoia, Paolo, *Cosmesi e chirurgia. Bellezza, dolore e medicina nell'Italia moderna* (Milan: Editrice bibliografica, 2017).

Stolberg, Michael, *A Cultural History of Uroscopy, 1500–1800* (Aldershot: Ashgate, 2015).

Stolberg, Michael, 'A sixteenth-century physician and his patients: the practice journal of Hiob Finzel, 1565–1589', *Social History of Medicine*, 32, 2 (2019), 221–40. https://doi.org/10.1093/shm/hkx063.

Stolberg, Michael, '"You Have No Good Blood in Your Body": oral communication in the Sixteenth-century physicians' medical practice', *Medical History*, 59 (2015), 63–82.

Verheyen, Egon, *The Palazzo del Tè in Mantua: Images of Love and Politics* (Baltimore: Johns Hopkins Press, 1977).

Welch, Evelyn, 'Art on the edge: hair and hands in Renaissance Italy', *Renaissance Studies*, 23 (2009), 241–68.

Witcombe, Christopher L. C. E., *Copyright in the Renaissance. Prints and the Privilegio in Sixteenth-Century Venice and Rome* (Leiden and London: Brill, 2004).

Zerner, Henri, *École de Fontainebleau. Gravures* (Paris: Arts et métiers graphiques, 1969).

Zorah, Rebecca, *Blood, Ink, Milk, Gold: Abundance and Excess in the French Renaissance* (Chicago: University of Chicago Press, 2005).

7

SUFFERING THROUGH IT

Visual and textual representations of bodies in surgery in the wake of Lepanto (1571)

Paolo Savoia

Introduction

In his essay *On schoolmasters' learning* (*Du pédantisme*, 1582), the sceptical relativist Michel de Montaigne wrote: 'Both in that martial government and in all others like it, examples show that studying the arts and sciences makes hearts soft and woman- ish rather than teaching them to be firm and ready for war. The strongest state to make an appearance in our time is that of the Turks; and the Turkish peoples are equally taught to respect arms and to despise learning'.[1] The orientalist image of Ottoman Turks—the way all the inhabitants of Ottoman lands were defined—as men having a hardened body, indifferent to learning, and remarkably resistant to all kinds of suffering was widespread in the sixteenth century. It was so widespread, in fact, that the Venetian intellectual, patriot, and publisher Francesco Sansovino, writing in a 1570 pamphlet addressed to 'Christian soldiers', felt the need to state that, after all, Ottoman 'Turks' were 'made of flesh and bones just like you are'.[2]

Concentrating on two illustrations from the 1583 Italian translation of a best- selling manual of surgery, Giovanni Andrea Dalla Croce's *Cirugia universale e perfetta*, first published in Latin in 1573, this chapter discusses a case history in the history of pain (Figures 7.1 and 7.2). One of the illustrations shows a Christian soldier heroically enduring pain as battlefield surgeons extract an arrow or a bullet from his chest. The second illustrates a Turkish soldier, his body contorted, in physical agony. While the Christian knight endures his pain as would a martyr, the Turk is represented as unable to suffer with dignity. After describing how pain manage- ment techniques were discussed by surgeons in sixteenth-century Italy, this chapter focuses on Venice and the representation of patients enduring pain in the aftermath of the battle of Lepanto (1571), between the Holy League (of which Venice was part) and the Ottoman Empire. In the aftermath of the defeat of the Ottoman fleet, along with millenarian hopes for a restoration of a Christian global Empire, a

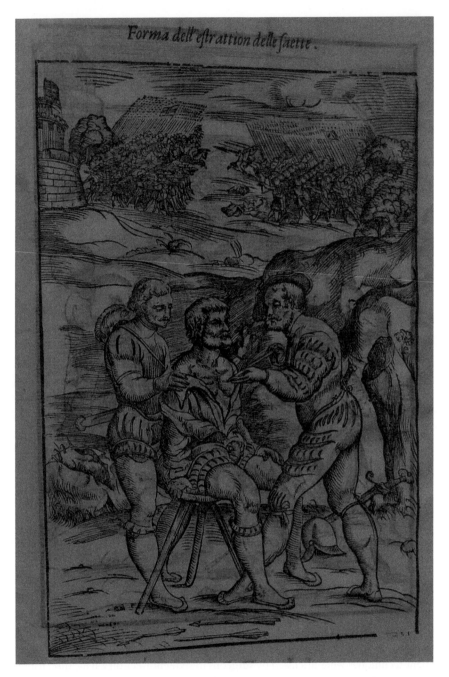

FIGURE 7.1 Giovanni Andrea Dalla Croce, *Cirugia universale e perfetta, Christian Soldiers*

Source: Biblioteca Comunale dell'Archiginnasio di Bologna

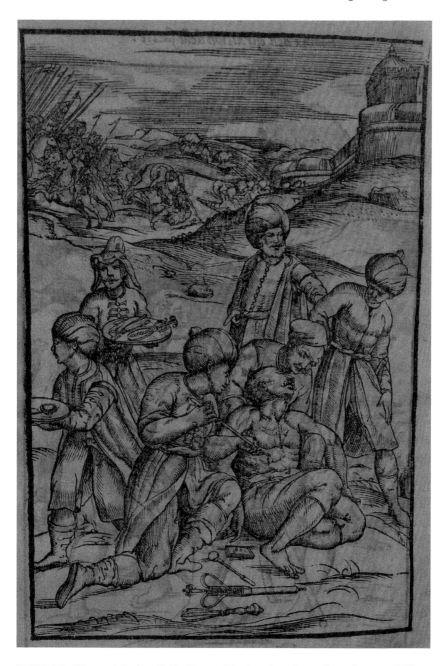

FIGURE 7.2 Giovanni Andrea Dalla Croce, *Cirugia universale e perfetta, Ottoman Soldiers*

Source: Biblioteca Comunale dell'Archiginnasio di Bologna

certain reassuring awareness that 'Turks' were not invincible but made of flesh and bones like Westerners was expressed in surgical imagery.

In Renaissance and early modern Italy, surgery was not just a medical specialty but part of a wider culture of suffering. This included visualizations of martyrdom and a celebration of Christianity, as well as discourses on bravery and the moral strength of patients. The illustrations in Dalla Croce's treatise should be understood in a broader context: the lack of a clear relationship between word and image in books written by barber-surgeons and especially by surgeons. Wordy descriptions mention pain and pain management techniques, while visual representations, such as anatomical images, suggest impassibility and abstractness. The history of these two illustrations indicates how popular images travel, and how their meaning changes over time, depending on different scientific and cultural communities. Finally, this case also shows the multiple relationships between the construction of the orientalist political and religious image of the 'Turk', on the one hand, and the moral contract between patients and surgeons regarding the painfulness of surgical procedures, on the other. By looking at and beyond the epistemic function of images in the history of early modern science and medicine, this chapter explores one of the 'material traces' extra-Europeans have left in European imagery, traces that 'offer key insights into the protracted and multiple ways in which European societies constructed a sense of themselves as a separate, coherent geographic unit distanced from entanglement with other peoples'.[3]

The status of surgery

The status of surgery in the multifaceted medical tradition called Galenism has always been very clear in theory, but less so in practice. In the Galenic humoral system, the entire edifice of medicine was divided into three branches: physic, pharmacy, and surgery. Galen and his followers emphasized the unity of the three parts. Physic, which can also be called learned medicine, focused on the inner and thus invisible parts of the body. From a therapeutic point of view, physicians were those who could prescribe oral medicaments: compounds of herbs and animal substances, but also food and drink (diet). Pharmacists were those who had the practical skills of composing medicaments and were experts in handling medical substances, but they were intellectually dependent upon the physicians. Finally, surgeons were those who dealt with ailments or diseases affecting the external parts of the body, including all kinds of swellings and skin diseases, but also wounds, fractures, eye conditions, tooth conditions, hernias, and bladder and kidney stones.

In the Galenic system, all surgical conditions, both those coming from within the body (ulcers, tumours, etc.) and those from without (war wounds, firearm wounds, etc.), were defined as 'diseases'. Though surgeons had to use their hands to practise, and mostly dealt with solid organs and the mechanics of bodily functions, the conditions they addressed were assigned causes that ultimately led back to humoral imbalances or corruptions of humours. Surgical diseases were attributed to either humoral imbalances (the case of ulcers and tumours) or a dissolution of continuity (the case of wounds and fractures); the latter, in turn, were considered diseases because they carried with them humoral imbalances manifested in a range of ways, including inflammation, gangrene, swellings, and corruption of humours.

Italy occupied a special place in the landscape of surgery in early modern Europe. Surgery had become an academic speciality in Italian universities, starting at least from the late thirteenth century, a tradition that developed steadily up to the sixteenth century.[4] Latin surgery books, written almost invariably by professors of medicine, were part of a textual tradition of representing bodies in a learned way, comparable to the scholarly representation of the body in anatomy books (Figure 7.3).

To see surgeons in action, we need to look instead at barber-surgeons' manuals (Figure 7.4). While anatomical books represent abstract and idealized bodies, immersed in almost metaphysical landscapes, and placed within symbolic contexts, barber-surgeons' books visually describe bloodletting as a collective activity involving surgeons, supervisors, assistants, and family members.[5] These images are idealized too, in that they are never gory and never show too graphically the painfulness of the procedures in question, but the patients are always represented as part of a more complex and more realistic choreography. No practitioner liked to have pain represented in his book, but all of them addressed the issue of how to manage it.

Pain management

Respect and concern for the patients' pain was common in sixteenth-century surgery books. Galen and tenth-century Persian physician Avicenna (Ibn Sīnā) had provided standard definitions and physiological models of pain, individuating its causes in humoral imbalance and in a 'dissolution of continuity' of the soft or hard parts of the body.[6] As shown by the Neapolitan Aristotelian philosopher Simone Porzio, professor of philosophy at Pisa in the 1540s and physician at the Medici court, there was a certain consensus about the nature and causes of pain. In a treatise on pain published in Florence in 1551, Porzio identified the three basic conditions that allowed for a human being to feel pain: the body needed to receive impressions and feel sensations; a sudden and violent mutation had to happen; and a change 'against nature' had to take place, one contrary to pleasurable feelings of the body.[7]

Medieval learned surgeons all dealt with the painfulness of surgical operations, agreeing on the precept that one of the most basic duties of surgeons was to minimize patients' pain.[8] The treatment of wounds, fractures, and ulcers and the more complex operations like the extraction of bladder stones and the elimination of cataracts were all accompanied by remarks on easing pain, cheering up patients with artful conversation, and preventing patients from moving, so as not to put their lives in danger.

Pain in surgery was considered to be a liability from a purely technical-medical point of view. Physicians and surgeons believed it was accompanied by dangerous inflammation and that it attracted bad humours to the damaged parts of the body.

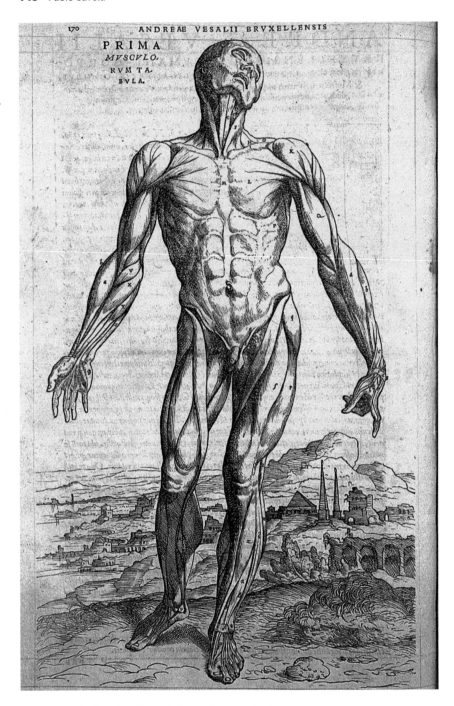

FIGURE 7.3 Andreas Vesalius, *De humani corporis fabrica*

Source: Biblioteca Comunale dell'Archiginnasio di Bologna

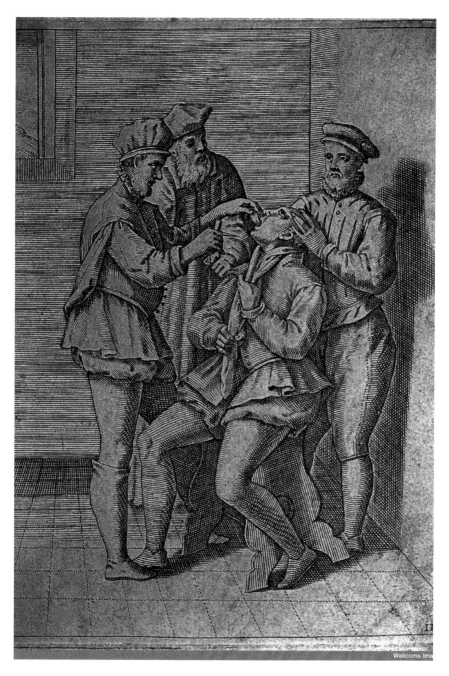

FIGURE 7.4 Pietro Paolo Magni, *Discorsi sopra il modo di sanguinare*

Source: Biblioteca Comunale dell'Archiginnasio di Bologna

Moreover, it was a symptom of the patient's weak state and inability to undergo treatment. In a few particularly serious cases, pain could even be the cause of death. As Dalla Coce wrote, summarizing surgical pain:

> When pain is powerful it attracts to the wounded part other materials and causes inflammation, and there is not a more powerful cause of the filtering of evil humors than pain; fever can cause a strong pain too, when it produces a sudden change in natural operations. . . . When pain is cruel, it weakens the vital virtue, corrupts digestion, hinders sleep, and sometimes causes death: for all these reasons it is commonly said that pain is an evil accident, and one must take care of it with great solicitude and before attending to other things.[9]

In the dominant physiological models of the sixteenth century, surgical pain weakened the patients' strength and could generate powerful responses, ranging from kicking and screaming to fainting. Typically, one or two strong male assistants were required for particularly painful procedures, and descriptions of their role abound in surgical literature. Ambroise Paré, when giving instruction on how to extract kidney stones, which was one of the most painful pre-anaesthesia surgical procedures, offered precise suggestions about how surgeons could make use of their assistants. In this case, there were four of them.

> You must place the patient on a stable table, the kidneys on a pillow, a folded cloth under the buttocks; he must be half-reclining, his tights folded, heels almost touching the buttocks: you must tie his feet at the height of his ankles with a resistant bandage three fingers wide, which must pass behind his neck two or three times; from there, his hands will be tied against his knees, as you see in this figure. Having placed and tied the patient in this way, you need four strong men, who are neither afraid nor shy: two of them have to keep the patients' arms, and the other two will block his knee and feet, so firmly that he will not be able to move his legs or his buttocks, but he will remain immobile.[10]

Though the author does not specifically mention pain in this passage, we can almost hear the patients screaming and see them writhing as they try to free themselves from the assistants' hold.

Sixteenth-century surgery books also included recipes, classifications of painkillers, and remedies to ease operatory pain, but much more often, they focus on post-operative and collateral pain. Little had changed from the times of Avicenna. The Persian physician explained that pain relief was based on the use of contraries. According to him, 'pain is relieved either by modifying complexional balance, or by eliminating the material which causes it, or by stupefying by destroying the power of sensation in the part'.[11] Some medicinal preparations had a relaxing effect, such as dill, linseed, melilot, chamomile, celery seed, bitter almond, especially when mixed with the gum of prunes, starch, lead carbonate, saffron, marsh mallow, cardamom, cabbage, turnip, and various kinds of oils. The most powerful of the stupefacients was opium, which was to be used with great caution, said Avicenna. Phlebotomy, cupping, poultices, and so on were also listed as remedies to ease pain. Avicenna additionally mentioned a series of psychological remedies: patients could be encouraged to 'walk about gently' and listen to 'pleasant songs', since, in general, being 'occupied with something that cheers you up removes the severity of pain'.[12]

Sixteenth-century health-care culture was not indifferent to pain, as surgery textbooks, remedy collections, and recipes all attest. Natural magician and experimenter Giovanni Battista Della Porta listed in the second edition of his *Magia naturalis* (1589) a series of sleep-inducing plants and recipes, explaining that such remedies 'are in high esteem among physicians, because with them they can soothe many pains'. These included mandrake, already described by the Greek botanist Dioscorides, poppy seeds, and a special essence gained by mixing together poppy, opium, mandrake, and hemlock juice into a device he described a 'little lead basket'. Once filled, it was placed under the nose of the patient or the sufferer.[13] At the beginning of the seventeenth century, surgeon Tarduccio Salvi da Macerata devoted several chapters of his vernacular surgery book to painkillers. Standard ingredients were 'seasoned olive oil, almond oil, egg yolk, milk, fatty butter, chicken fat, rabbit fat, duck fat, and similar things'.[14] Other resources were the 'stupefacient, which had a nature cold and dry in the fourth degree, and were used to induce sleep when pain became extreme'. There were strict conditions for this use: the patient had to have 'able virtue' in the entire body as well as in the affected part, he had to be purged, and the medicaments had to be of very modest quantity.[15] Standard remedies included oil of roses, egg white, several kinds of oils, lettuce, cabbage, turpentine (pine distilled raisin), and warm baths. Dalla Croce systematized the whole matter of painkillers as follows. They could be of three kinds: anodyne medicaments (the afore-mentioned oils and local agents and ointments), medicaments that acted on the cause of pain and altered the balance of humours (pharmacy and diet), and medicaments which made the painful part dull or insensitive. If the cause of pain was occult, or hidden, Dalla Croce suggested phlebotomy. Like all medieval and Renaissance surgeons, he warned that 'narcotic medicaments'—mostly compounds with opium—had to be used only in extreme cases of absolute necessity, since they could prove to be lethal.[16]

Ways of managing surgical pain

Surgical pain appeared in surgeons' books and acted as an event mediating the doctor-patient relationship in different ways, according to the different professional role of practitioners. Learned surgeons began to make an epistemic use of pain by taking note of what patients told them they were feeling, using their accounts to adjust surgical practice. This was particularly the case of areas in which there was room for innovation, such as the treatment of new types of wounds. Bartolomeo

Maggi and Ambroise Paré[17] both referred to their patients' painful sensations when they talked about new ways of managing firearm wounds. In his 1552 book on gunshot wounds, Maggi corrected the widespread view that harquebus balls were poisoned or heated, thus burning the flesh. In doing so, he advanced two claims. First, the pain felt by patients came from the bruises and lacerations caused by the bullet, not by its inherent heat. Maggi came to this conclusion by making use of his patients' accounts, gathered on the battlefield. 'I did not hear from any of the many wounded soldiers in the siege of Mirandola any complaints about suffering a burn or a feeling of heat when injured by harquebus, but rather they all said that they were feeling a sense of heaviness, like that coming from a severe bruise'.[18] Maggi then replied to an anticipated objection. It was well known that, according to Hippocrates, of two pains, only the stronger is perceived—in this case the stronger pain caused by the bruise would silence the less acute pain caused by the burning. Maggi replied that since the two pains were felt in the same place, the burning sensation should have been perceived before the second one kicked in, but this was not the case.[19] Second, Maggi combined his patients' narratives with an experiment. He explained that if you fired a bullet with a harquebus at a highly inflammable substance hanging from a tree (like straw or wool), this would not catch on fire, as one would expect from the Aristotelian theory of heat. Moreover, there were no signs of burning on the clothes and armour of the people who were shot.[20]

Pietro Paolo Magni's vernacular manual of phlebotomy (1584) provides an example of the barber-surgeons' view on pain. Magni devoted considerable attention to minimizing pain in cutting veins and to reassuring frightened patients, much more than his learned colleagues who wrote in Latin. Contrary to medieval writers on bloodletting, Magni addressed the issue of its inherent painfulness.[21] The barber-surgeon was eager to put into practice the Galenic prescription of performing painless, swift, and safe procedures. For example, when evaluating the tools of the trade—lancets—and making suggestions to the apprentice barber-surgeons, he argued that the lancets had to be 'very well sharpened, so that they do not inflict too much pain on patients.'[22]

Magni suggested that the barber-surgeon simply trick his patients whenever he realized that they were too afraid of pain and at risk of fainting. He told the story of one patient who was angry because a few barbers had tried to bleed him with no success, since he did not want them to use the lancet. Magni recounted that 'in a very friendly manner', he told the patient that he had no intention of using the lancet, but he only wanted to check his arm. In order for the patient to believe him, he gave him his case containing the lancets and said: '[Y]ou see? I don't have any intention to bleed you, and without these tools I couldn't even if I wanted to'. At this point, the patient relaxed and showed the barber-surgeon his arm, and the operator, who had a small lancet hidden in his robe, all of a sudden made the incision without the patient having the time to notice it.[23] Barber-surgeons had to become experts of the mind in order to manage fear and pain.

Finally, Leonardo Fioravanti can exemplify the empiric surgeon and the 'professor of secrets'. In general, he was highly sceptical about learned surgery, and he often exalted natural remedies learned from the wisdom of nature herself, as opposed to the complex, painful, and technologically advanced procedures of surgeons who had graduated from university. In his 1570 *Cirugia*, Fioravanti bitterly criticized the practice of perforating the skull, describing trephination as too 'artificial'. He wrote that he could not understand what reasons physicians could adduce to justify their treatment of skull fractures, which involved cutting and dilating the bones of the head. 'But I mostly marvel—he added—at how the wounded patients let themselves be tortured without any plausible reason'.[24] Patients should rebel against the pain which learned surgeons uselessly inflicted on them. Fioravanti argued for a treatment of the wounds of the skull with ointments and through application of external remedies, of his invention and sold by him. Nature was for him a process of self-healing, which the surgeon's art must second, while learned surgery inflicts unnecessary pain by focusing on solid organs.

Some surgeons addressed the question of pain as a matter of gender and ethics. This is how Gaspare Tagliacozzi commented upon the extremely painful procedure of repairing facial mutilations through skin grafting:

> We all know that extreme pain not only causes prostration, but also interrupts the normal functions of the body. I have yet to see this happen during my operation. But if by some change a patient were to faint, I would attribute it not to the violence of the procedure, but rather to the patient's abject soul. This type of effeminate and weak man (*molles, & effoeminatos*) is terrified at the prospect of suffering pain, and the only virile thing about him is the appearance. The cowardly man should not participate in this procedure.[25]

Tagliacozzi both denied that his procedure was extremely painful and argued that only morally defective men—men who were not masculine enough—were not able to endure it.

Andrew Wear has described three functions of surgical pain in early modern medicine: as a matter of negotiation between surgeons and patients, a diagnostic sign, and a practical concern to be integrated in the surgeons' operations and handy work.[26] The success rate of surgical operations in the past must be evaluated as historically and socially determined, rather than against modern standards. Sixteenth-century writers about surgery—in both Latin and vernacular, both university-trained and self-taught—had great respect for patients' pain and were deeply concerned by the inherent painfulness of surgical procedures. Some of them associated pain control with epistemic and technological innovation, others considered it a tool with which to attack competing professional categories, and still others believed that minimizing pain demonstrated a high level of professional proficiency. Being skilled in pain management was a shared value among the different kinds of experts of the human body. The empiric surgeon could accuse the learned surgeon of being cruel and inhumane, of inflicting torture-like treatment on patients for the sake of knowledge and prestige. In turn, the learned Latin-writing surgeon could accuse the empiric of treating wounds, fractures, and ulcers blindly, thus greatly damaging and hurting patients.

Pain never became the object of explicit focus, being confined to passing remarks and marginal sub-paragraphs, at best implicitly present and indirectly readable between the lines of descriptions of surgical operations. But painfulness and emotional reactions to perceived and expected pain were both to be taken into consideration and a result of weakened bodies and unbalanced temperaments. Moreover, in the Galenic tradition, pain was never a purely corporeal matter, separate from what we would call 'psychological' reactions and sensations. Besides considering pain—a phenomenon of the body and of the soul, or the imagination—elements like patients' social status, political opportunity, and the practitioner's professional reputation must be taken into account in order to paint an accurate picture of pain management in sixteenth-century surgery.

Writers on surgery in the sixteenth century presented pain as an element in a delicate balance that had death as a possible outcome or the impossibility of carrying on a normal life. A tacit moral contract between surgeons and patients implied a justification of severe pain only insofar as it was the only way to prevent death or of removing the causes that made living a normal life impossible. Paré explained very clearly the terms of this moral contract in the introduction to his complete works, published in 1575:

> To tell the truth surgical procedures cannot be performed without causing pain: indeed, how would it be possible to cut an arm, or a leg, or to make incisions on the neck of the bladder and put there several instruments without inflicting pain? . . . [There are also] other procedures that cannot be accomplished without causing great and often extreme pain. However, without the surgeon's help, people would die miserably. Is performing such operations enough to call surgeons cruel and inhuman, and to despise them?[27]

Striking a balance between bearing pain and living a relatively normal life is a more or less explicit and constant theme in the history of pre-modern surgery. Surgical patients shared with martyrs, anatomical models, and soldiers the fact that they could reveal some kind of truth by paying the price of being subject to violence; they needed to have their pain, fear, and endurance placed within meaningful contexts.[28] Pain must have a meaning in order for it to be tolerable.[29] The balance between death/impairment, on the one hand, and pain, on the other, had the function of legitimizing painful surgical procedures.

Patients, martyrs, criminals

Returning to the two images reproduced in Giovanni Andrea Dalla Croce's treatise, the representation of bodies in pain took a peculiar turn in the aftermath of the battle of Lepanto. Dalla Croce was an important surgeon and a Venetian public figure in the sixteenth century. The 1604 title page of the Venetian edition of

Vesalius's *De fabrica*, simply titled *Anatomia*, presents Dalla Croce discussing human anatomy around a dissection table with the likes of Valverde and Vesalius himself.[30] Despite not having a formal medical degree, Dalla Croce had been an important member of the College of Surgeons in Venice since the 1530s and became prior of the College between the late 1540s and the early 1550s, where he also taught human anatomy in both Latin and the vernacular. The College was a learned institution, different from the College of Physicians and also from the guild of barber-surgeons, whose members it supervised. He was fluent in Latin, and the Venetian Republic also employed him as a *condotto*.[31]

The first image shows a Christian soldier and battlefield surgeons extracting an arrow from his chest. The stoic patient sits upright, holding his chair with one hand and resting the other on his knee. An assistant holds the Christian steady with one hand on his shoulder, but there is evidently no need to forcibly restrain the figure. On the ground there are broken arrows and a *specillo*, a thin instrument used to check whether anything had been left behind in the wound. The second illustration shows a 'Turk', an Ottoman soldier, and surgeons extracting a bullet from his chest. On the ground is a *specillo* as well as a *cannulo con il terebro*, an instrument employed in extracting a bullet. The wounded soldier writhes indecorously on the ground and is clearly suffering, as seen from his open mouth and the wrinkles above his eyes. In the background the Ottomans are beginning to flee; the Christians have triumphed. In his impassive expression, the representation of the Christian closely recalls the images of martyrs being tortured, such as those in a 1591 visual catalogue of martyrdom by the Oratorian friar Antonio Gallonio.[32]

Connections between martyrs, executed criminals, and surgical patients could take many forms. For example, after the Council of Trent, medical post-mortem examinations of the bodies of prospective saints became stricter, and in several cases, the physicians and surgeons examining holy bodies found signs of impassibility and asceticism. Both Carlo Borromeo's and Ignatio de Loyola's corpses revealed, upon anatomical inspection, abnormally large kidney and bladder stones. In hagiographic terms, large stones served as proofs of the supernatural toleration of pain typical of a Counter-Reformation male saint.[33]

Religious, civic, and medical imagery shared other features. In late medieval and Renaissance Europe, handbooks containing instructions for the preparation of a good and Christian death became popular. One of the aims of this literary genre, known as *ars moriendi*, was to prepare criminals condemned to execution to confession and eventually absolution. This new concern was reflected in turn in the foundation, by the early fourteenth century, of confraternities devoted to ensuring a good death for criminals.[34] While in northern Europe these functions were administered by clerics, confraternities of laymen that gave themselves the task of assisting with religious care the condemned until the very moment they went to the scaffold began to appear in Italy in the same period. Very often, these companies of comforters also founded hospitals for the sick and the poor, who in turn became, by the sixteenth century, associated with medical instruction and began to provide bodies for public anatomical dissection.[35]

For example, in Bologna the brotherhood that was committed to this task, which was also in charge of managing the hospital of Santa Maria della Morte, was very much active and appreciated in the city. The fifteenth-century comforters' 'textbook' of Santa Maria della Morte explicitly tells the member of the confraternity to rouse the condemned to view himself and behave like a martyr. Besides singing and praying, the comforters presented those about to be executed with a tablet, a little board painted with the instruments of the Passion, that could show a depiction of the Crucifixion of Christ or of the martyrdom of a saint. One of the comforters had to keep these boards as close to the face of the condemned as possible, in order to keep his attention fixed on the image while he was on public display, focusing his mind on the virtuous and comforting examples of Christ and the martyrs just before the very act of the execution.[36]

The images and their printers

Battlefield images were not common in medicine and surgery books, while they occasionally appeared in geometry and applied mathematics books, showing tools useful for military purposes.[37] However, Dalla Croce's images of the two soldiers circulated widely across Europe and via various printers. They relate to the detailed representations of surgical instruments, specifically the different tools used for extracting arrows or bullets. According to the Venetian surgeon, there are two ways an arrow can be extracted: directly with a simple instrument, or, if the wound is more serious and the arrow more vicious, with the use of several instruments and over a longer period of time. Most probably, the image of the Christian represents the extraction of an arrow, while that of the Turk relates to the extraction of a bullet, given that the instruments seen near the latter figure recall those described in Dalla Croce's book for the treatment of firearm wounds. Moreover, in the 1573 Latin edition of Dalla Croce's book, the Christian soldier is placed before the section on the extraction of arrows and the 'Turk' before that on the treatment of harquebus wounds.

Dalla Croce's book was not the first publication to include the print of the knight heroically bearing pain on the battlefield; this had long circulated in Venice, particularly in books published by printer and publisher Vincenzo Valgrisi. For example, it appears in Giovanni Da Vigo's 1558 edition of the celebrated surgical textbook, where it served to represent the extraction of a 'balotta', a Venetian term for little ball or bullet.[38] That publication, in turn, borrowed the same image from Jean Tagault's *De chirurgica institutione*, published by Valgrisi in Venice in 1544.[39] Here, it appeared under a heading that reads 'how to extract a leaden ball' from a soldier, found in the middle of a chapter on how to extract arrows. More surprisingly still, the prototype for this Christian knight appears to be German, given that the illustration adorns Hans von Gersdorf's very famous surgery compendium of 1517;[40] it was also copied in the first Latin edition of Tagault, published in Paris in 1543. The German and French examples do not depict any battle between Christians and Ottomans, and the latter do not appear in the Venetian editions of

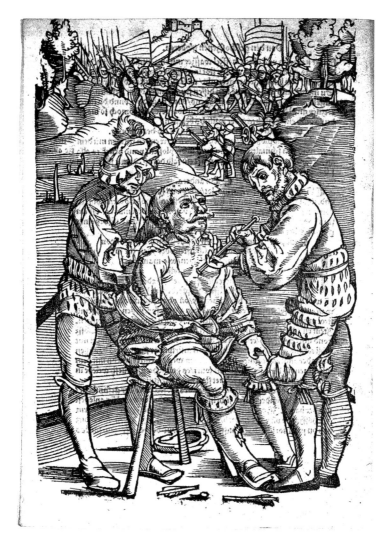

FIGURE 7.5 Hans von Gersdorf, *Feldtbuch der Wundartzney*

Source: Wellcome Collection

Da Vigo and Tagault. Only with Dalla Croce does the 'Turk' enter the picture (Figures 7.5, 7.6, and 7.7).[41]

The lives of the printers who include this image are closely intertwined. Giordano Ziletti, from Brescia, active between 1549 and 1583, the editor of both the Latin and the vernacular editions of Dalla Croce, married Vincenzo Valgrisi's daughter Diana in 1555. Valgrisi, who was French, was active in Venice, Rome, and Prague between 1539 and 1573, and he published Tagault's and Da Vigo's books, including the original

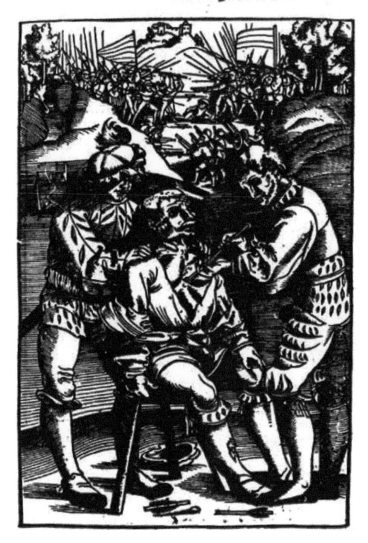

Quomodò plumbea glans, aut globus, à ferentarijs, & leuis armaturæ militibus emiſſus, extrahatur.

FIGURE 7.6 Jean Tagault, *De chirurgica institutione*

Source: British Library

image of the Christian knight. This explains how the image migrated from surgery book to surgery book, at least within the Veneto. Significantly, both the Valgrisi and the Ziletti families had problems with the Inquisition; the sons of Vincenzo Valgrisi, in particular, were suspects of sympathizing with the Protestant cause.[42]

&ʾ da tutti gli Jtromenti Jimili.

Figura oue ſi caua la ballotta.

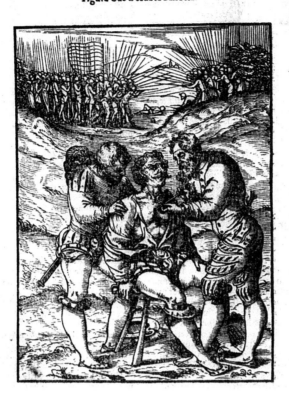

FIGURE 7.7 Giovanni Da Vigo, *Prattica utilissima*

Source: Biblioteca Comunale dell'Archiginnasio di Bologna

Venetians and Ottomans

The war of religion brings us back to the question of why one image should be associated with a Christian soldier and the other with a 'Turk', as they appeared in Dalla Croce's Latin book in 1573. Perhaps the answer lies with Valgrisi, a publisher who was suspected of heresy and of dealing in prohibited books. Moreover, the text appeared shortly after the battle of Lepanto, a time when messianic and prophetic meaning centred on the rebirth of a global Christian empire that the event carried with it.

Lepanto was a naval battle fought around the coastline of present-day Greece between the Holy League (the short-lived and litigious Catholic alliance of Venice, the Holy Roman Emperor, and the Pope) and the forces of the Ottoman Empire. The defeat inflicted on the 'infidels' was seen by many in the sixteenth century (and even today) as a sign of the imminent end of the 'Turks' and the long-standing threat they posed to the Christian lands. Indeed, Venice was taken by a certain celebratory frenzy after the battle.[43] The iconography of Lepanto is telling. Andrea Vicentino painted the battle in the Palazzo Ducale. The painting was commissioned to replace that by Tintoretto, destroyed in the fire of the building in 1577. Paolo Veronese is explicit in his depiction of the triumph of Christianity in his allegorical painting of 1573, commissioned by the Brotherhood of the Rosario for the Dominican church of Saint Peter Martyr. Here, the battle is in the background, while the scene of celestial glory includes St Peter, St Mark, St Jacob, and St Giustina.[44]

For his Venetian readers, Dalla Croce's image of the knight also recalled the extreme moral strength of the famous secular martyr Marcantonio Bragadin, captain of the Venetian army in Cyprus. His heroic deeds immediately circulated in a myriad of accounts: Bragadin was tortured and flayed alive by the Ottomans in Famagusta in the summer of 1571, and his skin was preserved as a relic in the Church of San Giovanni and Paolo in Venice (Figure 7.8).[45]

Fernand Braudel has written about a 'turcophobia' that extended to all of Western Europe and the Mediterranean by the second half of the sixteenth century.[46] Venice represented in this period the *limes* of Christianity facing the Turk. In the spring of 1573, however, the Republic of Venice signed a peace treaty with the Ottomans, seen by many contemporaries (first of all by the court of Philip II) as a capitulation to the 'Turk'. Venice chose commerce and economic vitality over the defence of Catholic identity. In this context, Dalla Croce's images appear as a deliberately propagandistic negative image of the Ottoman soldier. In reality, Christians' respect for the Turkish soldiers was widespread throughout the sixteenth century. The Janissaries, in particular, were considered examples of austerity, discipline, and self-restraint by Venetian diplomats and politicians. Moreover, the Western humanist tradition underlined their barbarism and savagery. Marino Cavalli, the Venetian ambassador in Constantinople, wrote in 1560 that 'the Turks are, in my judgment, the greatest fighters you can find in the world; if they had as much skillfulness as strength, it would be completely impossible to resist them'.[47] Ottoman Turks appeared more and more often in costume books by the second half of the sixteenth century, typically characterized by big turbans, also shown in Dalla Croce's illustrations. And in general, written and visual histories of the Turks and their way of life multiplied in the Venetian print market by this time.[48] It thus seems that Dalla Croce's volume aimed to emphasize the contrast between Christians and infidels by way of underlining the visual analogy between the Christian patient and the martyr, on the one hand, and, on the other hand, by exaggerating the unmanly behavior of the 'Turk'. In this way, the double image plays with a rhetoric that viewed the Turks as barbarians and half-savage beings, but they also exhibit a reactivation of ancient Greek and Roman descriptions of the Easterners as 'soft and effeminate'.[49] Bodies in surgery become political bodies through specific perceptions of how one should bear pain appropriately.

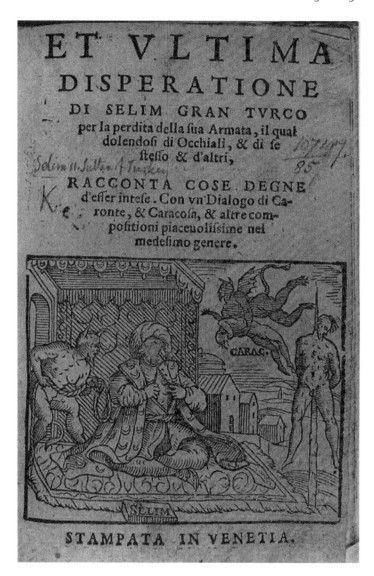

ET VLTIMA
DISPERATIONE
DI SELIM GRAN TVRCO
per la perdita della fua Armata, il qual
dolendofi di Occhiali, & di fe
ftefso & d'altri,

RACCONTA COSE DEGNE
d'efser intefe. Con vn Dialogo di Ca-
ronte, & Caracofa, & altre com-
pofitioni piaceuolifsime nel
medefimo genere.

STAMPATA IN VENETIA.

FIGURE 7.8 Anonymous, *Selim*

Source: British Library

Conclusion

Paintings shown to the condemned as they mounted a scaffold had a twofold purpose. One was to provide a model to emulate. The other was to have a sinner see
an exemplum of piety or Christ on the Cross just before he died, as a way of lessen-
ing to some degree the torture of eternal damnation. Perhaps surgical prints were

even shown to patients in surgery and retained at least the first function of religious images. Surgeons had to divert the minds of their patients from sad thoughts and images. Therefore, stimulating parallels with martyrs and knights would have been an uplifting strategy, just like the comforters showed pictures of martyrdom to those walking to the scaffold to be executed.

By looking at representations of bodies in surgery, this chapter argued that surgery was part of a wider culture of moralizing and gendering ways of bearing pain, which counted as exemplary models for surgical patients, martyrs, and knights. This is also significant because one of the techniques recommended by surgeons to ease surgical pain was to work on the patient's imagination. The epistemic function of these scientific images is inextricably intertwined with their political, religious, and therapeutic functions.

APPENDIX

The two images in the editions of Dalla Croce

0   1573, first Latin edition, published by Giordano Ziletti. The pictures of the Christian and the Turk are on p. 125 and p. 131, respectively. The Christian is placed immediately before the section devoted to the extracting of an arrow, the Turk before the text about 'gunshot wounds'.

1   1574, first vernacular edition, published by Giordano Ziletti. The image of the Turk is on p. 272, right before the section on gunshot wounds. The image of the Christian knight is on p. 260, right before the section on the extraction of 'weapons from the chest' in general. The image of the Turk contains a representation of a few instruments: a *specillo* (a thin instrument to check whether there are remnants in the wound) and a *cannulo con il terebro* (an instrument to pull the bullet off). The image of the Christian has broken arrows and only a *specillo*. The knight is kept still by the assistant, one hand holding the chair and the other his arm; the expression is almost impassible.

2   1583, second vernacular edition, published by Francesco Ziletti. The two images are the same, but this time they are placed at the very end of the book (and at the end of the *officina* section), one after another. This time the image of the Christian is accompanied by the title 'Forma dell'estrattion delle saette'. The transition from bullets to arrows is now complete, and the image now represents something different from its German and French progenitors. Also note that in the image of the Turk, the battle in the background has taken a clear pro-Christian turn: the Ottomans are beginning to flee. Also note that in the first of the three collective scene images, the patient is clearly suffering: open mouth, wrinkles above his eyes, and so on.

3   1596, second Latin edition, published by Roberto Meietti in Venice. The two images are placed one after the other at p. 54 and p. 55 of the *officina* book (the book illustrating the surgical tools). The Christian image is accompanied by the 'extraction of an arrow' heading, but now they both are placed at the beginning of the section on cauterization.

4   1661, third vernacular edition of the book, published by Niccolò Pezzana in Venice, has all the images of the tools and additionally an *antidotarium* by Jacopo Dondi, but the Christian/Turk scene has disappeared, as its cultural import waned.

Notes

1   Montaigne, *The Complete Essays*, 381.
2   Sansovino, *Informatione a Soldati Christiani*, A10. All translations in the chapter are my own, unless otherwise stated.
3   Johnson and Molineaux, 'Putting Europe in its place', 63.
4   This was not the case in most countries of northern Europe, where surgery was mostly an 'empiric' enterprise, practised by people who did not have academic training. On the early institutional and academic teaching of surgery in medieval Italian universities, see Siraisi, *Medieval and Early Renaissance Medicine*, 153–86; Pesenti, 'Professores chirurgie', 1–38; McVaugh, *The Rational Surgery of the Middle*. On early modern surgery, see Palmer, 'Physicians and surgeons', 451–60; Gentilcore, *Medical Charlatanism*, 182–87; Conforti, 'Chirurghi, mammane, ciarlatani', 323–40.
5   Harcourt, 'Andreas Vesalius and the anatomy of antique sculpture', 28–61; Carlino, *Books of the Body*; Park, *Secrets of Women*; Lincoln, 'Curating the Renaissance body', 42–61.
6   'I remember often saying that the two types of pain are the sudden change of temperament and the rupture of continuity': Galen, *Of the Affected Parts*, quoted by Cohen, *The Modulated Scream*, 88.
7   Porzio, *De dolore*, 7.
8   McVaugh, *The Rational Surgery*, 106–10.
9   Dalla Croce, *Cirugia universale*, 27r.
10 Paré, *Oeuvres completes*, 2, 478–79. On the history of lithotomy, see Wangensteen, Wangensteen, and Wiita, 'Lithotomy and lithotomists', 929–52.
11 Avicenna, *Canon*, 233 (1. 4. 5. 30); also see Aziz, Nathan, and McKeever, 'Anesthetic and analgesic practices', 147–51.
12 Avicenna, *Canon*, 234 (1. 4. 5. 30).
13 Della Porta, *Magia naturalis*, 150–51.
14 Salvi da Macerata, *Il chirurgo*, 155.
15 Salvi da Macerata, *Il chirurgo*, 155–56.
16 Dalla Croce, *Cirugia universale*, 89v–90r. Medieval and Renaissance surgeons were highly sceptical of opium-based narcotics, including the almost mythical *spongia soporifera*, since they believed them to be too dangerous and difficult to dose; see McVaugh, *The Rational Surgery*, 106–10; Cohen, *The Modulated Scream*, 108–10; De Moulin, 'A historical-phenomenological study', 559; Schalick III, 'To market, to market', 5–20.
17 Maggi, *De vulnerum*; Paré, *Oeuvres*, 2, 126–27.
18 Maggi, *De vulnerum*, 2v. On Maggi's life and work, see Gentili, *La vita e l'opera*.
19 Maggi, *De vulnerum*, 2v–3r. On the lack of incorporation of patients' pain narratives in scholastic medicine, see Salmon, 'From patient to text?', 373–95.
20 Maggi, *De vulnerum*, 3v–5r.
21 Gil-Sotres, 'Derivation and revulsion', 110–55.
22 Magni, *Discorsi*, 8.
23 Magni, *Discorsi*, 13.
24 Fioravanti, *La Cirugia*, 12r–v.
25 Tagliacozzi, *De curtorum*, 1, 83–84.
26 Wear, *Knowledge and*, 241–48.
27 Paré, *Oeuvres*, 1, 30–31.
28 The connection of pain representations with martyrs, anatomical models, and soldiers in the sixteenth century has been noted by Moscoso, *Pain*, 18–20; Cohen, *The Modulated Scream*; Park, 'The life of the corpse', 111–32.

29 Morris, *The Culture of Pain*, 36–37.
30 Giordano, 'Iconografia anatomica e cruciana', 164–65.
31 *Condotto* was a physician paid by towns and cities to treat the people for free. Giordano, 'Intorno a un chirurgo del '500', 156–63; Di Matteo and others, 'The Renaissance and the universal surgeon', 2523–528; Bamji, 'Medical care in early modern Venice', 483–509.
32 Touber, 'Articulating pain', 59–89.
33 Bouley, *Pious Postmortems*, 102–07.
34 Park, 'Birth and death', 33–34.
35 Edgerton Jr, *Pictures and Punishment*; Posperi, *Delitto e perdono*, 212–62 and 326–35.
36 Fanti, *Confraternite e città*, 171–73; Falvey, 'Scaffold and stage', 16–17.
37 Bennett, 'Geometry in context', 223–24. On battlefield representations in sixteenth century Italian art see Borgo, *Battle and Representation*.
38 Da Vigo, *Prattica utilissima*.
39 Tagault, *De chirurgica institutione*, 228.
40 Von Gersdorf, *Feldtbuch der Wundartzney*.
41 Andreoli, *Ex officina erasmiana: Vincenzo Valgrisi*, 209–15.
42 Borraccini and others, *Dizionario degli editori*, 1094–96 and 1037.
43 Gombrich, 'Celebrations in Venice', 62–68; Mammana, *Lepanto*.
44 Sindging-Larsen, 'The changes in the iconography', 298–302; Mìnguez, 'Iconografia de Lepanto', 255–84.
45 DeVries, 'A tale of venetian skin', 51–70. Around 170 poems were published in Venice in the sixteenth century to celebrate the martyrdom of Bragadin; see Gibellini, *L'immagine di Lepanto*, 35–40.
46 Braudel, *The Mediterranean*, 2, 844.
47 Alberi, *Relazioni degli ambasciatori veneti*, 270. See also Bardacci, 'Dopo Lepanto', 19–43. On the representations of the Ottoman Turks by the elite of Western scholars during the Renaissance, see Bisaha, *Creating East and West*; Zoli, 'L'immagine dell'Oriente', 70–82. On medical anti-Arabism, which left no trace in Dalla Croce, see Pormann, 'The dispute.'
48 Wilson, 'Reflecting on the Turk', 38–58.
49 Bisaha, *Creating East and West*, 48; Bettella, 'The marked body', 175. After Lepanto, Venetian ambassadors insisted more and more on the Ottomans' effeminacy: see Preto, *Venezia e i Turchi*, 63.

Bibliography

Primary sources

Avicenna, *Canon medicinae* (Venice: Juntarum, 1608).
Dalla Croce, Giovanni Andrea, *Cirugia universale* (Venice: Giordano Ziletti, 1583).
Da Vigo, Giovanni, *Prattica utilissima e necessaria di cirugia* (Venice: Valgrisi, 1558).
Della Porta, Giovanni Battista, *Magia naturalis libri XX* (Naples: Horatium Salvianum, 1589).
Fioravanti, Leonardo, *La Cirugia* (Venice: heredi di Melchior Sessa, 1570).
Maggi, Bartolomeo, *De vulnerum, a bombardarum, & sclopetorum globulis illatorum, & de eorum symptomatum curatione, & medicamenta ipsis ulceribus curandis idonea, in De sclopettorum et tormentariorum vulnerum natura, et curatione, libri IIII* (Venice: Guglielmum Valgrisium, 1566).
Magni, Pietro Paolo, *Discorsi intorno al sanguinar i corpi humani* (Rome: Bartolomeo Bonfadino & Tito Diani, 1583).
Montaigne, Michel de, *The Complete Essays*, trans., A. M. Screech (New York: Penguin Books, 2003).
Paré, Ambroise, *Oeuvres completes*, ed., Jean-François Malgaigne (Paris: Baillière, 1840).
Porzio, Simone, *De dolore* (Florence: Laurentium Torrentinum, 1551).

Relazione dall'Impero Ottomano di Marino Cavalli bailo a Costantinopoli nel 1560. In Relazioni degli ambasciatori veneti, serie III, *vol.* I, ed., Enrico Alberi (Florence: Tipografia all'insegna di Clio, 1840).

Salvi da Macerata, Tarduccio, *Il chirurgo* (Rome: Gio. Battista Robletti, 1643).

Sansovino, Francesco, *Informatione a Soldati Christiani* (Venice, 1570).

Tagault, Jacques, *De chirurgica institutione* (Paris: Wechel, 1543).

Tagault, Jacques, *De chirurgica institutione* (Venice: Valgrisi, 1544).

Tagliacozzi, Gaspare, *De curtorum chirurgia per insitionem* (Venice: Gasparem Bindonum, 1597).

Von Gersdorf, Hans, *Feldtbuch der Wundartzney* (Strasbourg: Schott, 1517).

Secondary sources

Andreoli, Ilaria, *Ex officina erasmiana. Vincenzo Valgrisi e l'illustrazione del libro a Venezia e Lione alla metà del '500* (unpublished PhD dissertation, University of Lyon and University of Venice, 2006).

Aziz, E., B. Nathan, and J. McKeever, 'Anesthetic and analgesic practices in Avicenna's Canon of Medicine', *The American Journal of Chinese Medicine*, 28, 1 (2000), 147–51.

Bamji, Alexandra, 'Medical care in early modern Venice', *Journal of Social History*, 49, 3 (2016), 483–509.

Bardacci, Marco, 'Dopo Lepanto. Il turco negli scritti politici italiani di fine Cinquecento, 1571–1607', *Il pensiero politico*, 41 (2008), 19–43.

Bennett, Jim, 'Geometry in context in the sixteenth century: the view from the museum', *Early Science and Medicine*, 7, 3 (2002), 214–30.

Bettella, Patrizia, 'The marked body as otherness in Renaissance Italian culture', in Linda Kalof and William Bynum (eds), *A Cultural History of the Human Body in the Renaissance* (Oxford and New York: Berg, 2010), 149–82.

Bisaha, Nancy, *Creating East and West: Renaissance Humanists and the Ottoman Turks* (Philadelphia: University of Pennsylvania Press, 2004).

Borgo, Francesca, *Battle and Representation in Cinquecento Art and Theory* (unpublished PhD dissertation, Harvard University, 2017).

Borraccini, Rosa Maria and others, eds, *Dizionario degli editori, tipografi, librai itineranti in Italia tra Quattrocento e Seicento* (Pisa and Rome: Serra, 2013).

Bouley, Bradford, *Pious Postmortems: Anatomy, Sanctity, and the Catholic Church in Early Modern Europe* (Philadelphia: University of Pennsylvania Press, 2017).

Braudel, Fernand, *The Mediterranean and the Mediterranean World in the Age of Philip II*, trans., Sian Reynolds (Berkeley: University of California Press, 1995).

Carlino, Andrea, *Books of the Body: Anatomical Ritual and Renaissance Learning*, trans., Anne C. Tedeschi and John Tedeschi (Chicago: The University of Chicago Press, 1999).

Cohen, Esther, *The Modulated Scream: Pain in Late Medieval Culture* (Chicago: The University of Chicago Press, 2009).

Conforti, Maria, 'Chirurghi, mammane, ciarlatani. Pratica medica e controllo delle professioni', in Antonio Clericuzio and Germana Ernst (eds), *Il Rinascimento italiano e l'Europa. Volume 5: Le scienze* (Treviso: Angelo Colla Editore, 2008), 323–40.

De Moulin, Daniel, 'A historical-phenomenological study of bodily pain in Western man', *Bulletin of the History of Medicine*, 48, 4 (1974), 540–70.

DeVries, Kelly, 'A tale of venetian skin. The flaying of Marcantonio Bragadin', in Larissa Tracy (ed), *Flaying in the Pre-Modern World* (Cambridge: D.S. Brewer, 2017), 51–70.

Di Matteo, Berardo and others, 'The Renaissance and the universal surgeon: Giovanni Andrea Della Croce, a master of traumatology', *International Orthopaedics*, 37, 12 (2013), 2523–528.

Edgerton Jr, Samuel Y., *Pictures and Punishment: Art and Criminal Prosecution during the Florentine Renaissance* (Ithaca: Cornell University Press, 1985).

Falvey, Kathleen, 'Scaffold and stage: Comforting rituals and dramatic traditions in Late Medieval and Renaissance Italy', in Nicholas Terpstra (ed.), *The Art of Executing Well: Rituals of Execution in Renaissance Italy* (Kirksville: Truman State University Press, 2008), 13–30.

Fanti, Mario, *Confraternite e città a Bologna nel medioevo e in età moderna* (Rome: Herder, 2001).

Gentilcore, David, *Medical Charlatanism in Early Modern Italy* (Oxford: Oxford University Press, 2006).

Gentili, Giulio, *La vita e l'opera di Bartolomeo Maggi (1516–1552)* (Bologna: Università di Bologna, 1967).

Gibellini, Cecilia, *L'immagine di Lepanto. La celebrazione della vittoria nella letteratura e nell'arte veneziana* (Venice: Marsilio, 2008).

Gil-Sotres, Pedro, 'Derivation and revulsion: the theory and practice of medieval phlebotomy', in Luis García Ballester (ed), *Practical Medicine from Salerno to the Black Death* (Cambridge: Cambridge University Press, 1994), 110–55.

Giordano, Davide, *Scritti e dsicorsi pertinenti alla storia della medicina* (Milano: Hoepli, 1932).

Gombrich, Ernst, *Studies in Renaissance and Baroque Art* (New York: Phaidon, 1967).

Harcourt, Glenn, 'Andreas Vesalius and the anatomy of antique sculpture', *Representations*, 17 (1987), 28–61.

Johnson, Carina L. and Catherine Molineaux, 'Putting Europe in its place: material traces, interdisciplinarity, and the recuperation of the early-modern extra-European subject', *Radical History Review*, 30 (January 2018), 62–99.

Lincoln, Elizabeth, 'Curating the Renaissance body (Pietro Paolo Magni's Illustrated Treatise "Discorsi Sopra Il Modo Di Sanguinare, Attaccar Le Sanguisughe, & Le Ventose, Far Le Fregagioni Vessicatorij a Corpi Humani")', *Word & Image*, 17, 1–2 (2001), 42–61.

Mammana, Simona, *Lepanto: rime per la vittoria sul Turco. Regesto (1571–1573) e studio critico* (Rome: Bulzoni, 2007).

McVaugh, Michael, *The Rational Surgery of the Middle Ages* (Florence: SISMEL/Edizioni del Galluzzo, 2006).

Mìnguez, Victor, 'Iconografia de Lepanto. Arte, propaganda, y representaciòn simbòlica de una monarquia universal y catolica', *Obradoiro de Historia Moderna*, 20 (2011), 255–84.

Morris, David B., *The Culture of Pain* (Berkeley: The University of California Press, 1991).

Moscoso, Javier, *Pain a Cultural History*, trans., Sarah Thomas and Pau House (New York: Palgrave Macmillan, 2012).

Palmer, Richard, 'Physicians and surgeons in sixteenth-century Venice', *Medical History*, 23, 4 (1979), 451–60.

Park, Katharine, 'Birth and death', in Linda Kalof (ed.), *A Cultural History of the Human Body in the Middle Ages* (Oxford: Berg, 2010), 19–37.

Park, Katharine, 'The life of the corpse: division and dissection in Late Medieval Europe', *Journal of the History of Medicine and Allied Sciences*, 50 (1995), 111–32.

Park, Katharine, *Secrets of Women: Gender, Generation, and the Origins of Human Dissection* (New York: Zone Books, 2007).

Pesenti, Tiziana, 'Professores chirurgie, medici ciroici e barbitonsores a Padova nell'età di Leonardo Buffi da Bertapaglia († dopo il 1448)', *Quaderni per la Storia dell'Università di Padova*, 11 (1978), 1–38.

Pormann, Peter E., *Islamic Medical and Scientific Tradition* (London and New York: Routledge, 2010).

Posperi, Adriano, *Delitto e perdono: la pena di morte nell'orizzonte mentale dell'Europa cristiana, XIV-XVIII secolo* (Turin: Einaudi, 2013).

Preto, Paolo, *Venezia e i Turchi* (Florence: Sansoni, 1975).

Salmon, Fernando, 'From patient to text? Narratives of pain and madness in medical scholasticism', in Brian Nance and Florence Eliza Glaze (eds), *Between Text and Patient: The Medical Enterprise in Medieval & Early Modern Europe* (Florence: SISMEL/Edizioni del Galluzzo, 2011), 373–95.

Schalick III, Walton O., 'To market, to market: The theory and practice of opiates in the middle ages', in Marcia Meldrum (ed.), *Opioids and Pain Relief: A Historical Perspective* (Seattle: IASP Press, 2003), 5–20.

Sindging-Larsen, Staale, 'The changes in the iconography and composition of Veronese's Allegory of the Battle of Lepanto in the Doge's Palace', *Journal of the Warburg and Courtauld Institute*, 19 (1956), 298–302.

Siraisi, Nancy, *Medieval and Early Renaissance Medicine* (Chicago: The University of Chicago Press, 1990).

Touber, Jetze, 'Articulating pain martyrology, torture, and execution in the works of Antonio Gallonio (1556–1605)', in Jan FransVan Dijkhuizen and Karl A. E. Enenkel (eds), *The Sense of Suffering: Constructions of Physical Pain in Early Modern Culture* (Leiden: Brill, 2009), 59–89.

Wangensteen, Owen H., Sarah D. Wangensteen, and John Wiita, 'Lithotomy and lithotomists: progress in wound management from Franco to Lister', *Surgery*, 66, 5 (1969), 929–52.

Wear, Andrew, *Knowledge and Practice in English Medicine, 1550–1680* (Cambridge: Cambridge University Press, 2000).

Wilson, Bronwen, 'Reflecting on the Turk in late sixteenth century Venetian portrait books', *Word & Image*, 19, 1–2 (2003), 38–58.

Zoli, Sergio, 'L'immagine dell'Oriente nella cultura italiana da Marco Polo al Settecento', in Cesare De Seta (ed), *Storia d'Italia. Annali, vol. 5: Il paesaggio* (Turin: Einaudi, 1982), 45–123.

8

ARTISTIC REPRESENTATIONS OF GOITRE IN EARLY MODERN ART IN ITALY

Danielle Carrabino

Introduction

An Italian proverb states that 'he who is born with a weak intellect and a goitre can never be cured'.[1] This statement offers a window into common perceptions about goitre and its association with low intelligence at a time when its cause and cure were unknown. According to the ancient humoral theory of medicine, goitre was defined as a cold abscess (*apostema frigidum*) in the neck caused by an accumulation of phlegm, for which there were several remedies but no definitive cure.[2] Sometimes accompanied by cretinism, which stunts physical and cognitive development, goitre was described in ancient and early modern texts alike as especially prominent, or 'endemic', among the low, labouring class living in the mountainous regions of Italy. Figures with goitre also appear frequently in art from the fifteenth to eighteenth centuries and have sparked great interest among endocrinologists, historians of science, medical professionals, and, in a few instances, historians of art. Long before its causes were known, goitre may have carried culturally coded meanings that would have been understood by contemporary viewers but have been lost to most modern viewers. It is for this reason that my main focus is on early modern perceptions of goitre, without making the assumption that the condition was understood then in the same way as it is now.

Today, we know that goitre is a pathology of the thyroid gland that causes swelling in the neck due to the lack of iodine, especially in older women. When iodine is present, the thyroid secretes hormones that regulate growth, heart rate, blood pressure, body temperature, and metabolism. In areas with little iodine, such as mountainous regions, residents are particularly prone to goitre. The thyroid gland, its functions, and its pathologies were not entirely understood until the nineteenth and twentieth centuries, when iodine was discovered. The artistic representation of an infirmity informs us about how it was perceived before its cause was known.

Modern scientific publications on the representation of goitre in art have contributed significantly to the literature on this subject by compiling a growing list of the occurrences of goitre observed in art, perceived or actual. Beginning with *The History and Iconography of Endemic Goitre and Cretinism* (1971) by Swiss surgeon Franz Merke, medical professionals became interested in tracing goitre in works of art.[3] In this comprehensive study, Merke argued that goitre appeared in art due to five 'artistic intentions': to create revulsion, mock, commiserate, document endemic regions, or 'give anecdotal verisimilitude to genre scenes'.[4] In 2011, Carol Z. Clark and physician Orlo H. Clark provided an updated version of Merke's study. Containing over 200 paintings, their book *The Remarkables: Endocrine Abnormalities in Art* (2011) differentiates between 'the goitre beautiful' and 'the goitre grotesque'.[5] Articles published in medical journals have also identified numerous works of art in which figures with goitre are purportedly present. Unfortunately, their diagnoses disregard the historical contexts in which images were created, leaving the reader wondering why such figures were depicted.

The present study examines early modern texts alongside a selected group of works of art containing figures with goitre within the contexts of humoral definitions of goitre as well as other cultural and historic contexts in which they were created. Rather than attempting the impossible and subjective task of accounting for reputed instances of goitre in art, as in previous studies, I will focus on works created in areas of Italy in which contemporaries recorded that goitre was endemic. Texts by artists such as Michelangelo and Leonardo da Vinci will be considered alongside other written sources, including theoretical writings on beauty. Close analysis of the sculptures at the Sacro Monte of Varallo, Caravaggio's *Crucifixion of Saint Andrew*, Neapolitan *presepi*, and Ribera's prints will expand on Merke's categories to demonstrate that the representation of goitre in this period was varied and complex. In some cases, as seen in the examples from the Alpine area of Varallo, goitre signalled low intelligence, animal-like nature, moral corruption, and poverty associated at the time with mountain-dwellers, eliciting repulsion and mockery. However, these same figures were also viewed with empathy and performed moralizing roles in the scenes represented. In other examples, such as in Caravaggio's painting and *presepi* created near the mountainous areas around Naples, figures with goitre carried more positive associations, such as humility and piety, evoking responses of empathy and wonder in the viewer. These individual examples illustrate how goitre carried different meanings in accordance with the function of the work. These figures share a common role of adding to the sentiment and significance of the works of art in which they appear.

Ancient and early modern texts

Before turning to specific examples of representations of goitre, it is useful to note how this condition was described in early modern medical literature, and in the ancient texts on which they relied. Hippocrates's *Epidemics* (400 BCE) provides one of the earliest textual descriptions of swelling of the neck.[6] According to this and later texts, goitre was thought to be caused by drinking snow water in mountainous areas. In his treatise, *Airs, Waters, Places*, Hippocrates defined endemic disease as particular to a certain place, whereas epidemic diseases did not have locally specific causes. Hippocrates also claimed that endemic diseases were due to both the drinking of local water and a locale's orientation to the winds and the sun.[7] By the sixteenth century, this notion was widely accepted.[8]

Goitre is endemic to mountainous areas, including the Alpine region, as was mentioned repeatedly in ancient and early modern texts. Pliny the Elder explicitly referred to the harmful waters of the Alps twice in his *Natural History* (*c.* 77 CE). In the first instance, he wrote, 'Only men and swine are subject to swellings in the throat, which are mostly caused by the noxious quality of the water they drink' (Book XI, 68).[9] He also described the amber necklaces worn in that area by women peasants, both as jewellery and as a remedy for tonsillitis and 'other affections of the pharynx', likely implying goitre (Book XXXVII, 11). In *On Architecture* (Book VIII, 169), Vitruvius, in the first century BCE, warned against construction in the Alps due to the local waters, which cause goitre. That goitre was caused by drinking snow water was a commonly held belief, prompting Juvenal, in *Satires* (XIII, 136), written in 127 CE, to quip, 'Who wonders at a swollen throat in the Alps?'

Ancient writings continued to be revived and elaborated throughout the Renaissance, often repeating and reinforcing certain beliefs concerning goitre. Swiss physician Paracelsus wrote that 'all goitrous persons are more disposed to foolishness than to cleverness'.[10] In his revival of the Vitruvian concept of building on sites that would foster good health, Renaissance humanist Leon Battista Alberti assumed the reader's familiarity with goitre when he stated, 'I shall not dwell here on the goitres and stones for which water may be responsible'.[11] The perception that people afflicted with goitre belonged to the lower classes and lacked intelligence is instead gleaned from *Book of the Courtier* written by Baldassare Castiglione, who mentions 'anyone gazing too intently with dull eyes after the manner of an idiot, or laughing as stupidly as those goitrous mutes in the mountains of Bergamo'.[12] In fact, the Bergamasque *Commedia dell'arte* character Zanni, who is comic and foolish, sometimes wore a mask fitted with a false goitre.[13] In seventeenth-century England, Shakespeare in *The Tempest* (Act III, Scene 3) referred disparagingly to 'mountaineers/Dew-lapp'd like bulls, whose throats had hanging at 'em/Wallets of flesh', while John Evelyn took note of people with 'monstrous gulets, or wens of flesh, growing on their throat' when he travelled through the Alpine Simplon Pass in 1646.[14] These references to goitre, whether fictional or factual, attest to the belief that people with goitre were considered beast-like, monstrous, and lacking intelligence.

While medical writings from the Renaissance did little to expand upon the ancient understanding of goitre, it was during this period that dissections led to a better understanding of the anatomy of the neck. Leonardo da Vinci produced the first accurate drawing of the human thyroid gland around 1500 for his treatise on anatomy (Fol. 3r, MS A), graphically indicating the correct position of the thyroid as well as its shape—two rounded half-moon lobes rather than the shield-like form Galen had proposed.[15] The thyroid gland is one of many parts of the body, both human and animal, included on the page along with the larynx, tongue, and pharynx, which Leonardo believed were all involved in the production of voice. Next to these anatomical drawings, Leonardo penned a few lines of explanation: 'These glands are made to fill up the space where the muscles are missing and to keep the trachea away from the clavicle'.[16] Present-day physicians, such as Fernando Vescia and Luigi Basso, have identified Leonardo's caricatures known as the 'grotesque heads' as 'real goitres'.[17] While it is tempting to relate Leonardo's anatomical studies to his fanciful drawings, we have no evidence that he recognized any correlation between the thyroid and his caricatures of figures with swollen necks.[18]

Caricature is the vehicle for another source of the definition of goitre in early modern Italy. In a celebrated letter penned by Michelangelo Buonarroti in 1509, the artist writes about the physical labour involved in painting the Sistine Chapel ceiling (Figure 8.1). In words and a quick sketch, he created a vivid image of himself straining to such an extreme extent that he claimed to have developed 'goitre'

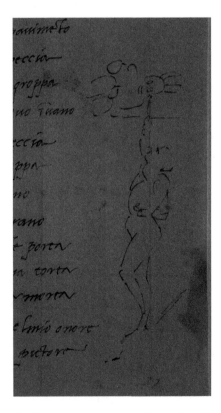

FIGURE 8.1 Michelangelo Buonarroti, *Sonnet to Giovanni da Pistoia and Self-Portrait of the Artist Painting*

Source: Casa Buonarroti, Florence; © Associazione Metamorfosi, Rome

(*gozzo*), 'such as water gives the cats in Lombardy'.[19] The artist thus draws on the popular beliefs that goitre was widespread in the sub-Alpine area of Lombardy and was contracted by drinking the water. Most probably, 'cats' here refers to a common nickname for peasants.[20] This poetic use of goitre is intended to demonstrate the artist's physical deformations, reducing the artist to a lowly, manual labourer.[21] To give visual form to his text, and to ensure great dramatic effect, Michelangelo sketched a caricature of himself to the right of his poem. This drawing contains an unmistakable protrusion in the neck. This is an example of what several modern scientific publications have identified as 'pseudogoitre',[22] which also includes thick necks and prominent Adam's apples.

This caricature and its accompanying poem of similes have erroneously led two physicians to take Michelangelo's self-description too literally, arguing that the artist actually suffered from goitre,[23] although there is no firm evidence that he suffered from this condition.[24] Some authors have even detected goitre in the Sistine fresco of *God Separating Darkness from Light*.[25] Nevertheless, Michelangelo's sonnet and sketch provide a secure example of an early modern artist intentionally and unmistakably representing goitre. Moreover, the sheet provides evidence for the popular conceptions of goitre in early modern Italy as an infirmity that was socially coded and associated with the labouring classes. Finally, it allows us to distinguish between the undeniable representation of goitre in the caricature with a swollen neck (or 'pseudogoitre') in the Sistine Chapel fresco.

Figures with goitre in the Sacro Monte of Varallo

Early modern visual evidence of goitre and its association with the labouring class appear in the art at the Sacro Monte of Varallo ('sacred mountain') in the Alpine region of Lombardy. Established in the last decades of the fifteenth century by Franciscan Observant friar Benedetto Caimi as a 'new Jerusalem', this mountainous site was intended to simulate the experience of pilgrimage to the Holy Land.[26] Visitors to this devotional site would be moved to 'imagination, emotional participation and identification'.[27] By the early seventeenth century, pilgrims were able to visit a series of forty-three chapels, each dedicated to individual scenes from the life of Christ, where they were inspired to meditate and pray. Formerly assumed to appeal only to the lower classes, these scenes were intended for audiences of all levels of society, local or otherwise.[28] The Alps stood in for the hilly topography of the original sites just as each chapel was richly decorated and the figures were painted and sculpted with a high degree of naturalism, so that the visitors could imagine themselves witnessing first-hand these historic events.[29] Figures with goitre appear at least twice in the Sacro Monte of Varallo, namely in the chapels dedicated to Christ on the Road to Calvary and the Calvary.[30]

The Sacro Monte chapels were decorated in various campaigns over more than a century. Architects, sculptors, and painters collaborated to re-create each scene in hyper-realistic fashion and on a life-sized scale. Among these artists was Lombard painter and sculptor Gaudenzio Ferrari, who is credited with the overall design of the Road to Calvary and Calvary scenes.[31] In the frescoed backgrounds and sculpted figures in these two chapels, Ferrari was influenced by Leonardo's 'grotesque' caricatures.[32] In total, more than ninety polychrome terracotta sculptures were adorned with clothing, real hair, and other accessories to make them appear life-like.[33] Often described as *tableaux vivants*, these scenes were not so much frozen as they were activated by visitors. With Franciscan guides to help chart their paths, pilgrims were allowed to wander through the spaces, fully immersing themselves in the scenes.[34] To add to the illusion that this scene is taking place in the viewer's own time and space, the figures with goitre, known to be mountain-dwellers, further stress the immediacy of the experience at Varallo.

Chapel XXXVI depicts Christ on the Road to Calvary with about forty painted terracotta figures (Figure 8.2). Standing to the left of the fallen Christ figure, an executioner with a large goitre tugs at a rope that is attached to a chain around Christ's neck. Kneeling between this figure and Christ is Veronica, with her veil on which Christ's face has just been imprinted. The juxtaposition of these two holy figures and the executioner with goitre is stark. The idealized faces of Christ and Veronica and their rich, detailed drapery are skilfully modelled. They

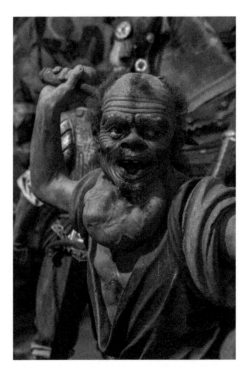

FIGURE 8.2 Giovanni Tabacchetti and Giovanni d'Enrico, *Christ on the Road to Calvary*, detail

Source: Santuario del Sacro Monte, Varallo

both appear stoic and inward-looking, in spite of their suffering. By contrast, the executioner is much more crudely sculpted, perhaps even indicating a different hand. His splayed stance with feet akimbo, arms flung open, and mouth agape to reveal a few missing teeth present an outwardly expressive figure that elicits a response of repulsion and fear in the viewer. Moreover, the executioner bares more skin than others in the scene, exposing his arms, legs, and chest. The viewer cannot miss his enormous goitre, which has been carved and painted with a great degree of naturalism, including veins and numerous nodes. His face is tracked by wrinkles and marred by moles and patchy hair. His eyes are wild and may indicate mental deficiency.

Similarly, in Chapel XXXVIII, a figure with goitre participates in the scene of the Crucifixion at Calvary (Figure 8.3). This figure, which has been compared to Leonardo's grotesques, holds the sponge, one of the instruments of the Passion of Christ.[35] This 'sponge-bearer' is positioned at the foot of the cross, holding up to Christ a long rod to which is attached a sponge soaked in vinegar, according to the Gospels of John and Matthew.[36] Similar to the figure in the Road to Calvary scene, the goitre is oversized and impossible to miss. He also shares with the figure in the Road to Calvary a short tunic, open at the chest to bare more skin, open mouth, and lack of hair. Underscoring his debased condition, soldiers surround him. Some are finely dressed in colourful and ornate armour and sit astride equally adorned horses, while the afflicted figure is set apart from the soldiers: he is perhaps associated with

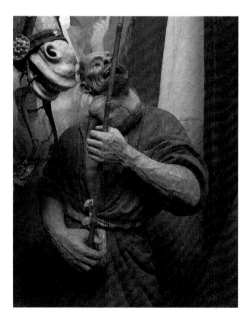

FIGURE 8.3 Gaudenzio Ferrari, *Crucifixion at Calvary*, detail

Source: Santuario del Sacro Monte, Varallo

the animals, given that one of the horse's heads is positioned extremely close to his face. Like the tormentor in the earlier scene, this figure also interacts directly with Christ to inflict pain, mockery, and suffering.[37] As such, they take on a moralizing role, reminding the viewers to practise kindness unless they should want to be physically marred.

These two figures in the Sacro Monte of Varallo seem to represent the human world, complete with its imperfections, unlike the saints and saviour nearby, who are idealized to correspond with their spiritual roles. Even the soldiers are portrayed as more noble than those whom they direct to inflict torture. Moreover, the deformed features of the executioner suggest that he suffers from cretinism, which resonates with the Christian notion that he knows not what he does.[38] Merke and others have rightly noted that figures with goitre indicated to the viewer that their physical disfiguration was a sign of their inherent evil character.[39] They play the role of the hated and bestial tormentors of Christ. Of course, not all tormenting figures in Varallo had goitre.[40] In these two cases, goitre was perhaps viewed not only as an expression of one's inner character but also as an outward disfigurement of that nature that evoked a response of disgust.

Though the figures with goitre appeared as repulsive and moralizing, they also may have inspired curiosity and wonder.[41] Allie Terry-Fritsch convincingly argues that the 'somaesthetic' experience at the Sacro Monte of Varallo produced a sense of wonder, or 'meraviglia', in pilgrims due in equal parts to the naturalism of the scenes and their artifice.[42] Early visitors to the site often commented on the naturalism of these figures. For example, in 1566 Francesco Sesalli remarked that 'they are so natural as if nature herself and not art had made them'.[43] Artist Federico Zuccari recorded his visit to Varallo in 1604 in his *Il passaggio per Italia* (1608); he noted that the painted and sculpted figures 'seem alive and true to life'[44] but also described the 'artifice of many chapels'.[45] The figures with goitre may have elicited empathy or repulsion in the viewer, but their physical malformations and the naturalistic way in which they were artistically portrayed were also a source of wonder, no matter how common the infirmity.

Caravaggio's 'crucifixion of Saint Andrew'

Goitre carried somewhat different meanings in art created in Naples, near another mountainous region where it was long known to be endemic. Michelangelo Merisi da Caravaggio painted the *Crucifixion of Saint Andrew* in 1607, in which the saint is depicted during his martyrdom (Figure 8.4). According to the *Golden Legend*, Andrew was martyred in Patras, where he was tied to an X-shaped cross, from which he continued to preach for two days.[46] The weary and aged Andrew occupies most of the canvas, his feet crossed in a subtle X-shape and his lips parted in the act of speaking. Four people have gathered at the foot of the cross to represent the purported thousands who listened to Andrew in the final days of his life. When the crowd pleaded with the Emperor Aegeas to end Andrew's suffering, he issued an order to release him from the cross. However, when the executioner,

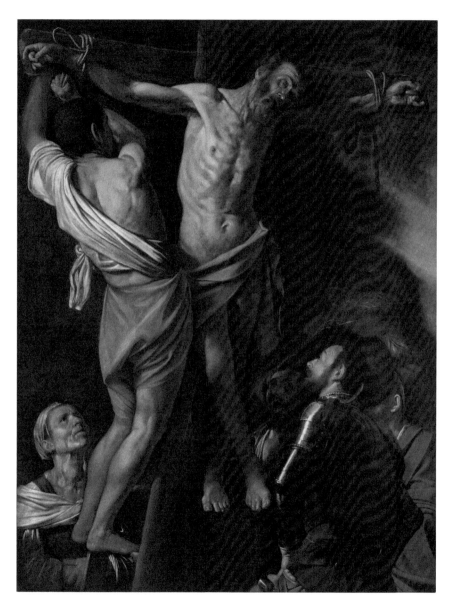

FIGURE 8.4 Michelangelo Merisi da Caravaggio, *The Crucifixion of Saint Andrew*

Source: The Cleveland Museum of Art, Cleveland

here seen on the left, attempted to untie the binding ropes, he suddenly was unable to proceed, leaving Andrew to fulfil his destiny as a Christian martyr. The flash of light from the right side of the canvas indicates the precise moment when the executioner was paralyzed and the last moments of the saint's life.

Caravaggio's painting is rare in its subject matter of depicting this miraculous moment of paralysis and Andrew drawing his final breath: two difficult states to render pictorially.[47] Also curious is the elderly woman with a goitre who stands by herself to the left of the cross and looks up at Andrew, her hands clasped at her waist. She wears seventeenth-century garb, is pushed close to the picture plane, and, like the viewer, bears witness to the scene. She is physically separated from the crowd, and her clothing identifies her as a peasant. Although her goitre is not as heavily caricatured as in the Varallo figures, the lump at her throat is pronounced. X-ray analysis of the painting reveals a *pentimento* precisely in the area of the woman's neck where her hands were originally joined in prayer. Her hands were later lowered and a large goitre was painted in their place.[48] This change indicates that initially, Caravaggio either did not paint the goitre or hid it behind the woman's praying hands so that it would have been decidedly less prominent than in the final composition. As such, the fully exposed goitre indicates a deliberate choice that necessitates further examination.

Scholars have often interpreted the old woman's curious presence in the scene in relation to Andrew's role as the patron saint of neck and throat ailments.[49] In their 1977 comprehensive study of the painting, Ann Tzeutschler Lurie and Denis Mahon described the woman as follows: 'Her enormous goitre unsparingly exposed injects a disturbing note of naturalism into the painting. As a rule, when goitres appear in art they are to be found in depictions from those regions—mostly mountainous—where they are common'.[50] This statement relies on Merke's study, recently published at that time, and has remained uncontested. While there does seem to be a correlation between the appearance of figures with goitre in art created in mountainous areas, the 'rules' governing the appearance of goitre in art are not fixed. Reducing the woman with goitre in Caravaggio's painting to an example of naturalism is to misunderstand the deeper implications of her presence in the scene. Similarly, a physician's diagnosis of the woman in the painting as exhibiting signs of 'metastatic thyroid carcinoma (rather than lymphoma of thyroid or cervical nodes)'[51] is of little use in explaining her role in the painting.

The lack of documents concerning this painting's patronage and original location or function makes it difficult to draw secure conclusions, but the context in which it was painted and the image itself provide important clues. Though she is significantly less threatening than the figures in Varallo, the woman may provide a counterpoint to the saint, and specifically to his preaching. Both have parted lips, but due to her goitre, the woman will not produce the same clear and melodious sound as the saint beside her. Though few people suffering from goitre lost their voice,[52] a growth of this size pressing against the larynx would have likely interfered with the woman's ability to speak.[53] I return here to Castiglione's observation of lower-class people with low intelligence from the mountains of Bergamo as 'goitrous mutes'.

In a treatise on the voice published between 1600 and 1601, just a few years before Caravaggio completed his painting, Giulio Casserio posited that the primary function of the larynx is to produce fluid that makes the voice more harmonious and pleasant.[54] Casserio cited the importance of voice in humans, providing ancient and biblical examples of great speeches that shaped history, including the examples of Christ's apostles, whose mission was to preach.[55] Thus, the subject of this painting becomes not so much about the martyrdom of Andrew but the miracle of his voice as he preached the word of God from the cross in his last two days of life. As the first apostle, Andrew's mission in life was to preach, an act to which he devoted himself in body and soul up to his final breath.

Caravaggio painted this work in Naples, not far from Amalfi, where Saint Andrew was patron saint and where his remains are housed in the cathedral of Sant'Andrea. The mountainous area around Naples has long been known to be endemic to goitre.[56] Scholars agree that the woman with goitre in the painting was likely a peasant native to the surrounding hills of Naples. The underlying assumption is that the artist painted the woman from life. Biographers of the artist, including Giovan Pietro Bellori, claimed that Caravaggio painted exclusively from the live model,[57] an idea that has sometimes been overstated and one that ignores his remarkable visual memory.[58] There is no firm evidence, technical or otherwise, that this figure was indeed painted from life or even that she had goitre, as the pentimento may demonstrate. Moreover, an old, unidealized woman closely resembling this figure but without goitre appears in other paintings by Caravaggio.[59] These figures typically evoke empathy, prompting this emotion in the viewer. The woman with the goitre who leads our eye upward towards the saint is therefore present in the scene to facilitate spiritual contemplation of Andrew's martyrdom.

This figure with goitre in Caravaggio's painting recalls Merke's category of this medical condition to inspire the viewer to empathize with humble subjects. Erin Benay argues convincingly that the woman's position at the foot of the cross on the left is typically reserved for the Virgin Mary in scenes of Christ's Crucifixion. By association, Caravaggio's woman with goitre may represent humility and piety.[60] As in Varallo, the figure with goitre provides the viewer with a model of humility and represents a typical person often seen in the area in which the work of art was created and viewed. She is an indication that this event is taking place in the viewer's time and place. However, unlike the figures with goitre in Varallo, this woman does not appear to lack intelligence or be the perpetrator of malfeasance. Her presence reinforces the devotional aspect of this painting and the miracle Caravaggio captured in the scene.

Presepe figures

Similar to the old woman in Caravaggio's painting, the *donna gozzuta* was a fixture in *presepi*, or nativity scenes, especially those created in Naples in the seventeenth and eighteenth centuries (Figure 8.5). Although not always women, these figures

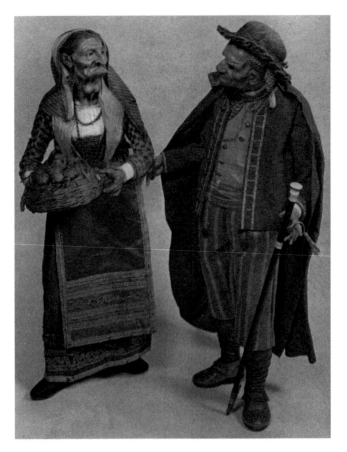

FIGURE 8.5 D. Tagliaferri, *Old Couple* (*Presepe* figures)

Source: Collezione Corrado Catello, Naples

were often elderly. The Neapolitan *presepi* are among the first and most studied of their kind, even though this tradition extends well beyond the Italian peninsula. Several publications have highlighted these figures, explaining their inclusion as related to the theme of the humility of Christ's beginnings.[61] As in Caravaggio's painting, the people afflicted with goitre represented in Neapolitan art signalled humility and inspired empathy. They are of the same lower strata of social class as the figures with goitre in Varallo, and are also mountain-dwellers, but share more with Caravaggio's old woman.

The figures with goitre in *presepi* are difficult to overlook. *Presepi* are often cast in the time in which they were created, providing a glimpse into everyday life. In *presepi*, such as the one illustrated here, vendors sell their wares, while others carry out their daily routines and occupations. In a remote corner of the composition, the Virgin Mary and Joseph adore the Christ child along with tradespeople and shepherds. This scene is dominated by the quotidian bustle of a town. This accessible and familiar scene may be a way to draw viewers into an extension of their own world, as in Varallo.

The old woman with goitre is usually dressed as a peasant, like many of the other figures that populate *presepi*. In some cases, she sells chestnuts or other produce. Gennaro Borrelli noted that this figure often appears in tavern scenes from the 1630s, largely due to the liturgical dramas from about a decade earlier on which *presepi* were based.[62] In fact, the earliest *presepi* were placed on top of the altar as backdrops for *sacre rappresentazioni*, or liturgical dramas, that recounted the nativity.[63] By the end of the sixteenth century, *presepi* became larger structures arranged in churches or private homes, particularly in southern Italy, for temporary display at Christmas. As at Varallo, the hilly settings of most *presepi* represent the Holy Land, in which these historic events took place, as well as the mountainous areas outside Naples, in which these people reside.

The *presepe* assemblages were often commissioned by upper-class patrons for whom such stereotypes would have reinforced their positions of privilege. In an age when caricature and theorized notions of beauty were coming to the fore, the woman with the goitre in *presepi* and other works of art created around this time should be considered as part of the larger body of images of the grotesque and the unusual, often low-class workers, that fascinated seventeenth-century Italy.

Theories of beauty

Texts by art critics and natural scientists alike featured definitions of beauty which may provide insight into how works of art featuring goitre could have been understood by contemporary viewers. As demonstrated earlier, goitre was recognized as a condition requiring medical attention, but, unlike other infirmities, it was not known to cause death. Perhaps the need to cure goitre had more to do with the unsightly swollen neck it caused than a life-threatening disease. As we have seen, bodies that were disfigured, misshapen, or 'ugly' were viewed with pity and disgust but also sparked wonder in early modern society. Understanding what constituted ugliness and its counterpart, beauty, further explains why goitre may have been cast in a pejorative light.

As we have seen, one of the first early modern artists who thought about beauty and the 'grotesque' in art was Leonardo da Vinci. While it is true that Leonardo was employed at the Sforza court at Milan for several years and probably had seen people with goitre, his 'grotesque' heads are not necessarily portraits of specific individuals. Similar to Caravaggio's old women, these caricatures constitute types that are the products of an artistic exercise that employed the creative powers of the artist.[64] Leonardo recorded his thoughts on beauty, stating:

> If the painter wishes to see beauties which will make him fall in love with them, he is a lord capable of creating them, and if he wishes to see monstrous things that frighten, or those that are grotesque and laughable, or those that arouse real compassion, he is their lord and their creator.[65]

Monsters were one source of curiosity that became popular over the course of the seventeenth century. Ulisse Aldovrandi's *Monstrorum historia* (1642) provided a compilation of a wide range of humans suffering from birth defects and other infirmities who he called 'monsters'.[66] Aldovrandi did not illustrate people with goitre in his study, but he did write about it as a cursed condition and one that resulted in a 'putrefying sensual humour lodged in the gullet'.[67] The current reception of visibly infirm people may also be gleaned from Giambattista della Porta's treatise on physiognomy in which he associated beauty with good proportions and ugliness with bestiality.[68] Thus, the negative reception of disfigured people in art, such as the two tormentors of Christ in Varallo, may have encouraged the viewer to adore the 'beautiful' holy figures beside them, further focusing their religious meditation as a juxtaposition of good and evil, saintly and terrestrial, or sacred and profane.

Art theorists continued to ponder these motifs in art throughout the Renaissance and beyond. For example, in *Trattato della pittura* (1607–15), Giovanni Battista Agucchi noted that ideal beauty could only be apprehended by a noble audience, while low-life subjects were suited to vulgar artists and viewers.[69] This may help explain the figures in the Sacro Monte of Varallo, which was a site accessible to all pilgrims. It is less helpful when considering Caravaggio's painting, probably intended for the viceroy of Naples or another viewer of similar repute. That said, Caravaggio was often viewed by contemporary art critics as vulgar, because his presentation of subjects in painting was 'somewhere between the sacred and the profane'.[70]

One of the staunch defenders of the representation of beauty in art was Caravaggio's biographer, Bellori. In his preface to the *Lives of the Artists* (1672), Bellori reiterated his speech championing the 'idea del bello', or the ideal of beauty in art, criticizing artists such as Caravaggio, whose works were 'too natural' because they were merely copied from nature.[71] Thus, to include a figure with goitre in a religious scene would have been unthinkable for Bellori. Yet, other artists took deformed or 'ugly' people as their subjects. Examples include Annibale Carracci's drawing of a young, nude hunchback boy (Chatsworth House, *c.* 1580–90), and his brother Agostino's painting of three physically or mentally disabled men (Capodimonte Museum, *c.* 1598–60).[72]

Jusepe de Ribera was another artist who took 'ugly' or misshapen figures as his subjects. As noted by Jonathan Brown, the man featured in the *Small Grotesque Head* (*c.* 1622) bears a strong resemblance to the executioner in the later *Martyrdom of Saint Bartholomew* print (1624).[73] This is particularly interesting in light of the role of the executioner, as seen in the Varallo example. All of these figures share rough, unidealized features to communicate their grizzly profession to the viewer.

Goitre has also been identified in Ribera's *Large Grotesque Head* (*c.* 1622), but not adequately explained.[74] The print shows the head of a man in profile with several warts or small tumours on his face and two large flaps of skin hanging from his neck. This does not appear to be goitre at all, but something more in the realm of fantasy.[75] Writing in the mid-eighteenth century, biographer Bernardo De Dominci noted 'alcune teste deformi intagliate per ischerzo' (some deformed heads, engraved as a joke) by Ribera; the quote may indicate that the then current perception of such an image was that it was produced for comic effect, reminiscent of the Bergamasque Zanni character.[76] This agrees with Barry Wind's observation that the figure wears a ruff and a hat, both typically associated with buffoons and fools from the *commedia dell'arte*.[77]

Artistic depictions of deformed bodies provoked both repulsion and curiosity for the seventeenth-century viewer.[78] As a print, it could be disseminated widely, indicating that such images may have filled a market niche. Craig Felton astutely noted that Ribera produced other 'grotesque' images of infirm or disabled bodies, as in the paintings of *Magdalena Ventura with Her Husband and Son* (1631, Museo Fundación Lerma) depicting a bearded woman, and the *Club-Footed Boy* (1642, Louvre).[79] For Edward Payne, the print by Ribera is not quite a caricature and was probably not created from life; rather, it belongs to a category of exaggerated and capricious images of 'ugliness' that sometimes elicit repulsion and at other times, pity.[80] Reactions to goitre were thus varied and complex and were intrinsically tied to contemporary perceptions of physical appearance at the time.

Conclusion

It is impossible to create a single explanation that applies to all images of goitre. As demonstrated by the preceding examples, each was created for a specific audience and had an intended function and meaning. Unfortunately, we know very little about how goitre was perceived in early modern Europe due to the lack of records. Until more evidence is gleaned, the secondary literature that mentions goitre and works of art that document its prevalence must suffice. The present study aims to contribute to ongoing research on the problem of goitre in art with reference to its particular historical and cultural context. The examples may help explain other works in which this condition is given visual form and the possible reasons for its inclusion.

From the tormenter figures in the Sacro Monte of Varallo and Ribera's prints to the peasants in Caravaggio's paintings and Neapolitan *presepi*, goitre carried many associations in early modern Italian art. While all of the figures in these examples were lower-class inhabitants of mountainous areas, they varied in the responses they possibly elicited, from mockery, to repulsion, to sympathy, to wonder. Written sources further substantiate the claim that peasants living in mountainous areas were viewed as unintelligent. Among others, Michelangelo supported this idea when comparing his 'goitre', which developed due to the labour involved in painting the Sistine Chapel ceiling. Drawing on the exaggerated features of Leonardo's grotesque caricatures, the tormenters with goitre in Varallo and in prints by Ribera are presented as ugly, animal-like, and evil. Their disregard for the torture they inflict on holy figures is made manifest in their goitres, whereby they take on a moralizing function. Less exaggerated goitres appear on the old woman in Caravaggio's *Crucifixion of Saint Andrew* painting and the peasants in the *presepi* of Naples, who are non-threatening and epitomize humility and piety.

Despite the different roles these figures play in their respective works of art, their goitre represents a deliberate choice made by the artist, not a detail required by the subject or artistic tradition. While it is true that each of these examples is a work of art created in the areas in which goitre was endemic, they are not mere studies in naturalism. Rather, the figures with goitre localize the scenes in with they are included and reinforce their narratives and devotional function. Regardless of their varied meanings, negative or positive, each figure with goitre appears to spark wonder in the viewer. Their physical malformation separates them from the unblemished bodies that often surround them, drawing further attention to their difference. As such, figures with goitre, in all of their complexity, may also be understood as the result of artistic embellishment and the power of the artist to re-create these stories pictorially to communicate with their viewers. To imagine these scenes without the figures with goitre, these Crucifixions, martyrdoms, and Nativities would lack the *varietà* that was so prized in art at the time.

Notes

1 *Chi nasce smemorato e gozzuto non ne guarisce mai.* This was first published as one of Franco Sacchetti's tales that focused on the gullibility of goitrous peasants. Sacchetti, *Novella*, 267.
2 Merke, *History and Iconography*, 127.
3 Merke, *Geschichte und ikonographie.*
4 Merke, *History and Iconography*, 288–300.
5 Clark and Clark, *The Remarkables.*
6 Craik, *The Hippocratic Treatise*, 7.
7 Jouanna, *Greek Medicine*, 128.
8 Hermitte, *Il gozzo*, 136.
9 Medvei, *History of Endocrinology*, 59.
10 Merke, *History and Iconography*, 196.
11 Alberti, *On the Art of Building*, 13.
12 Merke, *History and Iconography*, 258.
13 Merke, *History and Iconography*, 260.
14 Merke, *History and Iconography*, 259, 260.
15 Galen had identified the thyroid, described its shape as resembling a shield, and noted its function to lubricate respiratory passageways, including the larynx (or 'voicebox'), which he located just behind it. Merke, *History and Iconography*, 84.
16 O'Malley and Saunders, *Leonardo da Vinci*, 386.
17 Vescia and Basso, 'Goiters', 29.
18 Merke, *History and Iconography*, 315; Vescia and Basso, 'Goiters', 29; Clark and Clark, *Remarkables*, 14, 26, 73; Hermitte, *Il gozzo*, figures 49 and 50; Sterpetti, De Toma, and De Cesare, 'Thyroid swellings', 591–96; and Martino and Vitti, 'Leonardo da Vinci', 781.
19 Merke, *History and Iconography*, 154.
20 The Florentine poet Burchiello (1404–49) also employed 'gatti' to refer to peasants. Saslow, *The Poetry of Michelangelo*, 70–72, note 2.
21 Merke, *History and Iconography*, 155.
22 Merke, *History and Iconography*, 296; and Vescia and Basso, 'Goiters in the Renaissance', 29.
23 Martino and Mariotti, 'Michelangelo', 1081.
24 Gil and others, 'The mystery', 1–5 and Tamargo and Suk, 'Concerning the concealed anatomy', E503–05.

25 Bondeson and Bondeson, 'Michelangelo's Divine Goitre', 609–11, and Bondeson and Bondeson, 'The creator', 189–92.

26 Göttler, 'The temptation of the senses', 394. Bram de Klerck noted that Carlo Borromeo visited this site days before his death in 1584, and referred to it as 'nuova Gerusalemme'; the Latin inscription over the entrance gate also qualified it as such. Klerck, 'Jerusalem in Renaissance Italy', 281.

27 Klerck, 'Jerusalem in Renaissance Italy', 232.

28 See Nova, '"Popular" art'. Kühnel also argues that the Sacri Monti were often not considered high art by art historians and, as such, have only attracted more attention recently. Kühnel, 'Virtual pilgrimages', 244.

29 Lasansky, 'Body elision', 252.

30 Merke, *History and Iconography*, 300–03; Dionigi and Dionigi, 'Iconography of goitre', 1301–04; Leatherbarrow, 'Image and its setting', 120.

31 Hood, 'The *Sacro Monte* of Varallo', 294.

32 Agosti and Stoppa (eds), *Il Rinascimento*, 101–03 and 109–20.

33 Klerck, 'Jerusalem in Renaissance Italy', 219.

34 Terry-Fritsch, 'Performing the Renaissance body', 123–24.

35 Göttler, 'The temptation of the senses', 411.

36 Jordan, 'The last tormentor of Christ', 21.

37 William Chester Jordan notes that the sponge-bearer was often represented in art as a Jew, usually physically deformed, impoverished, or in other manners to indicate his wickedness. See Jordan, 'The last tormentor of Christ'.

38 Giampalmo, 'Il gozzo endemico', 101.

39 Merke, *History and Iconography*, 303; and Clark and Clark, *The Remarkables*, 76.

40 For example, the executioner figure in Chapel XXXII pulls Christ by a rope. This figure's face is riddled with wrinkles, moles, and a dropping eyelid, and his hair is dishevelled but he does not have goitre. See Agosti and Stoppa (eds), *Il Rinascimento*, 32.

41 Göttler notes the women and children respond to the sponge-bearer with expressions that are 'a mix of curiosity and compassion'. Göttler, 'The temptation of the senses', 411. For Luigi Sena, figures with goitre created reactions of either wonder or fear in the viewer. Sena, *Arte e tiroide*, 17.

42 Terry-Fritsch, 'Performing the Renaissance body', 126.

43 Göttler, 'The temptation of the senses', 411.

44 'vive et vere paiono'. Göttler, 'The temptation of the senses', 444.

45 'artificio di molte capelle'. Göttler, 'The temptation of the senses', 413.

46 de Voragine, *The Golden Legend*. See also Pedro de Ribadeneyra, *Flos Sanctorum o Libro de las vidas de los Santos* (1601, Italian translation from 1604–05) as cited in Lurie and Mahon, 'Caravaggio's *Crucifixion of Saint Andrew*', 13.

47 In her recent comprehensive study of this painting, Erin Benay noted that Ippolito Scarsellino's *Martyrdom of Saint Andrew* (Verona, San Massimo all'Adige) also includes a figure with goitre who witnesses the scene. In his youth, Caravaggio might have even seen this work in its original location, the church of San Pietro al Po. See Benay, *Exporting Caravaggio*, 55; and Askew, *Caravaggio's Death of the Virgin*, 315.

48 This pentimento was left more visible in the most recent conservation of the painting by Dean Yoder at the Cleveland Museum of Art. See Benay, *Exporting Caravaggio*, 118.

49 For the somewhat tenuous identification of Saint Andrew as patron saint of throat ailments, see Lurie and Mahon, 'Caravaggio's *Crucifixion of Saint Andrew*', 18, n. 59. Although it appears that this saint is popularly associated with infirmities of the neck and throat, there is no textual evidence to suggest that this was the case when Caravaggio painted his picture.

50 Lurie and Mahon, 'Caravaggio's *Crucifixion*', 18.

51 Ferriss, 'The *Crucifixion of St. Andrew*', 518.

52 I thank Michael Stolberg for this observation.

53 Benay's argument differs slightly from mine. She notes that the saint and the man with the open mouth are rendered mute; Benay, *Exporting Caravaggio*, 38.

54 Casserius, *The Larynx*, 18–19.

55 Casserius, *The Larynx*, 13.
56 The School of Salerno was the earliest place where treatment was available for goitre. Merke, *History and Iconography*, 84.
57 Bellori, *Le vite*, 249.
58 Carrabino, '*Ascondersi per la Sicilia*', 118–19.
59 Many Caravaggio scholars have noted the recurrence of this figure in his paintings, including Lurie and Mahon, 'Caravaggio's *Crucifixion*', 18; Carrabino, '*Ascondersi per la Sicilia*', 69; and Benay, *Exporting Caravaggio*, 40.
60 Benay, *Exporting Caravaggio*, 40
61 Merke, *History and Iconography*, 323–24; Martino, 'Woman of Naples', 300; and Sena, *Arte e tiroide*, 272.
62 Borrelli, *Il presepe*, 43.
63 Berliner, 'The Origins', 260.
64 Payne, 'Ribera's grotesque heads', 89.
65 McMahon, ed. and trans., *Treatise on Painting*, 35.
66 Biancastella, *Animali e creature mostruose*.
67 Wind, *A Foul and Pestilent Congregation*, 53.
68 della Porta, *Della fisionomia*, 97–98, first published in 1677.
69 McTighe, 'Perfect deformity', 78.
70 Paleotti, *Discourse*. For the significant influence of Paleotti's text, see Schildgen, 'Cardinal Paleotti'.
71 Panofsky, *Idea*, 155–75.
72 Wind, *A Foul and Pestilent Congregation*, 19–48.
73 Brown, 'Jusepe de Ribera', 169.
74 Merke, *History and Iconography*, 315 and figure 156. See also Wind, *A Foul and Pestilent Congregation*, 53.
75 Craig Felton, Personal communication, August 16, 2018.
76 Payne, 'Ribera's grotesque heads', 98.
77 Wind, *A Foul and Pestilent Congregation*, 53.
78 Much of the modern literature related to Ribera's print has diagnosed the man depicted as suffering from von Recklinghausen's disease or multiple neurofibromatosis. Brown, 'Jusepe de Ribera', 169.
79 Felton and Jordan, *Jusepe de Ribera*, 211.
80 Payne, 'Ribera's grotesque heads', 99–100.

Bibliography

Primary sources

Alberti, Leon Battista, *On the Art of Building in Ten Books*, trans., Joseph Rykwert, Neil Leach, and Robert Tavernor (Cambridge, MA and London: MIT Press, 1988).

Bellori, Giovan Pietro Bellori, *Le vite de' pittori, scultori e architetti moderni*, ed., Evelina Borea (Turin: G. Einaudi, 1976).

Buonarroti, Michelangelo, 'To Giovanni da Pistoia' (1509), in James M. Saslow (ed), *The Poetry of Michelangelo: An Annotated Translation* (New Haven and London: Yale University Press, 1991), 70–72.

Casserius, Julius, '*The Larynx, Organ of the Voice* (1600–1601), trans., Malcom H. Hast and Erling B. Holtsmark', *Acta oto-laryngolgica*, 68, Supplement 261 (1969), 9–33.

della Porta, Giambattista, *Della fisionomia di tutto del corpo humano* (1586), ed., Francesco Stelluti (Rome, 1637).

de Voragine, Jacobus, *The Golden Legend Readings on the Saints* (c. 1260), trans., William Granger Ryan (Princeton: Princeton University Press, 2012).

Hippocrates, *On Glands*, ed. and trans., Elizabeth M. Craik (Leiden and Boston: Brill, 2009).

Leonardo da Vinci, *Codex Urbinas Latinus 1270*, trans., A. Philip McMahon (Princeton: Princeton University Press, 1956).

Sacchetti, Franco, '*Novella* CLXXIII (1399)', in Thomas Benfield Harbottle and Colonel Philip Hugh Dalbiac (eds), *Dictionary of Quotations French and Italian* (New York: Swan Sonnenschein and Macmillan Company, 1901).

Secondary sources

Agosti, Giovanni and Jacopo Stoppa, eds, *Il Rinascimento di Gaudienzo Ferrari* (Milan: Officina Libraria, 2018).

Askew, Pamela, *Caravaggio's Death of the Virgin* (Princeton: Princeton University Press, 1990).

Benay, Erin E., *Exporting Caravaggio: The Crucifixion of Saint Andrew* (Cleveland: Cleveland Museum of Art, 2017).

Berliner, Rudolf, 'The origins of the crèche', *Gazette des Beaux-Arts* 30 (1946), 248–78.

Biancastella, Antonino (ed), *Animali e creature mostruose di Ulisse Aldovrandi* (Milan: Motta Editore, 2004).

Bondeson, Lennart and Anne-Greth Bondeson, 'The creator separating light from darkness: a new self-portrait of Michelangelo?', *Konsthistorisk Tidskrift, Journal of Art History*, 70, 3 (2001), 189–92.

Bondeson, Lennart and Anne-Greth Bondeson, 'Michelangelo's Divine Goitre', *Journal of the Royal Society of Medicine*, 96, 12 (2003), 609–11.

Borrelli, Gennaro, *Il presepe napoletano* (Rome: De Luca—D'Agostino, 1970).

Brown, Jonathan, 'Jusepe de Ribera as Printmaker', in Alfonso E. Pérez Sánchez and Nicola Spinosa (eds), *Jusepe de Ribera, 1591–1652* (New York: Metropolitan Museum of Art, 1992), 167–73.

Carrabino, Danielle, '*Ascondersi per la Sicilia*': *Caravaggio and Sicily* (unpublished PhD dissertation, Courtauld Institute of Art, 2011).

Clark, Carol Z. and Orlo H. Clark, *The Remarkables: Endocrine Abnormalities in Art* (Berkeley: University of California Medical Humanities Consortium, 2011).

de Klerck, Bram, 'Jerusalem in Renaissance Italy: The holy Sepulchre on the Sacro Monte of Varallo', in Jeroen Goudeau, Mariëtte Verhoeven, and Wouter Weijers (eds), *Imagined and Real Jerusalem in Art and Architecture* (Leiden and Boston: Brill, 2014), 215–36.

Dionigi, Gianlorenzo and Renzo Dionigi, 'Iconography of goitre: four refined examples in the Sacred Mountain of Varese, Italy', *Thyroid*, 23, 10 (2013), 1301–04.

Felton, Craig and William B. Jordan, eds, *Jusepe de Ribera, lo Spagnoletto, 1591–1652* (Fort Worth: Kimbell Art Museum, 1982).

Ferriss, J. Barry, 'The *Crucifixion of St. Andrew* by Caravaggio', Letters to the Editor, *Thyroid*, 16, 5 (2006), 518.

Giampalmo, Antonio, 'Il gozzo endemico nelle raffigurazioni dell'arte', *Medicina nei secoli: arte e scienza, giornale di storia della medicina* 8, 1 (1996), 85–103.

Göttler, Christine, 'The temptation of the senses at the Sacro Monte di Varallo', in Wietse de Boer and Christine Göttler (eds), *Religion and the Senses in Early Modern Europe* (Leiden and Boston: Brill, 2013), 393–451.

Hermitte, Guido Barbieri, ed, *Il gozzo: storia, leggenda, aneddotica* (Venosa: Osanna Venosa, 1996).

Hood, William, 'The *Sacro Monte* of Varallo: Renaissance art and popular religion', in Timothy Gregory Verdon (ed), *Monasticism and the Arts* (Syracuse: Syracuse University Press, 1984), 291–311.

Jordan, William Chester, 'The last tormentor of Christ: an image of the Jew in ancient and medieval exegesis, art, and drama', *The Jewish Quarterly Review*, 78, 1–2 (1987), 21–47.

Jouanna, Jacques, *Greek Medicine from Hippocrates to Galen: Selected Papers*, eds., John Scarborough, Philip J. van der Eijk, Ann Ellis Hanson, and Joseph Ziegler, trans., Neil Allies (Leiden and Boston: Brill, 2012).

Kühnel, Bianca, 'Virtual pilgrimages to real places: The holy landscapes', in Lucy Donkin and Hanna Vorholt (eds), *Imagining Jerusalem in the Medieval West* (Oxford: Oxford University Press, 2012), 243–64.

Lasansky, Medina D., 'Body elision. Acting out the Passion at the Italian *Sacri Monti*', in Julie L. Hairston and Walter Stephens (eds), *The Body in Early Modern Italy* (Baltimore: Johns Hopkins University Press, 2010), 249–73.

Leatherbarrow, David, 'Image and its setting: a study of the Sacro Monte at Varallo', *RES: Anthropology and Aesthetics*, 14 (1987), 107–22.

Lurie, Ann Tzeuchtschler and Denis Mahon, 'Caravaggio's *Crucifixion of Saint Andrew* from Valladolid', *Bulletin of the Cleveland Museum of Art*, 64, 1 (1977), 2–24.

Martino, Enio, 'Woman of Naples countryside', *Journal of Endocrinological Investigation*, 25, 3 (2002), 300.

Martino, Enio and Stefano Mariotti, 'Michelangelo, goitre and . . . cats', *Journal of Endocrinological Investigation*, 27, 11 (2004), 1081.

Martino, Enio and Paolo Vitti, 'Leonardo da Vinci "design of Lady with Graves' disease" (1452–1519)', *Journal of Endocrinological Investigation*, 37, 8 (2014), 781.

McTighe, Sheila, 'Perfect deformity, ideal beauty, and the "imaginaire" of work: the reception of Annibale Carracci's "Arti di Bologna" in 1646', *Oxford Art Journal*, 16, 1 (1993), 75–91.

Medvei, Victor Cornelius, *History of Endocrinology* (London: MTP Press, Ltd., 1982).

Merke, Franz, *Geschichte und Ikonographie. des endemischen Kropfes und Kretinismus* (Berne: Hans Huber, 1971).

Merke, Franz, *History and Iconography of Endemic Goitre and Cretinism*, trans., D. Q. Stephenson (Berne: Hans Huber, 1984).

Nova, Alessandro, '"Popular" art in Renaissance Italy: Early response to the Holy Mountain at Varallo', in Claire Farago (ed), *Reframing the Renaissance: Visual Culture in Europe and Latin America, 1450–1650* (New Haven and London: Yale University Press, 1995), 112–26.

O'Malley, Charles D. and J. B. de C. M. Saunders, *Leonardo da Vinci on the Human Body: The Anatomical, Physiological, and Embryological Drawings of Leonardo Da Vinci* (New York: H. Schumann, 1952).

Panofsky, Erwin, *Idea, A Concept of Art Theory*, trans., Joseph J. S. Peake (Columbia, SC: University of South Carolina Press, 1968).

Payne, Edward, 'Ribera's grotesque heads: Between anatomical study and cultural curiosity', in Andrei Pop and Mechtild Widrich (eds), *Ugliness: The Non-Beautiful in Art and Theory* (London and New York: I. B. Tauris, 2014), 85–103.

Schildgen, Brenda Deen, 'Cardinal Paleotti and the *Discorso intorno alle imagini sacre e profane*', in Gail Feigenbaum and Sybille Ebert-Schifferer (eds), *Sacred Possessions: Collecting Italian Religious Art 1500–1900* (Los Angeles: Getty Research Institute, 2011), 8–16.

Sena, Luigi, *Arte e tiroide, gozzuti nelle scene di natività e nei presepi* (Turin: Aracne, 2013).

Sterpetti, Antonio V., Giorgio De Toma, and Alessandro De Cesare, 'Thyroid swellings in the art of the Italian Renaissance', *The American Journal of Surgery*, 210, 3 (2015), 591–96.

Tamargo, Rafael J. and Ian Suk, 'Concerning the concealed anatomy in Michelangelo's sistine *Separation of Light from Darkness*', *Neurosurgery*, 69, 2 (2011), 503–05.

Terry-Fritsch, Allie, 'Performing the Renaissance body and mind: somaesthetic style and devotional practice at the Sacro Monte di Varallo', *Open Arts Journal*, 4 (2014–2015), 112–32.

Vescia, Fernando G. and Luigi Basso, 'Goiters in the Renaissance', *Vesalius: Acta Interantionales Historiae Mediicinae*, 3 (1997), 23–32.

Wind, Barry, *'A Foul and Pestilent Congregation'. Images of 'Freaks' in Baroque Art* (Aldershot and Brookfield, VT: Ashgate, 1998).

Ziv, Gil and other, 'The Mystery of Michelangelo Buonarroti's Goitre', *Special Issue on Differentiated Thyroid Carcinoma—Rambam Maimonides Medical Journal*, 7, 1 (2016), 1–5.

PART IV

Saints and miraculous healing

9

INFIRMITY IN VOTIVE CULTURE

A case study from the sanctuary of the Madonna dell'Arco, Naples

Fredrika Jacobs

Believed to have been commissioned as a votive offering, Giovanni Lanfranco's *St Luke Healing the Dropiscal Child* (Rome, Galleria Nazionale d'Arte Antica, *c.* 1622–23) unusually represents Luke as the 'beloved physician' of Colossians 4. 14. Lanfranco underscored Luke's role as *medicus* by prominently positioning in the foreground a bound volume of Hippocratic writings and, beside it, Luke's legendary portrait of the Virgin Mary, an image credited with healing the infirm.[1] Together, the medical text and the miracle-working image can be seen as a visualization of the remedial options available to those seeking good health and well-being in early modern Italy. Lanfranco's *St Luke* is not singular in this regard. So, too, do the texts and images of popular votive culture. Miracle books (*libri dei miracoli*) routinely record a 'desperate' supplicant's turn to a miracle-working image following a physician's failure to ease the votary's suffering. Popularly offered panel paintings (*tavolette votive*) left at shrine sites by or on behalf of supplicants visually affirm the efficacy touted in miracle books. But how much do these paintings—Lanfranco's *St Luke* and anonymously painted *tavolette votive*—actually disclose about the therapeutic landscape of early modern Italy? This chapter considers the question in the contexts of votive culture and the medical discourse, focusing first on Lanfranco's canvas and then on a distinctive group of seventeen votive panels preserved in the Neapolitan Sanctuary of the Madonna dell'Arco, which, in contrast to the vast majority of *tavolette*, represent the votary symptomatically and, in some cases, attended by a doctor and/or a priest.

Introduction

In his Letter to the Colossians, St Paul called Luke the Evangelist 'the beloved physician'.[2] Echoing Paul's words, Eusebius (*c.* 260—*c.* 339 CE) went on to describe Luke's legacy as a practitioner of medicine in *Historia ecclesiastica*. Cognizant that

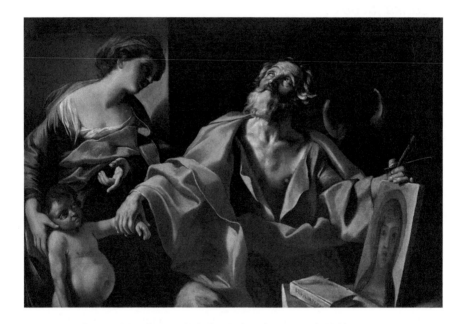

FIGURE 9.1 Giovanni Lanfranco, *St Luke Healing the Dropsical Child*

Source: Rome: Palazzo Barberini, Galleria Nazionale d'Arte Antica (courtesy of the National Galleries of Ancient Art—Bibliotheca Hertziana, Max Planck Institute for Art History/Enrico Fontolan)

both the body and the soul suffer pain and are desirous of alleviating affliction, Luke 'left us, in two inspired books, [one his Gospel, the other the testamentary Acts of the Apostles] proofs of the spiritual art of healing'.[3] Later writers, including Jacobus da Voragine (*c.* 1229–98), offered amplification. In his widely read compendium of saints' lives, *The Golden Legend, c.* 1260, Voragine noted that Luke, who was a physician, 'prescribed a very healthful medicine for us', which is of three kinds. The first, penance, cures 'all spiritual sickness'. The second, an observance of counsel, 'increases good health', while the third, the avoidance of sin and iniquity, is a safeguard against spiritual illness and decay.[4] But Luke's 'two inspired books' were not all that attested the Evangelist's capacity to heal. So, too, did the legendary portraits of the Madonna he purportedly painted. Voragine, who described Luke as both 'a physician and a distinguished painter (*arte medic' e pictor egregious*), provided an example of the latter ability in his biography of Pope Gregory I (papacy 590–604). Seeking to dispel the fetid air of plague that had settled on Rome, Gregory organized a penitential procession. Holding aloft 'a perfect likeness' of the Virgin 'painted by St Luke', the pontiff led the repentant Romans through the polluted warren of city streets.[5] When, in the procession's wake, the air turned from foul to pure, it was evident to all that the sacred images Luke painted were as efficacious as the hallowed words he wrote.

By the mid-sixteenth century, some ninety editions of Voragine's *Golden Legend* had circulated the story of Luke's wondrous portrait of the Virgin Mary throughout Europe. Concurrently, miracle-working images of the Madonna proliferated. Some were Lukan icons imported from the East, others replicated the authentic archetype, and still others acquired cultic status independently, their ability to move, speak, rescue the endangered, and heal the infirm having been attested by the faithful and verified by ecclesiastical review.[6] As word-of-mouth and print media spread reports of miraculous happenings, countless representations of the Madonna became focal points of votive devotion, beckoning pilgrims in search of spiritual salvation and physical well-being.

Although Lukan icons were well and widely known by the eighth century, portrayals of Luke actively engaged in painting the Virgin Mary's true likeness began to multiply significantly only in later centuries. Following a surge in popularity during the fifteenth and sixteenth centuries, depictions of St Luke as *pictor* slowed in the seventeenth century, responding, perhaps, to the 'word-oriented devotional culture' of Protestantism and the Catholic call for the curbing of 'superstitious offenses' perceived to be taking place with and around sacred images. Predictably, representations of Luke reflected the din of critical voices. Increasingly, Luke 'the biblical author of God's word' was emphasized over Luke the 'distinguished painter' celebrated by Voragine.[7]

With attention focused on Luke as either *scriptor* or *pictor*, we might ask where during this period was the physician beloved by St Paul? Arguably, the answer is that he was omnipresent, at least implicitly. As Eusebius, Voragine, and others acknowledged, Luke was a safeguard against sickness to all who heeded the words he wrote and venerated the portraits of the Virgin he painted. That said, Luke's identity as a physician was rarely foregrounded in works of art. I know of only one

example: Giovanni Lanfranco's *St Luke Healing the Dropsical Child*, a striking painting believed to have been a votive offering commissioned by Orazio Falconieri
(1579–1664) and his wife of seven years, Ottavia Sacchetti (1590–1645).[8]

Lanfranco's St Luke, who is identified by the shadowed presence of his symbol-
izing ox, is an expansive figure. Facing forward, arms spread wide, head tilted back,
eyes turned heavenward, and with his face illumined by divine light, he is at once in
spiritual communion with God and in palpable contact with humanity. Focused on
the truths emanating from heaven and with fingers gently yet carefully positioned
to measure the strength and rapidity of his young patient's pulse, Luke cradles the
wrist of the sick child being urged forward by a young woman, most likely the boy's
mother.[9] With his other hand, he distractedly steadies the portrait of the Virgin Mary
perched upright on the table before him. Lying on the table is a closed book; the
name 'Hippocrates' is legible on its spine. Clearly, Lanfranco took care to arrange
the Virgin's portrait and the volume of Hippocratic writings parallel to one another.
Equally clear is the attention he took in visualizing the physical manifestations of the
child's sickness, namely the discolouration of skin, puffiness around bulging eyes, and
distended abdomen. Notwithstanding the artist's assiduousness, art historians have
not discussed the significance of the Madonna's portrait in relationship to either the
Hippocratic text or the child who suffers from an illness that, despite twenty-first-
century attempts at diagnosis, continues to elude undisputed identification.[10]

In contrast to other depictions of the Evangelist, in this painting Lanfranco
imparted all of Luke's defining capabilities.[11] The intensity with which Luke listens
to the divine directives that will help him heal the child identifies him as the con-
veyer of God's will and word, the *scriptor* who penned the third canonical Gospel
and recorded the Acts of the Apostles. Concomitantly, the brushes and palette he
holds distractedly in his left hand make clear that he is also the *pictor* who painted
the conspicuously displayed portrait of the Madonna. As for Luke *medicus*, Lanfranco's detailed depiction of a child rife with signs of sickness points to the 'beloved
physician' of Colossians 4. 14. The stricken child and his concerned mother are
not, however, all that signals Luke's capacity to assist the unwell. The volume lying
on the table indicates the Evangelist's familiarity with a corpus of ancient writings
renowned for thoughtful observations concerning illness and disease.[12] In con-
cert with other pictorial elements, the medical text can be seen to represent one
of several remedial options in a seventeenth-century quest for well-being. The
prominently displayed painting with which the volume is so purposefully aligned
pointedly proffers a second.

In seventeenth-century Italy, as elsewhere throughout Europe, individuals confronted by the ineludible reality of disease faced an array of different services to
deal with the many and varied effects of what contemporaneous sources generally
refer to as *infirmità*. Physicians and apothecaries offered the sick and enfeebled
therapies founded on observations and practices recorded in learned texts. Folk
healers tendered remedies rooted in popular wisdom that had been passed from one
generation to the next, while the Roman Catholic Church presented holy relics
and sacred images to the frail and afflicted with the caveat that votive behaviours

stay within monitored channels of orthodoxy.[13] To illustrate what was then commonplace, David Gentilcore mapped these options—medical, popular, and ecclesiastical—as three interlocking and overlapping circles. This model 'allows us to give due attention, where possible, to the attitudes and actions of both healers and the sick', something that is of critical importance in the context of votive culture.[14] As Gentilcore and others have argued, seeking succour in one sphere of care did not preclude efforts to procure it from another. Similar to the prominent juxtaposition of text and image within Lanfranco's *St Luke Healing the Dropsical Child*, coexisting entries in miracle books assert this fact. For example, in the miracle book of the Sanctuary of the Madonna dell'Arco, which was compiled by the Dominican friar Arcangelo Domenici and inscribed with the date 1608, we read that in 1593 one Francesco Cola di Ruzo was treated at the Ospedale dell' Incurabili dell'Annunziata in Naples before seeking curative care from the munificent Madonna dell'Arco, whose shrine is located about twelve kilometres northeast of the city in the town of Sant'Anastasia.[15] A similar but more detailed example is provided by the case of one Bartolomeo di Selvestro as it was described by Tomaso Bandoni. As sacristan of Viterbo's Sanctuary of the Madonna della Quercia, Bandoni began to compile a miracle book for the sacred site approximately a dozen years after Fra Arcangelo dated his book celebrating the many miracles performed by the Madonna dell'Arco.[16]

According to Bandoni, Bartolomeo earned his living mining alum, a mineral used to remove the natural oils from wool and fix dyes. On or about 8 March 1510, Bartolomeo became embroiled in an argument with two of his co-workers. The squabble soon escalated from offending words to injurious violence. Having received several 'deadly wounds', Bartolomeo was 'left for dead' by his assailants. Despite the severity of his injuries, he solicited holy aid from the Madonna della Quercia, saying, 'I commend my soul to you and I forgive my companions'. Having professed his dedication to the Madonna della Quercia, Bartolomeo received a visitation from a 'woman dressed in white', a vision that accords with other avowed sightings of the Virgin Mary. According to the miracle book narrative, which was based on the inscription attached to a modest votive figure fashioned of wax and wood in the Viterban shrine, 'the woman dressed in white' helped Bartolomeo to his feet, told him to maintain his faith in her, and then promised to restore his health. Although reassured, Bartolomeo apparently thought it wise to hedge his bets. Following the Madonna's departure from the scene of the crime, he had himself 'brought to the surgeon (*cerusico*) in Tolfa, [where] he was quickly looked after'. It was only on the following day and with the realization that he was 'safe and sound' that Bartolomeo 'came to give thanks to the Madonna'.[17]

Written at the same time as *St Luke Healing the Dropsical Child* was painted for Ottavio Falconieri, Bandoni's entry in the miracle book of the Madonna della Quercia verbalized the same message Lanfranco visualized in the 1620s and Gentilcore was to diagram several centuries later. The sick had recourse to—and clearly took advantage of—various remedial options. With its prominent juxtaposition of sacred image and venerable medical text, Lanfranco's *St Luke* can be viewed as a visual variant of

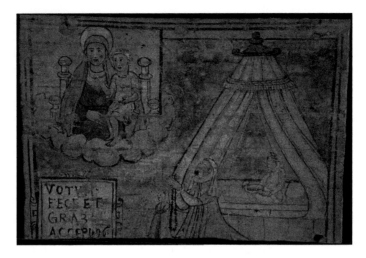

FIGURE 9.2 Anonymous, *Votive Panel Painting of a Seated, Bedridden Man Vomiting Blood*

Source: Credit: Sanctuary of the Madonna dell' Arco, Sant'Anastasia, NA

miracle book passages like those cited previously.[18] Moreover, and significantly, the votive image Lanfranco so masterfully painted for Orazio Falconieri and Ottavia Sacchetti is not singular in its visualization of remedial options. So, too, do seventeen *tavolette* comprising a distinctive group of votive panel paintings in the Neapolitan sanctuary of the Madonna dell'Arco, each one painted by an unnamed artist for an unidentified patron and all lacking the arresting virtuosity seen in Lanfranco's work.

As with Lanfranco's *St Luke*, identifying the depicted illness in most votive panels seems to be all but impossible. Certainly, the Madonna dell'Arco panels considered here resist retrospective diagnosis. Indeed, the shrine's miracle book suggests that the striking symptom of people emitting 'a great and highly dangerous flux of blood . . . from the mouth' was the result of one of two opposing states of health;[19] it either signalled the imminence of death or heralded the moment of crisis that marks the beginning of recovery.

Votive panel paintings and the votive context

Bartolomeo di Selvestro's choice of a wood-and-wax figure as a votive offering to the Madonna della Quercia was wholly in keeping with the time of its donation. By 1510, workshops located near Viterbo's Marian shrine had been producing figures of this type for more than thirty years.[20] Soon, however, a new votive form would begin to appear among the accretion of objects offered to the Madonna in grateful acknowledgement of an act of divine intervention.[21] Indeed, by the century's end, *tavolette votive*—which in general are small in size, rudimentary in style, and, at the time Lanfranco painted *St Luke Healing the Dropsical Child*, were produced principally for an open market—had gained widespread popular currency.[22]

These humble offerings can be divided roughly into two groups. One comprises illustrations of a life-threatening situation: a child falling into a well, a man engaged in military combat, a pregnant woman thrown from her horse, and a ship tossed on turbulent seas. The other references an illness or condition of infirmity. Despite an economy of means and an obvious reliance on convention, paintings in the first group communicate clearly their *raison d'être*. Rarely can the same be said about a painting in the second group. Whether or not this reflects the difficulty of depicting, for example, a fever or the failure of an internal organ, a *tavoletta* offered by a sick supplicant, whether he was soliciting divine assistance or acknowledging its receipt, seldom goes beyond equating *infirmità* with being bedbound.[23]

There are, to be sure, some striking exceptions to the rule. The collection of *tavolette* at the Sanctuary of the Madonna dell'Arco includes scenes in which a woman bares her breast to surgeons, a man props his ulcerated leg on a chair, a doctor confronts the risky challenge of attending a breech birth,[24] and, in one particularly remarkable case, a body is distorted by swelling.[25] Far more typically votive panel paintings in the second grouping represent the afflicted simply sitting or lying in bed, sometimes with a rosary clutched in hands that are positioned palm-to-palm in a gesture of prayer. Lacking an inscription, a viewer cannot know the cause or course of the ailment that consigned the votary to his bed. Even a prognosis cannot be surmised unless the pictured scene includes a priest administering last rites. Given that these stock images were available for purchase in shops located near shrine sites or by vendors attending fairs associated with the honouring of local saints, *tavolette* featuring the bedbound are so formulaic and vague that it is impossible to differentiate those suffering one infirmity from those vexed by

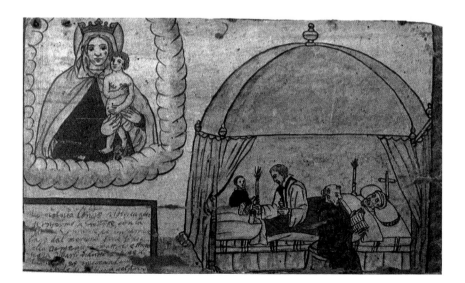

FIGURE 9.3 Anonymous, *Votive Panel of Tarquinio Longo Receiving Last Rites*

Source: Credit: Sanctuary of the Madonna dell' Arco, Sant'Anastasia, NA

another. This prompts an obvious question: was the specific nature of the ailment a matter important for the votary or, rephrased for a votive context, was it sufficient to convey a general state-of-being when the objective was to either solicit intercession or thank God and the saints for received grace?

What, then, do votive paintings—and this includes fine works of art like Lanfranco's *St Luke Healing the Dropsical Child* as well as rudimentary *tavolette* by unknown craftsmen—tell us about *infirmità* in early modern Italy? In considering the question, this chapter turns to a distinctive group of seventeen popularly donated votive panel paintings in the Sanctuary of the Madonna dell'Arco. In striking contrast to the hundreds of early modern *tavolette* that depict the infirm asymptomatically at both this site and elsewhere throughout the Italian peninsula, this particular group of paintings presents viewers with a graphically horrific presentation of disease. The bedbound cough, vomit, or heave and spit blood into a basin. Some votive panels in this group are further distinguished by the conspicuous bedside presence of doctors. It is a presence that runs counter to a sentiment that is repeated with regularity in miracle books as well as inscribed on some votive plaques and paintings. Normally, despaired and abandoned by doctors, the gravely ill are said to have turned to God, who, through His community of steadfast saints, succeeds where those equipped with medical knowledge faltered and failed.[26] It is not surprising that prayer should emerge in this context as the most efficacious of medicaments.

While the doctor's role in healing the sick was routinely verbalized as ineffective, visual evidence offers a more measured assessment. In this sampling of seventeen works, 38 per cent include one or more medical practitioners. By contrast, a priest

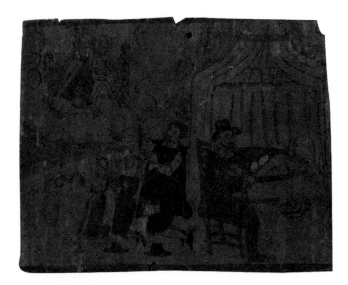

FIGURE 9.4 Anonymous, *Votive Panel Painting of a Doctor Attending a Sick Woman While Her Family Prays*

Source: Credit: Sanctuary of the Madonna dell' Arco, Sant'Anastasia, NA

unaccompanied by a doctor is represented in only 3 per cent. What is perhaps more notable is that doctors were represented at all. If learned medicine was seen to be ineffectual, at least in the votive context, then why bother depicting doctors at a patient's bedside? As I hope to demonstrate, the answer is found when the early modern medical presence is viewed in conjunction with the depicted symptom and both are considered in the context of the remedial options available to the *popolo*.

A case study

In addition to its large holding of sixteenth- and seventeenth-century *tavolette votive*, the Sanctuary of the Madonna dell'Arco lays claim to a miracle book twice inscribed with the date 1608.[27] The fortunate happenstance of preservation holds out the tantalizing prospect of analysing the visual in light of the textual and vice-versa. Unfortunately, the selectivity of the miracle book's author, Fra Arcangelo Domenici, a member of the conventual community tasked with caring for the sanctuary, coupled with the disappearance of popularly donated votive panel paintings from what was surely a significantly larger collection make this all but impossible. Indisputable matches between an entry in Fra Arcangelo's *Compendio dell' historia, miracoli e gratie* and a *tavoletta votiva* in the sanctuary's collection are few, and those that can be made, such as one that pictures three men, each accompanied by a member of a lay confraternity, being led to their execution, or 'good death',

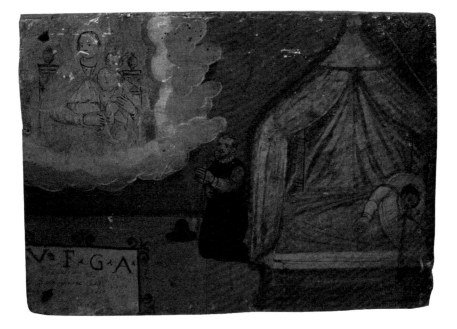

FIGURE 9.5 Anonymous, *Votive Panel of a Sick Man*

Source: Credit: Sanctuary of the Madonna dell' Arco, Sant'Anastasia/NA

reflect the *frate*'s obvious predisposition to the dramatic.[28] Even a cursory reading of Fra Arcangelo's *Compendio* reveals its author's preference for exorcisms, rescues from moral decay, last-minute conversions, and brutal assaults over cases of 'fever' and ill-defined infirmity. There are, for example, six entries citing a liberation from demonic possession as the reason for votive donation, but only one that points explicitly to tertiary fever (malaria), one that cites catarrh (an inflammation of the mucous membranes), one that mentions leprosy, and two that name *febre pestifera* (pestilential fever) as the reason for their offering.[29] As for the many cases that reference *infermità* without further explanation, Fra Arcangelo's brief and uninformative statement concerning Scipione Pasquale can be read as representative of the vast majority of the nearly 150 miracles he chose to include in the sanctuary's miracle book. The entry reads simply, 'Finding himself infirm and in complete despair of doctors, [he] made a vow to the Madonna dell'Arco [and . . .] received grace, July 3, [15]97'.[30]

It can be argued that entries like that of Scipione Pasquale, which use stock phrases, mirror Fra Arcangelo's sources. As the *frate* noted, he obtained information for the *Compendio* in several ways. In a manner similar to that which the sacristan of Viterbo's Sanctuary of the Madonna della Quercia would do approximately a dozen years later, he examined the long-established visual vocabulary of votive paintings and read inscriptions on votive plaques that were on display throughout the sanctuary.[31] He spoke directly with a supplicant on only two recorded occasions.[32] When it came to infirmity, Fra Arcangelo seems to have gathered whatever information there was available from the objects and images that were readily at hand.

There are other aspects of the votive record to be considered, one of which is that material objects and whatever inscriptions were cited as accompanying them do not account fully for the paucity of informative detail in the Madonna dell'Arco miracle book. In full accordance with other books of its kind, the compiled entries tend to be terse. No less bounded by convention, the sanctuary's surviving *tavolette* adhere to a visual vocabulary employed throughout Italy. Put simply, individualizing detail is scarce. For example, votive paintings that represent interrogation by the rope hoist (*strappado, fune,* or *corda*) at the Church of the Madonna del Monte in Cesena as well as those in the collection of the Madonna dei Miracoli just south of Verona look much the same as those in Naples' Sanctuary of the Madonna dell'Arco. Likewise, the infirm—the prayerful bedridden—were pictured uniformly. This is not to say that Fra Arcangelo's entries are unvaryingly brief and consistently uninformative, nor that *tavolette* representing the bedridden impede all efforts to distinguish an individual suffering one type of illness from a person enduring the agonies of another.

Concerning the first point, namely how much or how little is revealed in miracle book entries, consider the example of Stefano Gargano. As recorded in Fra Arcangelo's *Compendio*, Stefano was 'infirm with a great and highly dangerous flux of blood that issued from his mouth. He made a vow to the most holy Madonna dell'Arco and received grace. June 25, 1598'.[33] While the details in the inscription transcribed by Fra Arcangelo may be few, they are nonetheless notable, especially when compared to a relatively similar entry concerning one Agustino Cascano.[34] As was the case with Stefano, Agustino suffered from 'a most grave infirmity [*una infermità gravissima*]', and he too lost a significant amount of blood, so much so that 'he was left for dead'. The critical difference between these two entries comes down to a single and telling detail. Stefano Gargano lost blood through his mouth (*la bocca*). Unfortunately, this *Compendio* entry cannot be matched definitively with one of the extant votive paintings in the Madonna dell'Arco collection. It nonetheless has a notable number of visual counterparts.

Before considering these counterparts, it is important to state a few facts and acknowledge some generalizations about *tavolette votive*. First, although three of the seventeen panel paintings in the Madonna dell'Arco group have legible dates—1596, 1601, and 1613—we can only hazard a guess for the remaining fourteen. On rare occasions, an approximate date can be established by comparing the style of an undated work to one that is dated. In other instances, clothing provides the only clue. Regardless, the dating of *tavolette* is notoriously problematic. It must be said, therefore, that the number of panels comprising the group under consideration may be slightly greater or smaller than seventeen. In light of this, the tallied numbers and calculated percentages cited below come with a healthy dose of equivocation. Second, it is important to keep in mind that unlike Lanfranco's *St Luke Healing the Dropsical Child*, *tavolette* are not fine works of art painted by a well-known master artist with an eye to detail. They are popular offerings that were almost always produced by unnamed artisans for unidentified purchasers. Third, the detrimental effects of production short-cuts, which include painting on raw wood rather than on a prepared surface, were worsened by practices of display. Votaries often nailed their *tavoletta* over another. Combined, these aspects of making and display have in some cases caused paint to flake and panels to fracture. Consequently, it is often difficult and sometimes impossible to read an image, let alone decipher its details. The general challenge of this situation is compounded by the all-too-common absence of an inscription. Of the seventeen panels considered here, only one has an inscription and even this is not fully legible. From what is discernible, we learn that the panel's unnamed donor suffered symptoms similar to those endured by Stefano Gargano and Agustino Cascano, as noted in the sanctuary's miracle book. The donor of this panel, we read, spent six days and nights bleeding through his nose before he received grace and was restored.[35] With this information, the following observations and computations are put forward.

First, the percentage of panels in the Madonna dell'Arco collection depicting the bedridden with blood flowing liberally from their mouth, nose, or both comprise roughly 2.5 per cent of the total number of the extant early modern panels at this site, or roughly 5 per cent of those that acknowledge a miraculous restoration of health. Second, of the seventeen paintings in this group, thirteen appear to feature a male sufferer, four a female, and none depicts a young child. Third, with one exception, all of the afflicted are bedbound. Although all expectorate blood into a basin, half do so from a seated position. Apparently too weak to sit, the other half lie prone and lean over the bedrail. Fourth, beyond the numinous presence of the intercessor, the afflicted are unattended in just one panel. In the remaining sixteen scenes, the individuals assembled around the sickbed vary.[36] In nine of the painted scenes, one or more family members offer prayers to the Madonna dell'Arco, whose efficacy is sometimes redoubled by the presence of one or more other saints. In eight others, the family is joined or replaced by a priest, a doctor, or both. In one scene, a priest seated by the sick man's bedside offers instructive counsel. As the stricken man's wife prays, the priest points towards the cloud-ensconced Madonna and St Cyrus, his gesture indicating that it is through God-given grace that suffering is eased and anguish diminished. In comparison to priests, who are pictured in roughly 12 per cent of the panels, doctors, who can be identified by their clothing,[37] have a notable presence in this group of panels, appearing in roughly 30 per cent of the scenes. Curiously, in contrast to other scenes that include doctors, here the role of doctor parallels that of a priest. Most often, he provides comfort. Within this sampling of paintings, a doctor actively administers aid, dislodging something from his patient's mouth, in only one instance. Finally, on one *tavoletta* two doctors as well as a priest are pictured tendering care. Although the inscription VOTUM FECIT GRACIAM ACC[E]PIT suggests well-being was ultimately restored to the

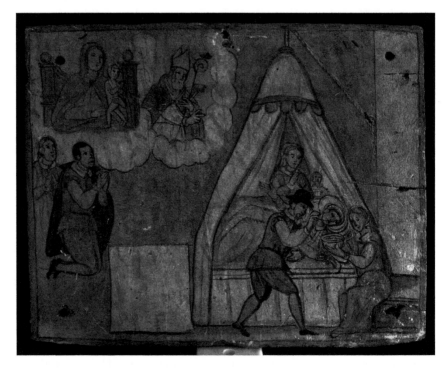

FIGURE 9.6 Anonymous, *Votive Panel Painting of a Doctor Actively Attending a Sick Man*

Source: Credit: Sanctuary of the Madonna dell' Arco, Sant'Anastasia, NA

sick through an act of divine intervention, it is important to note that the imagery does not discount the value of human efforts, both ecclesiastical and medical.[38]

Depicting a disease or representing a miracle?

What did the depiction of this coughing, spitting, and vomiting of blood signify to pilgrims wandering through the vast interior of the Sanctuary of the Madonna dell'Arco in the first decades of the seventeenth century? Although significantly earlier in date, the necrology of the Venetian convent of Corpus Domini compiled between 1395 and 1436 by Sister Bartolomea Riccoboni suggests a possible answer. Her text describes the piety of the nearly fifty women who died within the convent's walls and details to varying degrees the final days endured by each of the sisters before joining Christ in heaven.[39] In three cases Sister Bartolomea specified the illness as the wasting condition of 'consumption', as the cause of death. Sister Orsa Fraganesi 'remained ill with consumption (*inferma de tisego*) for a long time. When she reached the end [on 21 November 1426], she received all the holy sacraments and rested in peace'.[40] Nine months later, on 8 August 1427, Sister Benedetta Rosso followed Sister Orsa to her own grave. 'For a long time, she had severe tremors; then she became consumptive (*deventò etiga*) and often threw up globs of blood'.[41] The infirmity that sent Sister Eufrasia Minio to the tomb on 30 June 1432 is similarly labelled. For eighteen years, Eufrasia endured 'wasting fever and consumption' (*la se infermò e diventò etiga e tisegosa*). When she died at the age of thirty-five, she was 'extremely thin' (*tanta magrezza*).[42] In a fourth case, that of Sister Diamante, Sister Bartolomea did not put a diagnostic label on the illness, but the recorded symptoms that sent the suffering Diamante to her death in 1405 resemble those that killed Sister Orsa more than two decades later. She is described as having fallen ill with a 'terrible infirmity (*terribile infermità*)' that caused her to 'vomit a lot of blood (*buctò molto sangue*) with horrendous agony and without any remedy, with such tremors and fainting that it was a pity to see her'.[43] Had Sister Bartolomea been among those gazing at the Madonna dell'Arco *tavolette* depicting the infirm vomiting 'globs of blood', which she had witnessed Sister Benedetta Rosso doing, she would have understood by experienced observation that an expectoration of this kind could mean only one thing. Death was imminent. Centuries of learned medicine seem to validate her conclusion.

A symptom with many names: phthisis, tabes, morbo tisico

When entries in the Corpus Domini necrology are juxtaposed, it appears that the label 'consumptive' (*tisego* or *tisico*) was used loosely. Like the English word 'consumption', the Italian term 'was neither precise nor exclusive' until the pathological anatomy of the nineteenth century revealed the 'causation, course, and consequence' of the disease we now call pulmonary tuberculosis.[44] Nonetheless, by the mid-sixteenth century, at least some of the symptoms Sister Bartolomea Riccoboni placed under the rubric 'consumptive' (*tisico*) were understood as 'lung failure' (*guasto il pulmone*).[45] In fact, an ulceration of the lungs had been implicated with a general wasting away of the body since antiquity. In *Of the Epidemics* (410–400 BCE), Hippocrates described bluntly the grim progression of *phthisis* (from the Greek *phthiein,* φθίσιν, or 'wasting away'), a usually fatal illness that weakened the lungs with fever and ravaged the body until it 'wasted away'. His description of its signs and symptoms is dispassionately thorough, his advice candid to both students and colleagues. Those suffering the last phases of this consuming affliction run high fevers, experience constant sweats, endure cold extremities, suffer bowel and urinary disorders, and are plagued by continuous coughing accompanied by the violent 'spitting of crude matters'. Because death is inevitable, Hippocrates advised physicians to avoid treating anyone presenting these symptoms lest they jeopardize their good reputation.[46]

Some four centuries later, Celsus (14 BCE–50 CE) concurred. If the condition is 'long standing it is not readily overcome'. However, if treated early, the ill effects of the malady that he termed *tabes* could be mitigated. Best translated as physical deterioration brought about by disease or a lack of nourishment, *tabes* was the overarching name Celsus gave to three distinct conditions, *phthisis* being 'the most dangerous by far'.[47] Unlike the systemic 'corruption' of the body that occurs in cases of *atrophia* and *cachexia*, the presentation of *phthisis* is localized. 'The malady', Celsus wrote, 'usually arises in the head, then drips into the lung', causing ulceration. This, in turn, produces a frequent cough attended by the expectoration of blood-stained sputum. Although Galen (130–210 CE) was less decisive about differentiating *phthisis* from *atrophia*, he likewise maintained that the bloody sputum coughed up by patients originated in the lungs, specifically in *phûma*, a word that corresponds with our terms 'abscess' and 'tubercle'.[48]

Having been printed first in Florence in 1478, Celsus's *De medicina* soon circulated in other Italian printings: Milan, 1481, Venice, 1493 and 1497, as well as in numerous editions issued elsewhere throughout Europe.[49] There can be little doubt that a copy of one ended up in the hands of the Veronese physician, poet, astronomer, and mathematician Girolamo Fracastoro (*c.* 1478–1553), who discussed *phthisis* twice in his *De contagione* of 1546. Under the heading 'contagious phthisis' (*De phthisi contagiosa*), Fracastoro pointed to a glaring omission by 'those writers who have hitherto dealt' with the disease. Observing that his learned forbears maintained that the origin of *phthisis* is 'in an efflux [*aut ex defluxionibus*], which is carried to the lungs, or in the rupture of certain blood vessels, or in a deposit of matter after pleurisy or after pneumonia and similar maladies', he went on to note that 'none or very few of them thought of it as contagion'.[50] Without denying the validity of Celsus's claim, namely that the disease can arise when a 'pituitous discharge descends into the lungs', Fracastoro shifted focus. His concern was not with how the infirmity arose within the body but, rather, how it was contracted from external sources. Regardless, he asserted that the course of the disease is the same. What 'we call *tabes*, a term which, like the Greek *phthisis*, is generally applied to the consumption (*consumptione*) of the body, is more properly speaking a corruption of the lungs'. Here, as in his review of possible remedies for the condition, Fracastoro described the distinctive symptom depicted in seventeen votive paintings in the collection of the Sanctuary of the Madonna dell'Arco, as well as in approximately two dozen other votive panels preserved at other shrine sites. 'Tiny particles of the lung itself are thrown up in the patient's sputum'.[51]

Although the most telling symptom of Celsus's *phthisis*, or *morbo tisico*, was recognized as a sign of fatal illness by the advent of the fifteenth century, as Sister Bartolomea Riccoboni's necrology indicates, it was neither specifically nor consistently associated with the wasting away of the body that came to be a hallmark of 'consumption'. Indeed, following Fracastoro's discussion of *phthisis*, more than two hundred years passed before the malady became the sole focus of a medical tract. Reflecting concerns about the precipitous rise of the disease across Europe, Matteo Salvadori's *Del morbo tisico, libri tre*, 1787, distinguished different forms of the illness, devoting an entire chapter to the symptom that Galen, Sister Bartolomea, Fracastoro, and others had associated with the final phases of the disease, namely the expectoration of blood.[52] Can we, or should we, view the distinctive group of seventeen *tavolette* depicting this symptom with the deadly *Mycobacterium tuberculosis*, which was identified only in 1882, or is it better to shift focus? The lack of agreement among contemporary physicians concerning the illness depicted in Giovanni Lanfranco's *St Luke Healing the Dropsical Child* should caution us against retrospective diagnosis. More to the point, those living at the time Lanfranco put brush to canvas did not automatically interpret the vomiting of 'globs of blood' as a sure sign of impending death. An expectoration of this type was also understood to signal a crisis that was the beginning of a restoration of health. How we choose to understand the imagery of these works must be informed by the votive function each performed.

Crisis as miracle

Since antiquity, 'acute diseases were held to have a crisis, or turning point, which usually took the form of a sudden excretion of "bad humors"'.[53] Galen had argued the point in two treatises: *On Crisis* and *On Critical Days*. His ideas were subsequently taken up by Muslim medical authors and then developed further by Latin scholastic medicine. The long-practised procedure of bleeding a patient was a medical attempt to trigger just such a crisis, or turning point. In the absence of medical intervention, a heavy sweat during a fever, a bout of vomiting, or an attack of diarrhoea was understood to be an indicator of impending crisis. Far from being feared as presaging death, these dramatic expurgations were regarded as the start of the recovery process. Viewed from this perspective, as opposed to that recorded in the Corpus Domini necrology, the imagery on the seventeen Madonna dell'Arco *tavolette* under consideration can be seen to capture the miraculous transition from one state of being—illness—to another—wellness. Put simply, and contextualized in votive practice, these *tavolette* visualize the miracle as an excerpted scene from an unfolding narrative, and they do so with the same dramatic verve seen in *tavolette* depicting wolf attacks, falls down flights of stairs or from treetops, and ships tossed in the wave swells of tempestuous seas.

But did the people who purchased these *tavolette* in market stalls and shops catering to pilgrims understand expurgation in light of Galenic medicine? In all likelihood they did, at least in a popularized form. In recent years, historians have shown that by the seventeenth century, 'Galenism [had] found its way into all strata of society, where the precepts of the School of Salerno on regimen and the preservation of health were transformed into well-known and oft-repeated proverbs'.[54] Additionally, a wide range of popularizing medical books, health manuals, and collections of medicinal recipes were in wide circulation.[55] Admittedly, the material covered in popularly published sources varied. Some recorded magical remedies, others the medieval Salernitan tradition. Regardless, all illness narratives reveal a populace that assumed responsibility for its own well-being in an era of medical pluralism. Above all, this included choosing a curative course of action among available remedial options. Numerous entries in miracle books make it abundantly clear that selecting one option did not preclude taking advantage of another. Hence, Bartolomeo di Selvestro visited a surgeon before fulfilling his vow to the Madonna della Quercia, while Francesco Cola di Ruzo sought treatment at the Ospedale dell'Incurabili before turning to the Madonna dell'Arco. And so, it might seem with this distinctive group of *tavolette votive* except for the fact that of the ten doctors depicted, only one actively applies his skill. Typically, when doctors are represented on votive panels they are shown

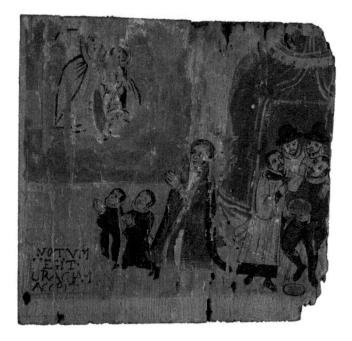

FIGURE 9.7 Anonymous, *Votive Panel Painting of Doctors and a Priest Attending the Sick*

Source: Credit: Sanctuary of the Madonna dell' Arco, Sant'Anastasia, NA

performing the surgical procedures ascribed to barber-surgeons. This is not the case here. Why?

There are, I think, a couple of possible answers. One relates the Madonna dell'Arco *tavolette* to *St Luke Healing the Dropsical Child*, or to be more specific, the prominent inclusion of a volume of Hippocrates in Lanfranco's painting. Closed, the book signals, perhaps, the ineffectuality of human intervention compared to the divine. Alternatively, the Hippocratic volume may point to the long-advocated integration of ecclesiastical and medical spheres that was mandated by papal bull in 1566. Although compliance 'may have been minimal', medical practitioners were informed that henceforth they 'would have to ensure that the sick had made confession before they began treatment'.[56] Arguably, this may be what we see in a *tavoletta* that pictures both doctors and a priest attending the afflicted. Perhaps more to the point of the votive culture in which this and all other *tavolette* operated, this group of *tavolette* can—and should—be seen as visually amplifying the inextricability of body and soul advanced by directive and embraced by medical ethicists such as Giovan Battista Codronchi.[57] If confession cleansed the soul through the purging of sin, then expectorating blood, whether by administered purgation or of itself, the body could be released from disease. In this sense, these votive paintings depict not one miracle but two. Through purgation—bloodletting, vomiting, sweating—health is restored to the physical body. It is a miraculous physical recovery worthy of thanks to God and his saintly agents *per grazia ricevuta* (grace received). And through a purgation of 'all spiritual sickness', which is one of the three types of healing prescribed to us by St Luke, the door for passage into the world of salvation is opened. This, too, is a miracle deserving of thanks *per grazia ricevuta*.

Reading the imagery of the Madonna dell'Arco panels in this manner points all too obviously to the absence of a similar signifying sign in other *tavolette*. Was this the happenstance of confluence, the imaging of a symptom of *infirmità* that could function as metaphor? Perhaps. Certainly, the Italian word for *consumptive*, *tisico*, as well as its cognates *tisicùccio* and *tisichezza*, was used metaphorically and, in notable contrast to the eighteenth- and nineteenth-century aestheticization of 'consumption', negatively. Baldassare Castiglione declared that princes who descended into a life of vice were *ftisici nella infirmità*.[58] Approximately fifty years later, Giorgio Vasari praised the vigour and boldness of Pontormo's style, juxtaposing it with a certain wasting of creative invention (*un certo tisicume e tedio*) visible in works by later artists. In the following century, Carlo Cesare Malvasia described the works of Pellegrino Tibaldi similarly. In this chapter, it is enough to reiterate that while illness is individually experienced, the concept of illness is a collective construct reflecting an 'intricate mix of circumstances that define life and social value'.[59] If, in the context of early-seventeenth-century votive culture, the hallmark symptom of *phthisis* could illustrate the inextricability of body and soul, then by the eighteenth century, the physical and emotional stresses of 'consumption' would expand in countless images and texts that articulate the binding of the body not only to the soul but also to the psyche.

Notes

1 Despite dispute concerning the nature of the depicted infirmity, Lanfranco's painting is here referred to by the title given on the wall text in the Palazzo Barberini.
2 Colossians 4. 14; Hornik and Parsons, *Illuminating Luke*, 11–14; Murray, 'St. Luke'.
3 Eusebius, *Ecclesiastical History*, III. 4. 85.
4 Jacobus, *Golden Legend*, 2, 251–52; Jacobus, *Legenda*, 103r–104v.
5 Jacobus, *Golden Legend*, 1, 174; Jacobus, *Legenda*, 1531, 29v. 'In the case of Gregory I's procession, Voragine may have combined facts with ancient legends: the earliest Byzantine precedent of a Marian icon being invoked to protect the city of Constantinople, is documented in A.D. 626 . . . An additional source for Voragine could have been the account of a ninth-century plague procession by Leo IV'. Boeckl, 'The Legend of St. Luke the painter', 14–15, no. 14. Also see Belting, *Likeness and Presence*, 57–59. Representations of Luke as a painter are numerous and the scholarly literature long. See, for example, Klein, *St. Lukas der Maler der Maria*; and Bacci, *Il pennello dell'Evangelista*, 151–64; 250–80; and for the dissemination of the icon throughout Italy, see 287–320.
6 Published in complete form in 1672 through the efforts of the Jesuit Wilhelm Gumppenberg, *Atlas Marianus, quo sanctae Dei genitrices Mariae imaginum miraculosarum origins duodecim historiarum centuriis explicantue* indexed 1200 Marian miracle-working sites worldwide. Christin, Flückiger, and Ghermani, *Marie mondialisée: L'atlas Marianus*. The literature on miracle-working images of the Madonna has grown in recent years. See, among others, Thunø and Wolf, *The Miraculous Image*; Holmes, *The Miraculous Image in Renaissance Florence*; Garnett and Rosser, *Spectacular Miracles*, 63–159.
7 Giorgio Vasari's *St Luke Painting the Virgin*, 1565, which was painted for the Accademia del Disegno's chapel in SS Annunziata, Florence, is illustrative of Luke as 'distinguished painter'. Giovanni Lanfranco's *St Luke and the Angel* (Piacenza, Musei Civici Palazzo Farnese, 1611) and Domenichino's fresco of Luke in one of the pendentives in S. Andrea della Valle, Rome, 1621–28, illustrate the privileging of the spiritually enraptured *scriptor* over the perspicacious *pictor*. Although Guercino's *St Luke Displaying a Painting of the Virgin* (Kansas City, Nelson-Atkins Museum of Art, 1652–53) foregrounds Luke as a painter, in contrast to Vasari's portrayal, the presence of the ink well and pen points to Luke's two creative roles. More significantly, the prominent inclusion of the angel identifies the divine as the creative source. Boeckl, 'The Legend of St. Luke the painter', 33.
8 The couple wed in 1615. Ottavia Sacchetti was the younger sister of Marcello and Giulio Sacchetti, who in 1622–23 hired Lanfranco to decorate their family chapel in San Giovanni dei Fiorentini, Rome. *St Luke Healing the Dropsical Child* was described together with other paintings by Lanfranco in the Falconieri palace, Rome, in eighteenth-century guidebooks, such as those written by Ridolfino Venuti (1767) and Nicola Roisecco (1765). For the painting, now in the Galleria Nazionale d'Arte Antica di Roma, Palazzo Barberini, Rome, see Crispo, 'Un inedito San Luca che risana un fanciullo idropico di Giovanni Lanfranco', 103–04 and the following.
9 Wallis, 'Medicine and the senses', 144–45. Galen wrote 'numerous treatises on pulse diagnosis'. The 'actual counting of the beats per minute was rare until the nineteenth century', see Duffin, *Medical Miracles*, 125.
10 Heyne, 'Lanfranco's Dropsical Child', 1–4. In conversation and by email, 13 March 2018, John E. Nestler, William Branch Porter Professor of Internal Medicine, Virginia Commonwealth University, suggests the child has 'anasarca due to kidney disease, more specifically to nephrotic syndrome—perhaps due to acute glomerulonephritis'. The relevancy of a specific diagnosis to the painting's function remains questionable as well. In a votive context it is enough that the child is obviously ill. On the challenges of retrospective diagnosis, see Michael Stolberg in this volume.
11 For other paintings of Luke by Lanfranco, see Schleier, *Giovanni Lanfranco*, 104–05, cat. no. 5; and 350–51, cat. no. D2.
12 The Hippocratic collection contains some sixty treatises composed between the late fifth and early fourth centuries BCE. See Park, *Doctors and Medicine in Early Renaissance Flor-*

ence, 194–95; Siraisi, *Medieval & Early Renaissance Medicine*, 1–16. Notably, Lanfranco's painting is not the sole example of a provocative juxtaposition. In *St Luke Painting the Virgin* (Rennes, Musée des Beaux-Arts, *c.* 1553), Maarten van Heemskerck placed an open book on human anatomy at the Virgin's feet while using statues from the Sassi Collection throughout the background.

13 O'Neil, *Sacerdote ovvero strione*.

14 Gentilcore, *Healers and Healing*, 3. The 'three concentric and permeable rings . . . refer not only to the types of healers and sources of healing, but to aetiological categories'.

15 Domenici, *Compendio*, 141, no. 1.

16 Adams, *Il Libro dei Miracoli*, 47–48. The 222-page-long illustrated miracle book (ASMQ 113) was initiated by Bandoni, sacristan between 1602–05; 1607–09; and 1619–59, in an attempt to record the votive effigies that were deteriorating in the shrine. His text relies on what he observed in the sanctuary and, more importantly, the dedicatory inscriptions attached to votives throughout the church. Basing miracle books on votive inscriptions was a typical practice. See, for example, Bertani, *Historia della Gloriosa Imagine della Madonna di Lonico*, 35; and Domenici, *Compendio*, 148.

17 For the complete passage, see Carosi and Ciprini, *Gli ex voto di S. Maria della Quercia*, 167. Aspects of the illustration accompanying Bandoni's text indicate that Bartolomeo's ex-voto was an effigy. This would have been wholly in keeping with one of the book's principal function, which was 'to serve [*ceraiuoli*] as a guide for future repairs to the statues'. Adams, *Il Libro dei Miracoli*, 133.

18 I am most grateful to Erich Schleier, who at the time of the writing of this chapter was preparing a detailed study of Lanfranco's painting, for sharing unpublished information about the work.

19 The cited language comes from an example in the Madonna dell'Arco's miracle book. Domenici, *Compendio*, 158, no. 43; 'Stefano Gargano, infermo con flusso di sangue grandissimo et pericolosissimo che gli usceva della bocca, fece voto alla Madonna santissima dal' Arco et ha ricevuto gratia, li 25 giugno [15]98'.

20 Adams, '*Il Libro dei Miracoli*', 34. Custodians of the Viterbo's Marian shrine approved the establishment of a *bottega della cera* on 8 December 1468.

21 For a description, see Nelli, *Origine della Madonna della Quercia*, 6v–7r. For additional examples, see Jacobs, *Votive Panels and Popular Piety*, 35–40.

22 Today, the Sanctuary of the Madonna della Quercia preserves 206 panels, most dating to the later fifteenth and sixteenth centuries.

23 In this respect, *tavolette* bear comparison with *Libri dei morti* kept by some cities such as Florence, which, in about 50 per cent of cases, either fail to identify a cause of death or ambiguously attribute it to 'infirmity' or a 'fever'. In 1439, for example, 33.9 per cent of deaths were undiagnosed, 6.9 per cent were said to be due to 'infirmity,' and 10 per cent were attributed to 'fever'. See Carmichael, *Plague and the Poor*, 95.

24 For two examples, see Jacobs, *Votive Panels and Popular Piety*, figs 41 and 42.

25 Sanctuary inventory nos 28/1516 (breast cancer); 29/1559 (ulcerated leg); 49/2702 (extreme swelling).

26 Common phrases include *disperato da medici* and *essendo abbandonata dal medico*. For the power of God's healing hand, see Gregory of Tours, *Liber vitae partum*, 15. 3. 272, as cited in Brown, *Cult of Saints*, 107.

27 Fra Arcangelo Domenici's miracle book is published in both print and facsimile versions in Miele, *Le origini della Madonna dell'Arco*. The 1608 miracle book was preceded by *Libro nel quale si notano giornalmente tutti li mobile, come sono voti d'argento, tovaglie et ogni altra sorte di paramenti*, ms. Madonna dell'Arco, 1592–93, cited in Lavan, 'Recording miracles', 204, note 29.

28 Domenici, *Compendio*, 152, no. 11; and, for the panel painting, original file inv. no. 175.

29 Domenici, *Compendio*, 167, no. 88; 136, no. 8; 152; no. 16; and 164, no. 65.

30 Domenici, *Compendio*, 155, no. 31.

31 Domenici, *Compendio*, 171, no. 106 (*parole scritte in una tabella*); and 149, no. 3 (*. . . come si vede nella sua tabella*).

32 Domenici, *Compendio*, 154, no. 25 'come egli stesso testificò di propria bocca quando portò la sua tabella'; 158, no. 42, Domenici also spoke with Paolo Lezzura, a *cavagliero*, who had suffered interrogation with the rope hoist, 'portò la sua tabella depinta con questo mistero et sopra detta scrittura, li 29 aprile [15]97'.

33 Domenici, *Compendio*, as quoted earlier in note 19.

34 Domenici, *Compendio*, 164, no. 66.

35 The partially legible inscription is written in the lower-left corner of figure 5. 'V.F.G.A. bella ma . . . come p [per] seje [sei] giorni e note li sangue il naso—1601[?]'.

36 The fragmentary condition of one panel makes it impossible to determine who, if anyone, comforts the sick.

37 For comparative examples of how Neapolitan barber-surgeons, as opposed to physicians, dressed in this period, see the illustrated Tiberio Malfi, *Il Barbieri . . . Libri tre, ne' quai i si ragiona dell'eccellenza dell'arte e de'suoi precetti . . . Con figure anatomiche, etc.* (Naples, 1629).

38 A survey of similarly dated *tavolette* preserved in the Sanctuary of the Madonna del Monte, Cesena, proffers an interesting comparison. In contrast to the seventeen panels in the Neapolitan Sanctuary, not one of the nine Cesena panels includes a doctor, and a priest is present only as a solitary sufferer of disease. See Faranda, *Fides tua te salvum fecit*, cat. nos 38; 42; 107; 126; 128; 144; 150; 153; and 213. Interestingly, the collection at Lonigo's Sanctuary of the Madonna dei Miracoli, which is especially rich in the variety of depicted trials and tribulations, has no symptomatically comparable examples until the mid-seventeenth century. See Lora, *Le tavolette votive della Madonna dei Miracoli di Lonigo*, cat. nos 262 (dated 1636); and 275 (dated 1647). In the former a woman suffers alone; in the latter a wife prays on behalf of her stricken husband. Neither a priest nor a doctor is present in the sickroom. As a corollary it is important to recognize perceptions of priest as doctor and sin as a disease; see Peter Howard's 'The language of medicine in Renaissance preaching' in this volume.

39 Riccoboni, *Life and Death in a Venetian Convent*. For the text in its original Venetian dialect, see Dominici, *Lettere spirituali*, 259–330. I am indebted to Daniel Bornstein, who generously assisted me with this text, and to Sharon Strocchia, for pointing me in Sister Riccoboni's direction.

40 Riccoboni, *Life and Death in a Venetian Convent*, 96; Dominici, *Lettere Spirituali*, 325.

41 Riccoboni, *Life and Death in a Venetian Convent*, 97; Dominici, *Lettere Spirituali*, 326.

42 Riccoboni, *Life and Death in a Venetian Convent*, 99–100; Dominici, *Lettere Spirituali*, 328.

43 Riccoboni, *Life and Death in a Venetian Convent*, 71; Dominici, *Lettere Spirituali*, 301.

44 Day, *Consumptive Chic*, 2–3.

45 For example, see descriptions of Eleonora da Toledo's (1539–62) 'consumption', in Pieraccini, *La stirpe de' Medici di Cafaggiolo*, 2: 68.

46 Hippocrates. *Of the Epidemics*, bk. 1, chap. 13–14, 125–26.

47 Celsus, *De Medicina*, bk. 3, chap. 22, 326–27.

48 For recent studies charting the history of the disease, see Dyer, *Tuberculosis*; and Bynum, *Spitting Blood. History of Tuberculosis*.

49 By the mid-nineteenth century, forty-nine printings of the first-century text had been put into circulation. Donaldson, 'Celsus', 252–54.

50 Fracastoro, *De contagion et contagiosis*, bk. 2, chap. 9, 46v. I have used, but not relied wholly upon, the translation of Wright, *Hieronymi Fracastorii, De contagione et contagionis*, 119. Pliny's 'remedies for melancholy, lethargy and phthisis', which are cited several times by Fracastoro, are in *Natural History*, bk. 28, chap. 67, 230–31. Among the more interesting suggestions for relieving the symptoms of *phthisis* are burnt cow's horn administered with honey, inhaling the smoke from burnt cow dung, and drinking goat's milk, preferably directly from the animal's udder.

51 Fracastoro, *De contagione et contagionis*, bk. 2, chap. 9, 47.

52 Salvadori, *Del morbo tisico*, bk. 2, chap. 3, goes into the unpleasant details of *spum di sangue*. Day, *Consumptive Chic*, 2, notes, 'Beginning at the end of the eighteenth century, mortality from tuberculosis was on the rise, at its peak causing 25% of all deaths in Europe'.

53 Siraisi, *Medieval & Renaissance Medicine*, 135.
54 Gentilcore, *Health and Healing*, 6; Cavallo and Storey, *Healthy Living in Late Renaissance Italy*, 25.
55 Cavallo and Storey, *Healthy Living in Late Renaissance Italy*, 13–47 (chapter, 'Print and a Culture of Prevention').
56 Gentilcore, *Healers and Healing*, 11.
57 Codronchi, *De christiana ac tuta medendi rationi*, 48–49.
58 Castiglione, *Il Cortegiano*, bk. 4, chap. 47, 360.
59 Day, *Consumptive Chic*, 3.

Bibliography

Primary sources

Domenici, Giovanni, Maria Teresa Casella, and Giovanni Pozzi, *Lettere spirituali* (Friburg: Edizioni Universitarie, 1969).

Eusebius Pamphilus, *Ecclesiastical History*, trans., Christian Frederick Crusé (New York: Stanford & Swords, 1850).

Fracastorii, Hieronymi, *De contagion et contagiosis morbis et eorum curatione, libri III*, trans. and ed., Wilmer Cave Wright (New York and London: G. P. Putnam's Sons, 1930).

Fracastoro, Girolamo, *Il contagion, le malattie contagiose e la loro cura*, trans., Vincenzo Busacchi (Florence: Leo S. Olschki, 1950).

Jacobus de Voragine, *The Golden Legend: Readings on the Saints*, trans., William Granger Ryan (Princeton: Princeton University Press, 1993), vol. 2.

Jacobus da Voragine, *Legenda: opus aureum quod legenda Sanctorum vulgo nuncupator* (Lyon: Nicolai Petit et Hectoris Penet, 1531).

Miele, Michele and Arcangelo Domenici, *Le origini della Madonna dell' Arco. Il 'Compendio dell' historia, miracoli e gratie' di Arcangelo Domenici (1608): introduzione, testo, note e illustrazioni* (Naples and Bari: Editrice Domenicana Italiana, 1995).

Riccoboni, Bartolomea, *Life and Death in a Venetian Convent: The Chronicle and Necrology of Corpus Domini, 1395–1436*, trans., Daniel Ethan Bornstein (Chicago: University of Chicago Press, 2000).

Secondary sources

Adams, Jennifer, *Il Libro dei Miracoli: Intersections of Gender, Class and Portraiture in Italian Multimedia Votive Sculpture, 1450–1630* (unpublished PhD dissertation, Arizona State University, 2012).

Boeckl, Christine M., 'The Legend of St. Luke the painter: Eastern and Western Iconography', *Wiener jahrbuch für kunstgeschichte*, 54, 1 (2005), 7–38.

Crispo, Alberto, 'Un inedito San Luca che risana un fanciullo idropico di Giovanni Lanfranco', *Parma per l'arte*, Nuovo serie, 15 (2008/2009), 103–04.

Day, Carolyn A., *Consumptive Chic: A History of Beauty, Fashion, and Disease* (London: Bloomsbury, 2017).

Gentilcore, David, *Healers and Healing in Early Modern Italy* (Manchester and New York: Manchester University Press, 1998).

Heyne, Thomas F., 'Lanfranco's dropsical child: the first depiction of congenital heart disease?', *Pediatrics*, 138, 2 (2006), 1–4.

Hornik, Heidi J. and Michael C. Parsons, *Illuminating Luke: The Infancy Narrative in Italian Renaissance Painting* (Harrisburg, PA: Trinity Press International, 2003).

Jacobs, Fredrika, *Votive Panels and Popular Piety in Early Modern Italy* (Cambridge and London: Cambridge University Press, 2013).

Murray, T. Jock, 'St. Luke', in David K. C. Cooper (ed.), *Doctors of Another Calling: Doctors Who Are Known Best in Fields Other than Medicine* (Lanham, MD: Rowman & Littlefield, 2014), 1–7.

Schleier, Erich, *Giovanni Lanfranco. Un pittore barocco tra Parma, Roma e Napoli* (Milan: Electa, 2005).

Siraisi, Nancy, *Medieval & Early Renaissance Medicine: An Introduction to Knowledge and Practice* (Chicago: The University of Chicago Press, 1990).

Ulčar, Milena, 'Saints in parts: image of the sacred body in an early modern Venetian Town', *Sixteenth Century Journal*, 48, 1 (2017), 67–86.

10

INFIRMITY AND THE MIRACULOUS IN THE EARLY SEVENTEENTH CENTURY

The San Carlo cycle of paintings in the Duomo of Milan

Jenni Kuuliala

Introduction

This chapter will examine the ways the infirm body is depicted in the *Quadroni di San Carlo* (1603–10), a cycle of twenty-three paintings of San Carlo Borromeo in Milan cathedral.[1] I consider which aspects of illness or impairment are emphasized, how bodily suffering is illustrated before the miracle cure, and what the differences are between various infirmities depending on the patient's age, gender, and social status.[2] Saints and their miraculous deeds were a central part of the religious milieu of early modern Catholic Europe. Despite the stricter rules imposed on the verification of sainthood and miracles by the post-Tridentine Catholic Church, neither the occurrence nor the perceived significance of miracles vanished. Instead, there was an increase in the founding of new shrines and the writing and production of miracle collections.[3] The veneration of saints and the saints' miraculous actions thus continued to lie at the core of the lived religious experience, where institutionalized forms of veneration and theological ponderings intermingled with everyday occurrences and the meanings people invested in them.[4] Miracle narratives provided a framework in which people could interpret and make sense of their everyday lives. As a part of the lived, communal religious life of sixteenth- and seventeenth-century Italy, the popular veneration of images also increased.[5] Additionally, visualizations of the miraculous were used in various promotional contexts.[6]

The infirm body played a crucial role in all of this. Cults had to respond to the lay public's needs in order to succeed,[7] and so the suffering or functional hindrances of the future *miracolato* [miracle beneficiary] needed to be explicitly stated in a manner that was credible, relatable, and applicable to the devotees' everyday experience. Since the miraculous was a vital part of lived religion in the period, it was also a distinctly communal phenomenon. I therefore examine how the paintings were used to highlight this message. Most importantly, in the context of this chapter, a majority of the *Quadroni di San Carlo* present a cure that was also documented in written form in St Carlo's miracle collections and in his canonization inquest records. A selection of case studies offers a rare and remarkable opportunity to compare pictorial evidence with texts and therefore to address the broader question of the similarities and differences between the two media.

The *Quadroni di San Carlo* offer an illuminating example of the promotional use of images in the wake of Catholic reforms. Carlo Borromeo is unquestionably one of the most important and widely venerated saints of the Catholic Reformation era. Born in 1538 to a noble northern Italian family, he was made a cardinal in 1560 and appointed archbishop of Milan in 1564. Following his death in 1584, Carlo Borromeo's *fama sanctitatis* spread rapidly, prompting the initiation of canonization procedures.[8] After evaluating evidence from witnesses to his saintly life and miraculous deeds, Carlo was beatified by Clement VIII in 1602. A set of paintings commemorating his life was initiated a year later. In 1610, a group of twenty-three paintings depicting his miracles formed a cycle to honour his canonization by Paul V.[9] Several artists were involved in the project: Giovanni Battista Crespi, called il Cerano (six paintings), Giulio Cesare Procaccini (six paintings), Camillo Landriani, called il Duchino (five paintings), Carlo Buzzi (three paintings), Giorgio Noyers (two paintings), and Alessandro Vaiani (one painting). Five more canvases were added to the group in the later seventeenth century. Giorgio Bonola and Giacomo Parravicini each painted one work, while the three additional paintings were created by an anonymous artist. Altogether, the cycle includes paintings of twenty-eight miracles. Thirteen of these represent a male *miracolato* and fifteen a female beneficiary. Among the *miracolati* are five small children, five nuns, and one friar. In accordance with the evidence in Carlo Borromeo's *processo*, most of the beneficiaries represented in the *Quadroni* were well-off, but the poor are included as well.

Carlo Borromeo's cousin, Federico Borromeo (1564–1631), had been elected the archbishop of Milan in 1595. A patron of the arts and sciences, he was instrumental in commemorating the sanctity of his celebrated cousin. Federico was responsible for erecting the colossal *Sancarlone* statue in Arona and for initiating the painting cycle at the Duomo of Milan. In realizing the monumental project, Federico Borromeo relied on the canon of the Duomo, Alessandro Mazenta. A meeting of the cathedral chapter decided on initiating the first set of paintings in September 1602, when Mazenta was given the task to decide on the figurative form of Carlo's sainthood. Ernesto Brivio and Marco Rosci, who are responsible for comprehensive studies on the *Quadroni*, suggest that the pictorial programme was provided by Federico Borromeo. Rosci has also demonstrated that the choices made regarding the style and tone of the paintings stem from Cardinal Federico's artistic ideas. His view was that paintings were to be historically accurate and visually gripping in order to simultaneously move and inspire viewers.[10] This reflects the principal function of images during the Catholic Reformation. The Council of Trent had emphasized the traditional view, inherited from Gregory the Great, regarding the instructive use of images. Later on, the decrees on images were further developed in Cardinal Gabriele Paleotti's 1582 treatise *Discorso intorno alle immagini sacre e profane*. He offered an alternative to the secularized use of art, recognizing that images provide pleasure and confirming the view that art was supposed to teach, move, and delight (*docere, movere,* and *delectare*).[11] Paleotti argued that one should reach people's hearts by using 'affective' means. This would in turn direct them towards desired behaviour, as 'the control of emotions will result in a situation wherein emotions facilitate control'.[12]

The views of Paleotti—like those of Archbishop Borromeo—were not dissimilar from the prevailing ideas regarding the representation and purpose of miracles. In all the miracle narratives, whether in written or pictorial form, emotions and religious experience intermingle with a promotional and juridical purpose, and they also have a didactic role of fighting heresies and strengthening faith.[13] The miracles in the *Quadroni* are thus connected to the trend of promoting sainthood as a larger objective, as well as visually conveying an individual's sanctity with the post-Tridentine use of emotions to highlight the message and purpose of art. Those promoting or investigating sainthood—be they auditors of a canonization inquest, authors of miracle collections, or people like Federico Borromeo wishing to promote a certain cult—were interested in verifying professed miraculous experiences. At the same time, those reporting their miraculous experience were well aware of the existing patterns according to which their experiences needed to be formulated, as was the audience of written and pictorial miracle narratives. The painters depicting miracles had equally internalized these cultural patterns, which they narrated by the techniques of their art. Pain—and infirmity in general—experienced by the beneficiary had a crucial role in all of this, for it is able to stir a sympathetic response and sensuous suffering in the onlooker.[14]

Suffering and anomalies of the body

Marc'Aurelio Grattarola's collection of texts related to Carlo Borromeo's canonization records the miraculous cure of Aurelia degli Angeli, a Milanese woman. She suffered from an infirmity in her left leg referred to as *male del canchero* ('cancerous disease') at the beginning of the narrative and as *nerui offesi, et attratti* ('injured nerves/sinews') at the end. Typical of all pre-modern hagiographic material, the diagnosis is somewhat vague.[15] Nevertheless, Grattarola carefully notes the drastic consequences of this ailment: the leg emitted pus and stank, the rotted flesh made the patient appear repulsive, and the accompanying fever made the illness dangerous. There was no medical cure, and so in 1601, Aurelia invoked St Carlo in front of his image and was healed. Interestingly, the leg, having been dislocated due to the injured nerves/sinews, returned to its natural place.[16] Grattarola's narrative is a very straightforward—one could even say typical—account of a miraculous cure. It recounts the physical symptoms of the infirmity as well as the improved situation after the cure.

When comparing Grattarola's narrative with il Cerano's painting (Figure 10.1), it is obvious which aspects of the miracle narrative were considered crucial to the

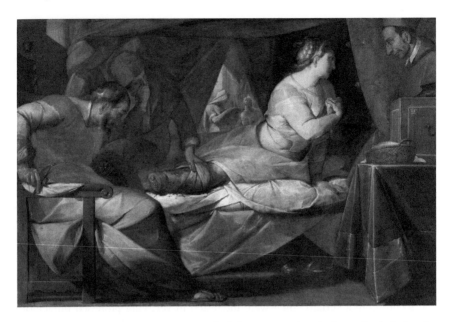

FIGURE 10.1 Giovanni Battista Crespi, called Il Cerano: *Miracolo di Aurelia degli Angeli*

Source: © Veneranda Fabbrica del Duomo di Milano, Milan

delivery of its primary message. Aurelia's cancerous leg is at the centre of the image, and the viewer's gaze is directed towards it, as it is examined and pointed out by two figures, at least one of them being a medical professional holding forceps or pincers. We will return to the role of physicians later, but here the curiosity, and even shock, of these two figures emphasizes the pus and wretched odour emitted from the leg. Horror or revulsion by other community members is not often portrayed in late medieval or early modern hagiography, but when it is referred to in texts, it usually relates to skin conditions. As a point of comparison, in the contemporary canonization dossiers of St Andrea Corsini from 1606, the witnesses—who reported cures of two beneficiaries with skin ailments also affecting the appearance of the face or afflicted member—related having feelings of shame or an inability to function properly in the community.[17] Similar remarks were made in late medieval *miracula* and canonization testimonies.[18]

During times of catastrophe in the early modern period, such as plagues, paintings and sculptures served as 'an instrument of healing and encouragement', without focusing on the horrors of the epidemic.[19] Rather than illustrating a shared catastrophe, the *Quadroni* depict the misfortunes of individuals, families, or other small communities, but the tone found in all the works is similar. Although the paintings make the beneficiary's suffering obvious to the onlooker, they do not dwell on the drastic physical symptoms but deliver their message in a less obvious manner. Grattarola's narrative does not refer to Aurelia being shunned from the company of others, but the image of a repulsive, stinking skin condition was well-known enough to stir the emotions of the onlooker. In contrast, 'health' in the early modern period referred to the ability to fulfil one's social role.[20] When the infirmity in question caused social and functional issues or disabilities—if we wish to use modern terminology—restoring the person's full functionality or social position was an even more powerful proof of the saint's power. In the *Quadroni di San Carlo*, the depictions of this aspect of the miraculous cure are very subtle. Traditional, medieval ways of portraying petitioners as walking on crutches, with a cane, or being led by others to a shrine are missing, and the portrayal of facial expressions, gestures, and performative bodies delivering the message of the much-needed cure is sensitive. Even in paintings portraying physical symptoms as straightforwardly as those seen in il Cerano's painting of Aurelia's cure, the focus is on the devotion and the solace provided by the saint. The message the paintings deliver is, obviously, the saint's healing power, but also hope and trust when facing a personal tragedy.

Undoubtedly, artistic choices informed the amount of detail each artist used to convey infirmity. Several paintings that represent nuns or children indicate that the depicted person's age, gender, and social status also had an important role in visual representations of infirmity. This idea can be traced back to the medieval period, when obviously disabled people were often represented as beggars. The San Carlo cycle includes the portrayals of the cures of five nuns: three by Carlo Buzzi,[21] and one each by Giulio Cesare Procaccini[22] and Alessandro Vaiani.[23] The religious women were reportedly cured of paralysis, dropsy, *catarro*, a 'crippled' leg, and *fibre etica*, respectively. The written forms of their miracles make their bodily suffering explicit. For example, the canonization protocols state that Sister Angelica Landriani's pain from dropsy was 'terrible'.[24] Giussani's narrative mentions that she was unable to walk without the assistance of others and that she could hardly stand.[25] In Vaiani's painting, the afflicted is portrayed leaning on a stick during her invocation to St Carlo, but nothing else hints at her medical condition. In the case of another nun, Donna Paola Giustina Casati, daughter of a renowned *medico*, Giussani's text states that due to her paralysis, she was unable to use her right hand, leg, or the whole side of her body.[26] In her own testimony, she added that she had to be lifted by two sisters to do her necessities.[27] Procaccini portrays her being assisted by another nun, but her body appears unaffected by paralysis (Figure 10.2). A similar trend is visible in paintings of the other nuns, as well as in il Cerano's painting of Fra Sebastiano da Piacenza, the only cleric whose miracle is portrayed in the series. He was cured of an unnamed illness that tormented his whole body with spasms and agitation for twenty-four years.[28]

In all these cases, the hagiographic texts specify the beneficiaries' drastic bodily symptoms, but the paintings only hint at them—if they depict them at all—and clearly the focus is on the moment of invocation. Because the same artists who were responsible for these works painted the ailing bodies in a more visible manner in their other *Quadroni*, they obviously chose to focus on certain aspects of the miraculous in the case of these *religiosi*. The social status of the *miracolata* undoubtedly had an influence on the appropriate manner of depicting their bodies, given that another painting in the same series carefully depicted the diseased leg of a

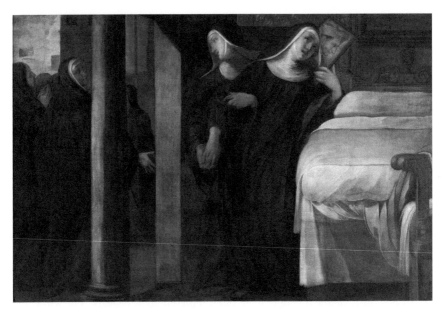

FIGURE 10.2 Giulio Cesare Procaccini: *Miracolo di suor Paola Giustina Casati*

Source: © Veneranda Fabbrica del Duomo di Milano, Milan

laywoman, Aurelia Degli Angeli. Moreover, the attention given to the cures of nuns in the painting cycle indicates a deliberate choice. Nuns had a very specific role in emphasizing and promoting the veneration of Carlo Borromeo, as seen by their frequent testimonies in his canonization inquests. In general, cloistered nuns were significant for the community, because while virtually invisible to the public, they had an important role as intercessors for the salvation and spiritual needs of Christians. Their devotion, which healed their ailments, was thus well suited for educating and inspiring the audience of the *Quadroni*.[29]

Moderation in depicting the infirm body of a woman is also visible in il Duchino's two portrayals of St Carlo's Polish miracles. Countess Anna Miskovviki Branika was cured of a severe infirmity that rendered her hands totally disabled. According to Giussani's graphic narrative, the pain was so severe that death seemed like a better option.[30] A woman called Marina Ferraro, for her part, suffered from dropsy (*idropisia*), especially of the stomach and face, which, again according to Giussani, 'made her monstrous'.[31] Il Duchino's paintings, however, focus solely on the invocation with the careful depiction of the altars, St Carlo's image, and the 'exotic', French clothing of the women. No physical condition is represented in these *Quadroni*, nor does the subjects' body language refer to pain.[32] According to Marco Rosci, the numerous miracles attributed to St Carlo in Poland, reported in a letter King Sigismund III sent to Pope Paul V, were important for the cult because Poland was the last refuge of many Italian Protestants and heretics.[33] Though the noble status of Countess Anna may have influenced il Duchino's decision not to

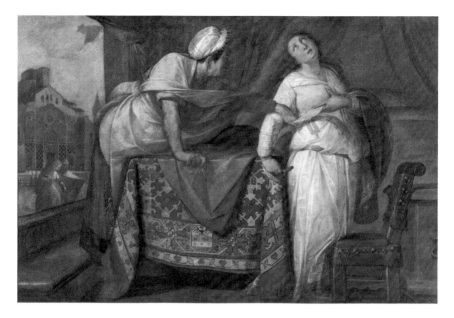

FIGURE 10.3 Giovanni Battista Crespi, called Il Cerano: *Miracolo di Beatrice Crespi*

Source: © Veneranda Fabbrica del Duomo di Milano, Milan

show her suffering, the wider religious and political significance of the Polish cures may have encouraged the artist to underline their foreignness and stress the Polish people's devotion to St Carlo.

Though most of the *Quadroni* focus on devotion rather than bodily torments, an ailing, infirm body provides the focus in one group of paintings. Among these works, different painters used a wide range of techniques to highlight physical ailments. For example, gestures are a dramatic mark of the physical infirmity in il Cerano's painting portraying the miracle of Beatrice Crespi (Figure 10.3). She had a great wound on her breast, which emitted 'a great quantity of corrupt material'. The girl was rendered 'crippled and humped' on her right side, a condition that caused her bones to dislocate.[34] Quite exceptionally for a Catholic Reformation painting, Beatrice's breast is visible, though she covers her nipple with her hand.[35] A servant woman is looking at her bare breast, and the young woman's eyes are turned towards the sky. Significantly, nothing in the work hints that Beatrice is 'crippled', nor is the wound portrayed. Despite the lack of physical signs of the girl's illness, the theatrical composition of the painting makes the point clear even to those viewers who have not read nor heard the miracle narrative. As is the case with many of the *Quadroni*, her infirmity and pain are made clear through gestures and expressions.[36]

The role of other people in the portrayal of a miracle is even more pronounced in il Cerano's painting of Margherita Vertua. According to Giussani's text, she fell ill 'at the end of the plague' (i.e. in 1577) and experienced a grave fever and other

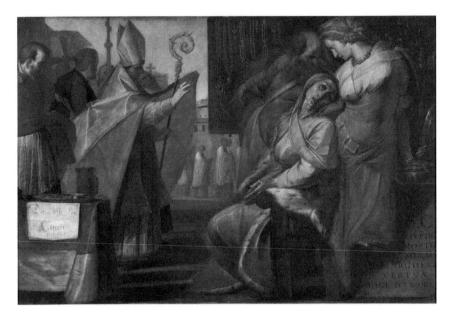

FIGURE 10.4 Giovanni Battista Crespi, called Il Cerano: *Miracolo di Margherita Vertua*

Source: © Veneranda Fabbrica del Duomo di Milano, Milan

ailments (Figure 10.4).[37] Despite the reference to the time period—catastrophes are a known marker of time in miracle narratives—the condition was not diagnosed as the plague, since it lasted for six months.[38] Il Cerano connects the scene to not only portrayals of St Carlo's activities during the Milanese epidemic but also his charitable actions. During Margherita's illness, her husband, the goldsmith Francesco della Guardia, asked for St Carlo's help. St Carlo told Francesco to bring Margherita to meet him near the *ospedale dei mendicanti* at Porta Varcellina during a procession on the Sunday of the Holy Trinity in 1578;[39] this hospital was one of the saint's charitable projects. He had founded it in the same year at the site of the Monastery of the Benedictines of Santa Maria della Stelle to house male and female beggars and obtained a plenary indulgence from the Holy See for this particular Sunday in order to persuade the Milanese to provide the hospital with substantial alms-giving.[40] With the help of some other women, Francesco followed St Carlo's advice, and when the procession passed by them, St Carlo blessed Margherita; she was subsequently healed.

Margherita's cure and the pictorial and written portrayals of it are a fine example of the communal significance of an infirm body in a city. In the painting, the living saint performing his charitable act is a central figure in a manner similar to the two *Quadroni* by il Cerano and il Duchino, which respectively depict St Carlo distributing his clothing and furnishings to the plague-stricken and St Carlo administering the sacraments to victims of the epidemic.[41] The painting of Margherita brings together St Carlo's charity with the devotional act of a married couple and the numerous onlookers, who often feature in late-sixteenth-century representations of processions;[42] here, healing a sick individual can be paralleled with Carlo Borromeo healing the city. At the same time, and in contrast to images of plague, in this particular painting the other central figure is the body of the future beneficiary. The ailing Margherita is sitting with a pained expression on her face. She is painted in monochromic, grey tones to mark her illness. The two people assisting Margherita, her husband and another woman, are looking down on her, while behind St Carlo we see the head of a man intensely gazing at the scene. The procession is ongoing, as a reminder of the public, communal significance of the miracle.

The St Carlo cycle contains few of the traditional images of disabled pilgrims, but one exception is Procaccini's painting of Girolamo Baio, who is pictured sitting on a stool at the shrine.[43] Giussani's narrative reports that he was completely paralysed to the point of resembling 'a cadaver'. He made a vow to St Carlo, promising to have himself carried to the shrine. Immediately, he began to feel somewhat better.[44] Procaccini's painting focuses on Baio's cure completed at the shrine. It is exceptional in the Quadroni that the man's torso is only half dressed, yet the stool is the only thing in the painting that clearly references the type of infirmity he suffered. Another, somewhat similar example is Giorgio Noyers's painting of Giacomo Lomazzo sitting on the ground at the shrine with a crutch at his feet.[45] The scarcity of images with miracle beneficiaries using mobility aids was probably an artistic choice, since many other *miracolati* had conditions that could have been portrayed in that way as well. At the same time, during the early modern period, a shift occurred in what kinds of miracle cures were favoured and chosen for investigation and representation. While in late medieval hagiography cures of long-lasting physical impairments were very common, early modern hagiographers, and especially those investigating and promoting canonizations, preferred cures of more acute conditions.[46]

Three of the *Quadroni* depict the cures of children with physical disabilities. Giorgio Noyers[47] portrays Margherita Monti, who was born, according to Grattarola's collection, with twisted feet looking like 'two mallets'.[48] When the girl was six years old, her mother took her to St Carlo's shrine. Despite Margherita's age at the time of her miraculous healing, Noyers portrayed her as a new-born child in her mother's arms. Her twisted feet are clearly visible. By contrast, il Cerano portrays Giovanna Marone, who was, according to both Grattarola and Giussani, born with 'crippled' legs and miraculously cured at the age of four, as an elder child (Figure 10.5). The texts further state that she was unable to walk, so she moved on her backside using a piece of soft leather as a cushion.[49] The focus on the details of a child's infirm body is further visible in il Duchino's painting of the cure of Melchiorre Bariola, a five-year-old boy (Figure 10.6). According to Giussani and Grattarola, the child had a life-threatening condition that made his stomach 'bloated like a balloon' (*gonfio come pallone*).[50] On the left side of the painting, the child is portrayed naked in bed. His stomach is indeed visibly bloated, but he also appears to have a scrofula-like condition on his neck. Undoubtedly, it was more

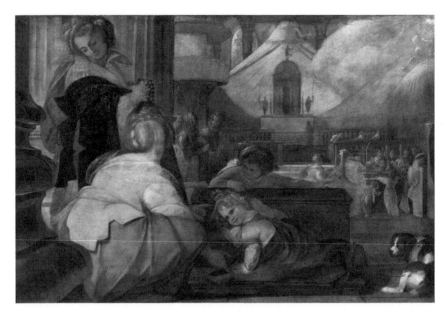

FIGURE 10.5 Giovanni Battista Crespi, called Il Cerano: *Miracolo di Giovanna Marone*

Source: © Veneranda Fabbrica del Duomo di Milano, Milan

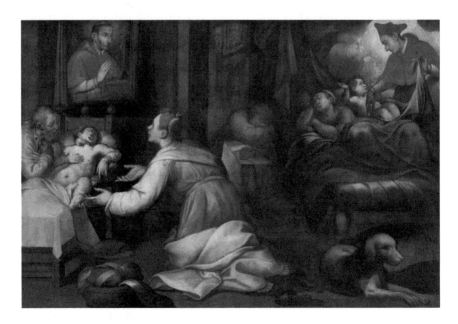

FIGURE 10.6 Paolo Camillo Landriani, called Il Duchino: *Miracolo di Melchiorre Bariola*

Source: © Veneranda Fabbrica del Duomo di Milano, Milan

appropriate to portray a young beneficiary naked than an adult man or woman. These two paintings are illuminating examples of the different levels of attention and detail focused on the suffering body in the *Quadroni*. The most extreme textual descriptions of illness and suffering are missing from almost every painting included in the series. In some works, however, the subtle movements and expressions and occasional portrayals of ailing body parts make infirm bodies the actual focus of the paintings, one that the viewer is forced to acknowledge.

Incurability and the cure

All forms of miracle narrative need to highlight unfortunate situations in order to give grounds and credibility to the miraculous. Visual representations of suffering are only the most obvious aspect of this need for proof. Additionally, in the culturally established narrative structure of a miracle, and in the theological and legal ideas of how to prove a miraculous cure true, it was essential to establish the incurability of a condition by earthly means. The most common way of doing this was to indicate futile medical treatment. Already the writers of the medieval miracle collections utilized their medical knowledge to convince their readers;[51] during the late Middle Ages, physicians testified often in the canonization inquests, giving the medical background to the cases under investigation.[52] A major shift occurred during the Catholic Reformation, with its need and drive to provide firmer proof for the miraculous. As a consequence, the role of physicians, and medical science in general, became increasingly important for the verification of miracles.[53]

Despite the importance of medical science during the Catholic Reformation, doctors are very rarely depicted in the *Quadroni*. The only examples where their presence is obvious are il Cerano's painting of Aurelia degli Angeli (Figure 10.1), and two anonymous paintings added to the series in the later seventeenth century, both depicting ailing legs.[54] Their portrayals of physicians examining the patients' legs clearly resemble il Cerano's composition. In all of these paintings, the physician is treating or inspecting the illness in awe, but while Aurelia degli Angeli's gaze is directed towards the saint, in the painting titled *Miracolo della gamba incancrenita*, the patient's dramatic facial expression forces the viewer to take the agitation seriously.

In these three paintings, the physicians direct the viewer's gaze while indicating and proving the severity and the incurability of the portrayed condition, thus highlighting the miraculous nature of the cure and Carlo Borromeo's power. But why did not artists depict physicians more often given the dramatic and understandable effect that their presence creates? One explanation may be that the miracles depicted in the *Quadroni* were already proven. Most of them were included in the *Relatio* of Carlo Borromeo's canonization process, in the canonization bull, or both;[55] the rest were reported elsewhere in his *vitae*, being established, approved parts of his *fama sanctitatis*.[56] In some of the depicted miracles, such as the two girls born with twisted feet, physicians played no role because the conditions were from the start considered to be incurable. According to Giussani's text, Giovanna Marone was not given medicine because 'she was born that way'.[57] The miracle narrative of

Margherita Monti is very cursory, but the canonization protocols state that she was given no medicine, except for an ointment administered by the midwife right after her birth.[58] These accounts and images provide interesting details about contemporary ideas of permanent impairment. Exactly how thoroughly internalized they were by the Milanese community is hard to deduce, but it is possible that on seeing a certain type of condition portrayed, the viewer of the period already recognized that earthly medicine could not help.

Though physicians rarely appear in the *Quadroni*, other figures—such as midwives or nurses—may serve a similar purpose. Their actions highlight the severity of the situation, thus suggesting the need for saintly assistance. For example, Giorgio Bonola depicted the miracle of Marco Spagniulo, who was suffering from a terrible flux. The bleeding itself is not visible, but the presence of two women—one of whom is holding a vessel near the head of the bed-bound patient, while the other is touching his forehead—indicates his dangerous condition.[59] In the image of the cure of Sister Paola Giustina Casati (Figure 10.2), another nun helps to support her when she makes her petition, which is a clear sign of her infirmity. The woman examining the breast of Beatrice Crespi can also be interpreted as being some kind of a caregiver.[60] Most of these assisting figures in the *Quadroni* are women, indicating the caregiving role of the female members of society. Their appearance in the paintings, usually at the moment of the successful invocation, highlights the communal nature of infirmity and the veneration of saints in particular. By depicting people with different roles, the painters also give the onlookers a chance to identify with the different characters of the narrations and to share and recognize their emotions.

In most paintings, including the five works by il Duchino, the ailing body is secondary to the invocation. Il Cerano, however, focused more on the infirm body itself. Moreover, the contributing artists used differing techniques to create the interplay between infirmity and communication with the sacred, such as asking for a saint's assistance. Girolamo Baio, as painted by Procaccini, sits paralysed on a chair at St Carlo's shrine and raises his hand and gaze towards the sky, while Marina Ferraro kneels down in front of an image. In il Cerano's painting, Aurelia degli Angeli appears almost unaware of the goings-on around her ailing leg. Instead of any facial expressions that would indicate pain, she is solely focused on St Carlo's bust. This is enough to illustrate the successive cure, and a healed body as a counterpoint is not necessary. In other words, the clearly portrayed devotional act of an infirm person already includes the promise of the miracle. This is evident in all paintings in the cycle, since the viewer of the period was well aware that they were depictions of a miracle. Similarly, even if the infirm body was not depicted in the painting, the onlookers knew that some kind of infirmity preceded the sacred moment.

The only two paintings depicting a clear symmetry between the infirm and the healed body are those of Giovanna Marone and Melchiorre Bariola. When Giovanna was four years old, she was carried by a servant and accompanied by her mother to St Carlo's grave, where she was healed.[61] Il Cerano's painting (Figure 10.5) illustrates these aspects: in the foreground, we see the child with adult women at the grave, her legs still twisted. In the background, St Carlo is performing his miracle with a heavenly light emanating from the sky. Even here, the girl's cured body is not the focus. The emphasis is placed on the interplay between the state of infirmity and the divine, thus creating a strong symmetry of the miraculous, as the two highlighted aspects are the girl's body and the saint and the light. In Melchiorre's case, the miracle narrative states that seeing her son in extreme pain, the 'poor mother' prayed in front of St Carlo's image in her room during the night. While she prayed, the boy fell asleep and woke up three hours later. He asked his mother if she was asleep and if she knew that he had been cured by the saint. The boy then recounted his vision of St Carlo touching his ailing body. The mother took a light, and upon examining her son, she found him cured.[62] Il Duchino portrays the healing scene with exceptionally fine attention to detail when compared to the other works of the *Quadroni*, including his other contributions to the series. On the left side of the painting (Figure 10.6), we see the mother praying near her infirm son in front of Carlo Borromeo's image. On the right side, the mother is asleep and the boy awake, with St Carlo standing next to him and touching his stomach.

The reason why the artists have chosen to depict the infirm and the cured body in such a specific manner in these two paintings may be the beneficiaries' young age. Typically, in miracles performed for the benefit of children, the narrative focuses on the devotion and sorrow of the parents, who were responsible for seeking a cure for their sick children.[63] Respectively, the miracle the saint granted also assuaged their woes.[64] Focusing on the child's infirm body and the miracle allowed the parents' devotional act to be highlighted. Given the fragility of children's lives, the audience of the period was certainly able to recognize and empathize with the emotions the painting aimed at stirring.[65] The *Quadroni* portray St Carlo's cult in different settings: in private chambers, on streets, in monasteries, and in these two paintings as a domestic, familial matter.[66] Showing the healed child also meant transmitting knowledge about the cult to the next generation.

At the same time, it is worth noting that the audience was not meant to see the paintings individually, but as a whole cycle at the same time. Therefore, they can also be approached as an entity in which the miraculous intermingles with but is presented as subordinate to or at least dependent on Carlo's *vita*, and the infirm body becomes a tangible yet fluid tool among the many good works of the saint. The selection of beneficiaries is also diverse, including people of different ages and social statuses. Some of the miracle paintings could even trigger a sensory experience in which the viewer could imagine the suffering of the future beneficiary, while others focus solely on veneration. Together, these paintings create a sense of the sacred and the miraculous, with the different aspects of each presented.

All of the *Quadroni* pay considerable attention to the role of the community. No *miracolati* appear alone, and most paintings include a significant number of people. Some of the community members perform a specific function, as caregivers or participants in the invocation of the saint. Some of them are there perhaps simply as markers of the communal nature of Carlo Borromeo's cult, as well as an essential part of the experience of infirmity. 'Infirmity', whether it was something we would label as an illness or a disability, was a very communal aspect of life. Every community must negotiate physical and mental difference,[67] and the role it plays is crucial in defining the severity of an infirmity, treating the illness, caring for the patient, and searching for a cure. In the *Quadroni*, the role of the community is further emphasized in creating the *fama* of the miracle, which is crucial for any cult. Miracles, along with the infirmity that required or received a miraculous cure, were part of this communally shared experience and memory. This is emphasized in the *Quadroni* not only in individual paintings but by the cycle as a whole. As noted by Angelo Turchini, the paintings create a vast theatre where the onlooker is accompanied by illustrations of Carlo's life and deeds until they reach his tomb.[68] The paintings have therefore continued to enhance and promote St Carlo's saintly reputation—as well as the *fama* of an infirm body that had been miraculously cured.

Conclusion

This chapter demonstrates that many similar principles hold true for written and pictorial forms of infirm bodies miraculously cured. Nevertheless, authors and artists have used different techniques to create the desired effect and to vary the emphasis of how infirmity and the miraculous are linked. Of course, the evident similarities are not a surprise given that the belief in saints' miracle-working abilities was culturally internalized and a vital part of the lived religion of the period; influences moved back and forth and created the dynamics around a cult. When a representation of a miraculous event had a clearly propagandist purpose, as was the case with the *Quadroni di San Carlo*, it was crucial that the aspects the paintings portrayed spoke to the viewers and delivered a comprehensible and relatable message.

The biggest difference between the *Quadroni* and the written versions of Carlo Borromeo's miracles, most of which were drawn from the canonization documents, is the level of descriptive detail used to portray the infirm bodies. With sporadic exceptions, the artists focused primarily on the moment of devotion and only hinted at the infirmity; in the majority of the few cases where the actual, bodily symptoms of the condition to be miraculously cured are depicted, the image is less graphic than the text. Similarly, only a couple of examples clearly illustrate the medical severity of the situation. Most likely, the fact that the miracles had already occurred and been confirmed reduced the need to depict any 'proof'. However, some examples in the series underline the severity of the conditions, mainly those portraying infirm children, a few laywomen, and Girolamo Baio, a paralysed man. Given that the *Quadroni* were meant to be seen as a complete collection, with paintings featuring Carlo Borromeo's *vita et miracula*, these variations gave versatility and colour to the cycle, with each work playing its own role in completing the visual programme and enhancing Carlo Borromeo's sanctity. The cycle can be seen as a part of the communal, lived religion of early-seventeenth-century Milan. As a part of lived religion, it provided a framework in which people could perform their social roles, find meanings for their own religious and bodily experiences, and encounter protagonists and events to identify with. Together with St Carlo's miracle collections, the *Quadroni* became a part of the dynamics of the miraculous, even if only temporarily, and they consequently enhanced St Carlo's importance in the Milanese community's lived religion and the role infirmity had in it.

Notes

1 Research for the present chapter was supported by the Academy of Finland post-doctoral grant 287483 and the Academy of Finland Centre of Excellence in the History of Experience(s) at Tampere University.
2 Late medieval and early modern vocabulary lacked a consistent umbrella term for ill health and disability, and it is often impossible to differentiate between the two. The most common terms used to denote the various bodily and mental afflictions that saints cured are *infirmitas* (Latin) *infirmità* (Italian); see for example Kuuliala, Mustakallio, and Krötzl, 'Introduction: *Infirmitas* in antiquity and the Middle Ages'.
3 Harline, *Miracles at the Jesus Oak*, 4–5.
4 For the concept of lived religion, see Katajala-Peltomaa and Toivo, 'Religion as an experience', 1–19.
5 Sangalli, *Miracoli a Milano*, 118.
6 For the importance of images in Carlo Borromeo's cult, see Turchini, *La fabbrica di un santo*, 40–44. Images were in general becoming increasingly important for Catholic Reformation canonization campaigns. In 1595, after the death of San Filippo Neri, 950 images were made and sold to interested parties, and more expensive images were reserved for those who could directly influence the process. Ditchfield, *Liturgy, Sanctity and History in Tridentine Italy*, 237–38. See also Ditchfield, 'Thinking with saints', 561–64, for the importance of images for the study of Catholic Reformation sainthood, and Noyes, 'On the Fringes of Center', for the Curia's control over the images of *beati moderni*.
7 Webb, 'Friends or the family', 188.
8 See Turchini, *La Fabbrica di un santo*, esp. 54–70. As a sign of the prevalence of the cult, in 1606 there were 1411 ex voto *tavolette*, 8019 silver votive gifts, and 8620 golden shields at Carlo Borromeo's shrine. Marcora, 'Il processo diocesano informativo sulla vita di S. Carlo per la sua canonizzazione', 79.
9 Rosci, *I Quadroni di San Carlo*, 130. The miracle collections were written by Giovanni Pietro Giussani, *Vita di S. Carlo Borromeo, prete cardinale del titolo di Santa Prassede* (1613), and the procurator of the canonization inquest, Marc'Aurelio Grattarola, *Successi maravigliosi della veneratione di S. Carlo* (1614). On the various *vitae* of Carlo Borromeo, see Turchini, *La fabbrica di un santo*, 31–33. On his canonization process and the sources, see Marcora, 'Il processo diocesano'.
10 Brivio, *The Life and Miracles of St Carlo Borromeo*, 22–24. See also Jones, 'San Carlo Borromeo and Plague Imagery in Milan and Rome', 65–96, for the paintings in the cycle where St Carlo Borromeo ministers to or helps plague-ridden Milan. Among the *Quadroni* depicting St Carlo's miracles, there are no cures of plague.
11 Levy, *Propaganda and the Jesuit Baroque*, 49.
12 Rietbergen, *Power and Religion in Baroque Rome*, 17.
13 Goodich, *Miracles and Wonders*, esp. 8–10.
14 Graham and Kilory-Ewbank, 'Introduction: visualizing sensuous suffering and affective pain in early modern Europe and the Spanish Americas'. For pain in early modern culture, see van Dijkhuizen and Enenkel (eds), *The Sense of Suffering*. For religious ideas of pain, see Jan Frans van Dijkhuizen, 'Partarkers of Pain' in the same volume.
15 See for example Sigal, *L'homme et le miracle dans la France médiévale*, 248.
16 Grattarola, *Successi maravigliosi*, 165: 'haveva la gamba sinistra molto guasta dal male del canchero, con alcuni buchi profondi in essa, per la carne e li nerui marciti, uscendo dalle inuecchiate piaghe di tre anni, insieme con molta copia di materia carognosa, tanto gran

fettore, che l'istesso cirurgico veniva quasi meno nel medicarla. La grauezza di questo male gli teneua adosso la febbre continua, non potendosi trouare medicamento veruno potente a sanarla. Onde ritrouandosi ella in malissimo stato, si voto l'anno 1601 al Beato Arciuescouo, e nell' inuocarlo in aiuto auanti una sua imagine, fù essaudita della sanita, con saldarsi le piaghe da se stesse, e ritornando la gamba al suo luogo naturale, che s'era ritirata assai per causa delli nerui offesi, et attratti'. Aurelia's miracle was also included in the canonization bull, making it one of St Carlo's most established miracles. Grattarola, *Successi maravigliosi*, 548.

17 Vatican City, Archivio Apostolico Vaticano (hereafter AAV), Riti Proc. 762, fols 168v, 192r.

18 The association of foul odours with hell, sin, and damnation is a medieval one; a sweet fragrance was its counterpoint as a marker of sanctity. See Rawcliffe, *Leprosy in Medieval England*, 134–35.

19 Mormando, 'Introduction: Response to the plague in early modern Italy', 2.

20 Gentilcore, *Healers and Healing in Early Modern Italy*, 185–86; for the significance of this in hagiography, see Kuuliala, 'Heavenly healing or failure of faith?'.

21 Rosci, *I Quadroni di San Carlo*, 212–17.

22 Rosci, *I Quadroni di San Carlo*, 186–87.

23 Rosci, *I Quadroni di San Carlo*, 218–19.

24 AAV, Riti Proc. 1682A, fasc. 13: 'id est difficultate respirandi tam graui corripiebatur, ut singulis momentis moritura sibi videretur, cum simul in omnibus iuncturis membrorum maximam sentiret doloribus'.

25 Giussani, *Vita di S. Carlo Borromeo*, 504.

26 Giussani, *Vita di S. Carlo Borromeo*, 517–18.

27 Cited in Turchini, *La Fabbrica di un santo*, 118: 'se tal volta era necessitate a levarmi per qualche bisogni o servicii io era sostentata e aiutata da due sorelle [. . .] e non mi potevo tener dritta che tutta che tutta languida e stenuata io cadeva con la testa giù e aveva la parte dritta che il braccio e la gamba con tutta quella parte era talmente morta'.

28 Rosci, *I Quadroni di San Carlo*, 138–39. See also Turchini, *La Fabbrica di un santo*, 102, for the case. Giussani, *Vita di S. Carlo Borromeo*, 407–08, records: 'essendo questo padre assalito e tormentato da diversi strani accidenti, i quali parevano quasi eccedere i termini della natura, non restando in lui parte veruna del corpo che non fosse con movimenti spasmodici e come fuori dell'ordine naturale mossa ed agitate con tanta veemenza e fierezza [. . .] Nè cassava mai questa crollatura e scuotimento del corpo, finchè non seguiva altro tormento più terribile, cagionato da quella crudele agitazione; ed allora egli strideva come un'anima tormentata per gl'insopportabili ed eccessivi dolori che pativa'.

29 See for example McIver, 'Introduction'. Though the canonization inquests investigated a few cures of nuns (and also other women) of possession, none of the *Quadroni* portray such a miracle. Though possession miracles occasionally appear in early modern canonization inquests, evidently they were not considered appropriate for a painted cycle. See Duffin, *Medical Miracles*, 103. On women witnesses and beneficiaries, see Turchini, *La Fabbrica di un santo*, 99–115.

30 Giussani, *Vita di S. Carlo Borromeo*, 425–26: 'Venne una infermità tanto grave nelle mani [. . .] che la privò affatto del vigore naturale, e uso di quelle, con gonfiezza grande, e attratione, e stupidezza delli diti, in maniera, che non se ne poteva servire in cosa alcuna [. . .] Oltre di ciò pativa dolori soprammodo acerbi ed atroci, i quali non le lasciavano aver riposo nè giorno, nè note, desiderando bene spesso che Dio nostro Signore la chimasse piuttosto a sè, che permetterle una pena tanto intollerabile'. For a shorter description of the same miracle, see Grattarola, *Successi maravigliosi della veneratione di S. Carlo*, 165–66. The extensive pain was also recorded in the canonization dossiers: AAV Riti Proc. 1682A, fasc. 17: 'manum morbo laborauit, cum doloribus adeo exessiuis ut potius mortem sapius optauerit quam illa tormenta pati: Digiti erant adeo contracti, ut illos extendere non posset: manus et digiti erant adeo tumidi ut illorum usus penitus esset impeditus'.

31 Giussani, *Vita di S. Carlo Borromeo*, 430: 'Avendo partorito Marina [. . .] fu assalita da un gran febbre accompagnata da idropisia, gonfiandosele in guisa tutte le parti del corpo, massime il ventre e la faccia, che la rendeva monstruosa'.

32 Rosci, *I Quadroni di San Carlo*, 200–03.

33 Rosci, *I Quadroni di San Carlo*, 200.

34 Giussani, *Vita di S. Carlo Borromeo*, 409: 'Si converti poi finalmente in una gran piaga che le passava dentro nell'interiore; dalla quale usciva grandissima quantità di materia corrotta con tanto gagliardo vento, che avrebbe spento ogni lume. [. . .] restò tutta storpiata e gobba dalla parte destra, essendosele smosse sino le ossa dal proprio luogo'.

35 Turchini, *La Fabbrica di un santo*, 50.

36 For gestures communicating pain, see Bourke, *The Story of Pain* esp. 159–61.

37 Giussani, *Vita di S. Carlo Borromeo*, 383–84.

38 For this phenomenon, see Archambeau, 'Healing options during the plague: survivor stories from a fourteenth-century canonization inquest'. The 1576–1577 plague of Milan was so essential to Carlo's *fama sanctitatis* that it became to be known as 'Carlo Borromeo's Plague'. Jones, 'San Carlo Borromeo and Plague Imagery', 65.

39 ASV Riti Proc. 1681, f. 41r; Giussani, *Vita di S. Carlo Borromeo*, 383–84.

40 Giussani, *Vita di S. Carlo Borromeo*, 417–18; see also Pena, *Relatione sommaria della Vita di S. Carlo Borromeo* 12.

41 See Jones, 'San Carlo Borromeo and Plague Imagery', 66–72, on these paintings.

42 For the processions, see Black, *Church, Religion, and Society in Early Modern Italy*.

43 Rosci, *I Quadroni di San Carlo*, 178–79.

44 Giussani, *Vita di S. Carlo Borromeo*, 512.

45 Rosci, *I Quadroni di San Carlo*, 222–23.

46 See Duffin, *Medical Miracles*, for these changes. In Carlo Borromeo's canonization inquests most of the infirmities to be cured lasted between six months and three years. Conditions affecting mobility are also quite common. See Turchini, *La Fabbrica di un santo*, 96, 98. For the proportions of various conditions in sixteenth-century French cases, see Burkardt, *Les Clients des saints* 5, 192–95, 207–11, 229–35.

47 According to Rosci, the painter's identity is only known through receipts of the payment he received; he is not included in any artist biographies. Rosci also notes the painting's modest artistic level and the possible influence of G. Cesare Procaccini's workshop. Rosci, *I Quadroni di San Carlo*, 222.

48 Grattarola, *Successi maravigliosi*, 164: 'havendoli aggroppati a guise di due mazzuole'.

49 Giussani, *Vita di S. Carlo Borromeo*, 410; Grattarola, *Successi maravigliosi*, 165.

50 Giussani, *Vita di S. Carlo Borromeo*, 422–23; Grattarola, *Successi maravigliosi*, 165.

51 Wilson, 'Conceptions of the miraculous'.

52 Ziegler 'Practitioners and saints'.

53 Duffin, *Medical Miracles*; Pomata, 'The devil's advocate among the physicians'.

54 Rosci, *I Quadroni di San Carlo*, 230–31.

55 Grattarola, *Successi maravigliosi*, 590–605.

56 For *fama sanctitatis*, see Krötzl, '*Fama sanctitatis*'.

57 Giussani, *Vita di S. Carlo Borromeo*, 672: 'non facendole i parenti rimedio alcuno, per essere nata in quel modo'.

58 ASV, Riti Proc. 1681, fol. 46v: 'nullis adhibis medicamentis, quibusdam exceptis unctionibus, tempore natiuitatis ab obstetrice frustra adhibetis'. See also AAV Riti Proc. 1682A, fasc. 18: 'unctionibus tamen nihil profuerunt et ideo mater nullum aliud remedium adhibuit'.

59 Rosci, *I Quadroni di San Carlo*, 226–27.

60 In the diocesan hearing of St Carlo, Beatrice's father testified that various medical procedures had been used to treat the girl but they had only aggravated her condition. Turchini, *La Fabbrica di un santo*, 119–20.

61 Giussani, *Vita di S. Carlo Borromeo*, 410–11.

62 Giussani, *Vita di S. Carlo Borromeo*, 422–23.

63 Haas, *The Renaissance Man and His Children*, 162; Kuuliala, *Childhood Disability*, esp. 106–48.

64 Kuuliala, *Childhood Disability*, esp. 106–48.

65 On parental emotions at the time of children's illnesses, see Newton, *The Sick Child in Early Modern England*, 121–60.
66 For devotion in the domestic setting, see Brundin, Howard, and Laven, *The Sacred Home in Renaissance Italy*.
67 See for example Smith and Wells, 'Introduction: Penelope D. Johnson, the Boswell Thesis, and negotiating community and difference in Medieval Europe'.
68 Turchini, *La Fabbrica di un santo*, 51.

Bibliography

Primary sources

Unpublished

Archivio Apostolico Vaticano, Riti Proc. 762
Archivio Apostolico Vaticano, Riti Proc. 1682A

Published

Giussani, Giovanni Pietro. *Vita di S. Carlo Borromeo, prete cardinale del titolo di Santa Prassede* (Brescia: Francesco Tebaldino, 1613).
Grattarola, Marc'Aurelio. *Successi maravigliosi della veneratione di S. Carlo* (Milan: l'Her. di Pacifico Pontio & Gio. Battista Piccaglia, 1614).
Pena, Francesco. *Relatione sommaria della Vita di S. Carlo Borromeo* (Rome: Stamperia della Camera Apostolica, 1610).

Secondary sources

Alexander, Gauvin and others, eds, *Hope and Healing: Painting in Italy in a Time of Plague, 1500–1800* (Chicago: University of Chicago Press, 2005).
Allen Smith, Katherine and Scott Wells, 'Introduction: Penelope D. Johnson, the Boswell Thesis, and Negotiating Community and Difference in Medieval Europe', in Katherine Allen Smith and Scott Wells (eds), *Negotiating Community and Difference in Medieval Europe: Gender, Power, Patronage, and the Authority of Religion in Latin Christendom*, Studies in the History of Christian Traditions 142 (Leiden: Brill, 2009), 1–16.
Archambeau, Nicole, 'Healing options during the plague: survivor stories from a Fourteenth-century canonization inquest', *Bulletin of the History of Medicine*, 85 (2011), 531–59.
Black, Christopher F., *Church, Religion, and Society in Early Modern Italy* (New York: Palgrave Macmillan, 2004).
Brivio, Ernesto, *The Life and Miracles of St. Carlo Borromeo: A Pictorial Itinerary in Milan Cathedral* (Milan: Veneranda Fabbrica Del Duomo, 1995).
Brundin, Abigail, Deborah Howard, and Mary Laven, *The Sacred Home in Renaissance Italy* (Oxford: Oxford University Press, 2018).
Burkardt, Albrecht, *Les Clients des saints. Maladie et quête du miracle à travers les procès de canonisation de la première moitié du xviie siècle en France* (Rome: École Française de Rome, 2004).
Ditchfield, Simon, *Liturgy, Sanctity and History in Tridentine Italy: Pietro Maria Campi and the Preservation of the Particular* (Cambridge: Cambridge University Press, 1995).
Duffin, Jacalyn, *Medical Miracles: Doctors, Saints and Healing in the Modern World* (Oxford: Oxford University Press, 2009).

Gentilcore, David, *Healers and Healing in Early Modern Italy* (Manchester: Manchester University Press, 1998).

Goodich, Michael, *Miracles and Wonders: The Development of the Concept of Miracle, 1150–1350*, 'Church, Faith, and Culture in the Medieval West' (Aldershot: Ashgate, 2007).

Graham, Heather and Lauren G. Kilory-Ewbank, 'Introduction: Visualizing sensuous suffering and affective pain in Early Modern Europe and the Spanish Americas', in Heather Graham and Lauren G. Kilory-Ewbank (eds), *Visualizing Sensuous Suffering and Affective Pain in Early Modern Europe and the Spanish Americas* (Leiden: Brill, 2018), 1–34.

Haas, Louis, *The Renaissance Man and His Children: Childbirth and Early Childhood in Florence, 1300–1600* (New York: Palgrave Macmillan, 1998).

Harline, Craig, *Miracles at the Jesus Oak: Histories of the Supernatural in Reformation Europe* (New Haven: Yale University Press, 2003).

Jones, Pamela M., 'San Carlo Borromeo and plague imagery in Milan and Rome', in Alexander, Jones, Mormando, and Worcester, *Hope and Healing*, 65–96.

Katajala-Peltomaa, Sari, 'Parental roles in the canonisation processes of Saint Nicola of Tolentino and Saint Thomas Cantilupe', in Katariina Mustakallio, Jussi Hanska, Hanna-Leena Sainio, and Ville Vuolanto (eds), *Hoping for Continuity: Childhood, Education and Death in Antiquity and the Middle Ages* (Rome: Institutum Romanum Finlandiae, 2005), 145–55.

Katajala-Peltomaa, Sari and Raisa Maria Toivo, 'Religion as an experience', in Sari Katajala-Peltomaa and Raisa Maria Toivo (eds), *Lived Religion and the Long Reformation in Northern Europe c. 1300–1700* (Leiden: Brill, 2016), 1–19.

Krötzl, Christian, '*Fama sanctitatis*. Die Akten der spätmittelalterlichen Kanonisationsprozesse als Quelle zu Kommunikation und Informationsvermittlung in der mittelalterlichen Gesellschaft', in Gábor Klaniczay (ed.), *Procès de canonisation au Moyen Âge. Aspects juridiques et religieux*, Collection de l'École française de Rome 340 (Rome: École Française de Rome, 2004), 223–44.

Kuuliala, Jenni, *Childhood Disability and Social Integration in the Middle Ages: Constructions of Impairments in Thirteenth- and Fourteenth-Century Canonization Processes*, Studies in the History of Daily Life 4 (Turnhout: Brepols, 2016).

Kuuliala, Jenni, 'Heavenly healing or failure of faith? Partial cures in later medieval canonization processes', in Sari Katajala-Peltomaa and Kirsi Salonen (eds), *Church and Belief in the Middle Ages: Popes, Saints, and Crusaders* (Amsterdam: Amsterdam University Press, 2016), 171–99.

Kuuliala, Jenni, Katariina Mustakallio, and Christian Krötzl, 'Introduction: *Infirmitas* in antiquity and the Middle Ages', in Christian Krötzl, Katariina Mustakallio, and Jenni Kuuliala (eds), *Infirmity in Antiquity and the Middle Ages: Social and Cultural Approaches to Health, Weakness and Care* (Aldershot: Ashgate, 2015), 1–15.

Levy, Evonne, *Propaganda and the Jesuit Baroque* (Los Angeles: University of California Press, 2004).

Marcora, Carlo, 'Il processo diocesano informativo sulla vita di S. Carlo per la sua canonizzazione', in *Memorie storiche della diocese di Milano*, 9 (Milan: Biblioteca Ambrosiana, 1962), 76–100.

McIver, Katherine A., 'Introduction', in Katherine A. McIver (ed.), *Wives, Widows, Mistresses, and Nuns in Early Modern Italy: Making the Invisible Visible Through Art and Patronage* (New York: Routledge 2016), 1–12.

Mormando, Franco, 'Introduction: Response to the plague in Early Modern Italy: What the primary sources, printed and painted, reveal', in Alexander, Jones, Mormando, and Worcester, *Hope and Healing*, 1–44.

Newton, Hannah, *The Sick Child in Early Modern England, 1580–1720* (Oxford: Oxford University Press, 2012).

Noyes, Ruth S., 'On the fringes of center: disputed hagiographic imagery and the crisis over the beati moderni in Rome ca. 1600', *Renaissance Quarterly*, 64, 3 (2011), 800–46.

Pomata, Gianna, 'The devil's advocate among the physicians: What Prospero Lambertini learned from medical sources', in Rebecca Messbarger, Christopher M. S. Johns, and Philip Gavitt (eds), *Benedict XIV and the Enlightenment: Art, Science, and Spirituality* (Toronto: University of Toronto Press, 2016), 120–50.

Rawcliffe, Carole, *Leprosy in Medieval England* (Woodbridge: Boydell & Brewer, 2006).

Rietbergen, Peter, *Power and Religion in Baroque Rome: Barberini Cultural Policies* (Leiden: Brill, 2006).

Rosci, Marco, *I Quadroni di San Carlo del Duomo di Milano* (Milan: Ceschina, 1965).

Sangalli, Maurizio, *Miracoli a Milano. I Processi informativi per eventi miracolosi nel milanese in età spagnola* (Milan: Nuove Edizioni Duomo, 1993).

Sigal, Pierre-André, *L'homme et le miracle dans la France médiévale (xie–xiie siècle)* (Paris: Les Éditions du Cerf, 1985).

Turchini, Angelo, *La fabbrica di un santo: il processo di canonizzazione di Carlo Borromeo e la Controriforma* (Turin: Marietti, 1984).

van Dijkhuizen, Jan Frans, 'Partakers of pain religious meanings of pain in early modern England', in Jan Frans van Dijkhuizen and Karl A. E. Enenkel (eds), *The Sense of Suffering: Constructions of Physical Pain in Early Modern Culture* (Leiden: Brill, 2009), 189–220.

van Dijkhuizen, Jan Frans and Karl A. E. Enenkel, eds, *The Sense of Suffering: Constructions of Physical Pain in Early Modern Culture* (Leiden: Brill, 2009).

Webb, Diana, 'Friends or the family: Some miracles for children by Italian Friars', in Diana Wood (ed.), *The Church and Childhood* (Oxford and Cambridge: Blackwell Publishers, 1994), 183–95.

Wilson, Louise E., 'Conceptions of the miraculous: Natural philosophy and medical knowledge in the Thirteenth-Century *miracula* of St Edmund of Abingdon', in Matthew M. Mesley and Louise E. Wilson (eds), *Contextualizing Miracles in the Christian West, 1100–1500: New Historical Approaches* (Oxford: The Society for the Study of Medieval Languages and Literature, 2014), 99–125.

11

EPILOGUE

Did Mona Lisa suffer from hypothyroidism? Visual representations of sickness and the vagaries of retrospective diagnosis

Michael Stolberg

Sick, ailing, and wounded bodies were represented visually in a variety of forms, genres, and contexts in the early modern period. We might expect medical text-books and treatises to be the privileged place for such images. However, while anatomists published scores of illustrations of the healthy body and its parts, images of sick bodies are relatively rare in early modern medical publications, and under-standably so. Most diseases that medical practitioners would encounter in their practice could not be diagnosed from their visible symptoms, and the few that did change the patient's appearance in a characteristic manner were usually too well known to call for an illustration. The most notable exceptions were visual repre-sentations of congenital malformations. When physicians published observations on children who were born with an additional limb or just one eye in the middle of the forehead, on conjoined twins, or people whose whole body was covered with hair, or on some other 'monstrosity', they sometimes added a picture of that specific, individual pathology, which illustrated their account and lent credibility to their claim.[1]

In a very different context, practical, surgical treatises, and manuals, occasion-ally offered abstract, idealized images of men with all kinds of wounds inflicted by different kinds of weapons.[2] Moreover, they sometimes showed patients on whom surgical practices, such as cupping or phlebotomy, were performed.[3] With the exception of plague victims whose buboes were opened, signs or symptoms of a specific disease were usually not depicted.

Visual representations of sick and infirm bodies were quite common, by contrast, in early modern art. As we can see from the contributions to this volume, these images appeared in a variety of contexts and served different purposes. Frescoes and paintings that showed the care of the sick and infirm in hospitals underlined the charitable pur-pose of these institutions. Images of saints caring for the sick, like those of St Elizabeth taking care of lepers, underscored the saints' humility and godliness. Frequently, Jesus or a saint can be seen in churches and monasteries performing miraculous cures. Votive images with a patient at the centre, whom the Virgin Mary or some other saint saved from a dangerous disease, must have been produced by the thousands. Some biblical figures and saints—Job or St Roch are well-known examples—were commonly shown as afflicted by disease. In the realm of secular art, Northern European genre painters, in particular, depicted numerous scenes of patients consulting a medical practitioner who feels their pulse or examines their urine.

Often, artists offered a generic image of an infirm, sickly body. In many contexts that was sufficient. Sometimes, however, they clearly sought to indicate a specific disease. It will be difficult, for example, to find a painting or a sculpture of St Roch without a prominent swelling, the plague bubo, on his thigh, towards the region of the groin. The bubo was his characteristic attribute. Contemporaries also hardly could have missed the huge swollen belly of the child in Giovanni Lanfranco's *St Luke Heals the Dropsical Child* in the Galleria d'Arte Antica in the Palazzo Barberini in Rome (Figure 9.1). And undoubtedly they would have noticed the large, protruding swelling on the neck of the old woman who witnesses the crucifixion of Saint Andrew in Caravaggio's painting, now in the Cleveland Museum of Art (Figure 8.4), and would have taken it for a goitre.[4]

The reasons why an artist decided to depict a specific disease are sometimes obvious. Images of St Roch with his bubo and his dog, for example, refer to a well-known legend. In other cases, things are quite complex. Before we look at the ways in which the underlying meaning might be fruitfully approached, we need to look at another group of works of art, however. These also have been taken to represent specific diseases, but, in this case, often only accidentally, without intending to do so.

Poor Mona Lisa

The study of the representation of disease in art is a booming business and one that seems to be growing evermore in recent years. Even a cursory bibliographical search unearths dozens of studies of early modern art which present a perspective very different from the one to which most historians of art and medicine are accustomed. Drawing on modern medical concepts and, in many cases, on their personal medical training and clinical experience, the authors diagnose diseases retrospectively, from personal portraits of known individuals or from representations of saints and other religious, mythological, or historical figures for which the artist presumably used a live model.

Professional historians of art and of medicine have not taken much interest in such efforts, but they would seem well advised to engage with them. Some of these claims have appeared in leading medical journals such as the *New England Journal of Medicine*, the *British Medical Journal*, and *The Lancet Oncology*, with a readership that far exceeds that of any historical journal. Moreover, such findings are popular with the mass media. Clearly, applying one's diagnostic skills to pre-modern visual representations is not only fun for those who practise retrospective diagnosis, it also satisfies the curiosity of a wider public.

The most spectacular example of a work subjected to retrospective diagnosis is Leonardo da Vinci's *Mona Lisa*, in the Musée du Louvre in Paris. There remains some doubt, but it is widely believed today that the painting represents a historical figure, Lisa Gherardini (1479–1542), who, in 1495, married the Florentine cloth and silk merchant Francesco Giocondo. The sitter's famous physiognomy has inspired a notable number of writers to confidently ascribe a remarkable range of diseases and pathologies to poor Lisa. Her famous smile has been attributed to the loss of her front teeth[5] but also to damage to her facial nerve.[6] Others have taken what they describe as a little raised area in the inner angle of her left eye for a so-called *xanthelasma*, a local deposit of fatty, lipoid matter. Taken together with the swelling that some believe they can see on her hands (and which others have taken for a sign of pregnancy),[7] some writers have suggested that she suffered from a severe hereditary lipoid disorder, which likely led to coronary heart disease and caused what was once believed to have been an early death (she actually died at the age of sixty-three). The most spectacular assertion, however, is that Lisa probably suffered from hypothyroidism, a malfunctioning of the thyroid. Even the renowned Smithsonian Institution recently endorsed this diagnosis.[8] It is based, in particular, on the appearance of her neck, which has been described as excessively heavy and as indicating a diffuse enlargement of thyroid. The colour of her skin has been described as yellowish. The thinned lateral parts of her eyebrows, her thin hair, and her receding hairline have all been taken for signs of hypothyroidism. Moreover, and most importantly, hypothyroidism can affect the muscle tone. Mona Lisa's enigmatic facial expression, we learn, was quite simply the result of her hypoactive facial muscles, due to an insufficient production of thyroidal hormones.[9]

The husband in Jan van Eyck's *The Arnolfini Wedding*, in the National Gallery in London, another famous painting featuring a figure with a strikingly enigmatic facial expression, has been explained in a very similar fashion, though not even a thick neck can be seen. The thin outer third of Giovanni Arnolfini's eyebrow, his heavy, lowered eyelids, what has been taken for a patch of discoloured skin, a *melasma*, on his forehead, and the fact that he is wearing heavy clothes while the cherries outside indicate the warm season, all have again been taken to indicate hypothyroidism.[10] In the absence of a distinct goitre, hypothyroidism has also been diagnosed just from a heavy neck in paintings of the Madonna by Antonello da Messina and other fifteenth-century artists.[11]

Others have drawn on their medical training to interpret a number of paintings which, they believe, show different types of rheumatoid diseases, like rheumatoid-like arthritis of the small bones of the hands[12] and a chronic inflammation of the temporal arteries,[13] or *scleroderma*, a rare disease that causes, among other manifestations, a hardening and shrinking of the skin.[14] Various writers have also diagnosed breast cancer from the strangely shaped area around the nipple of the left breast of Michelangelo's *Night* in the Church of San Lorenzo in Florence (see Figure 1.1).[15]

An obvious and fundamental problem with these and many other attempts at retrospective diagnosis is that the evidence is often insufficient or outright unconvincing. Attributing an enlarged thyroid to Mona Lisa and the various Madonnas whose necks strike us at most as somewhat fleshy, but do not even show the slightest protuberance in the area of the thyroid, seems far-fetched to say the least. As even some of these physician-authors concede,[16] the aesthetic ideals of the times favoured a somewhat more fleshy appearance of the neck and the female body in general. Contemporary ideals of beauty could very well also explain the thinning of the lateral parts of Mona Lisa's eyebrows and her receding hairline. Women at the time commonly plucked their eyebrows, and sometimes also their hair, in order to produce the impression of a higher forehead.[17]

Moreover, a neglect of the possibility of *pentimenti* and a lack of awareness of the effects of restorations and of the changes that can come with the degradation of pigments and varnish with age can lead to profound misunderstandings. In Maso da San Friano's *Allegory of Fortitude* (Figure 1.4), as we learn from Jonathan Nelson, the artist had originally painted a smaller breast, which started shining through with time. Mistaking the contours of that first, smaller breast for a lump, the authors of a recent paper in *The Lancet Oncology* declared that the painting provided some of the earliest evidence of breast cancer in Renaissance art.[18] The yellowish 'sickly' skin colour, in turn, that we see today in Leonardo's *Mona Lisa* and other portraits may well not be the original colour. Likewise, Mona Lisa's thin eyebrows may be due to the ageing of the painting and to repeated restorations. Giorgio Vasari's praise for the way in which Leonardo rendered her eyebrows may indicate that they were originally quite prominent and impressive.[19]

Moreover, stylistic preferences on the part of the artist can be mistaken for realistic representations. Fingers that seem excessively long and thin or hands with knuckled joints may be quite simply a means of artistic expression or reflect aesthetic conventions of the day. It would make little sense, for example, to understand Parmigianino's famous mannerist painting of the *Madonna with the Long Neck* in the Galleria degli Uffizi, Florence (*c.* 1534–40), as a representation of a cervical pathology.[20]

The highly speculative diagnostic conclusions and the outright nonsense that we find in many attempts at retrospective diagnosis have led some medical historians to reject retrospective diagnosis altogether. They have primarily textual sources in mind, but their argument would seem to apply equally to retrospective diagnosis based on visual evidence. Axel Karenberg and Ferdinand Peter Moog have described the practice as 'an historical anachronism and an extremely speculative exercise incapable of providing concrete results'.[21] According to Wolfgang U. Eckart and Robert Jütte, there is quite simply no place for retrospective diagnosis in professional medical historiography.[22]

However, as I have argued elsewhere,[23] such an approach risks throwing out the baby with the bath water. There is nothing intrinsically wrong with using modern terms and concepts. Historians do that all the time. After all, it is the historian's task to translate from one period and culture to another, to help their contemporaries understand the past in their own language. People in the early modern period did not speak of 'social control' or 'medicalization' either. In cases in which the historical account or the visual representation is sufficiently detailed and nuanced, we can safely assume that the sitter suffered, in modern—and sometimes even in contemporary—terms, for example, from hemiplegia, a goitre, or a cataract.

What is more, in certain contexts and for certain types of historical research, a retrospective diagnosis based on modern understanding and using modern terminology (and sometimes corroborated by palaeopathological findings) can be quite helpful or, indeed, inevitable. It would be preposterous to deny legitimacy, for example, to the efforts of historical demographers and epidemiologists, who want to study the spreading of the plague or the prevalence of goitre or leprosy at certain times and in certain areas from a modern perspective. Even retrospective diagnosis from the textual or visual representation of a historical individual, although inevitably more speculative, can at times contribute to our modern understanding of his or her works and actions. If it could be shown, for example, that Martin Luther contracted syphilis as a young man, this could hardly be shrugged off as irrelevant. Syphilis was not known in his day, but even Luther's own physicians suggested that he might suffer from the 'French disease', which, according to numerous contemporaneous accounts, caused many of the symptoms associated with syphilis today. Late-stage syphilis can come with festering bone tumours, severe headaches, and tinnitus—all of which plagued Luther—as well as affecting the brain and causing a profound personality change. Thus, a retrospective diagnosis of 'syphilis', which can severely affect the brain, might give a very different meaning to the ageing Luther's aggressive demeanour even towards close friends and followers as well as his notorious vitriolic polemics against the pope and the 'Jews'.[24]

In many cases, however, even when we are quite confident that we are faced with the representation of the typical signs of a specific disease, a second and crucial question remains: what is the point? In what way does it enhance our historical understanding, for example, to learn and accept that Canon Van der Paele in Jan van Eyck's *The Virgin with the Canon* in the Groeningenmuseum, Bruges (1436), may exhibit a rheumatic affection of the temporal arteries?[25] Or that the sitter of the portrait of the *Ugly Duchess* attributed to Quinten Metsys suffered from Paget's disease, which can cause massive and painful deformities of the facial bones?[26] Even the National Gallery in London now offers this interpretation.[27] Some proponents of a retrospective diagnosis from these and similar paintings have justified their enterprise as a means to prove that the disease in question already existed at the time.[28] This is a rather curious argument, especially coming from physicians. Modern medicine usually takes it for granted that the human body works according to very stable, unchanging biological laws. Obviously, the fact that a certain disease was only described and recognized as such, in modern terms, does not mean that the underlying pathological processes did not exist before.

Much worse, retrospective diagnostic labelling frequently fails to do justice to conventions of pictorial representations and to the profound differences in meaning, to the symbolic aspects, to the images and metaphors that were associated, at the time, with different diseases and their physical manifestations.[29] This almost inevitably results in a very narrow reading or, indeed, in blatant misinterpretation. Even if we accept that the sitter for the *Ugly Duchess* suffered from Paget's disease, this clearly was not what the painting was about. Art historians have argued convincingly that the budding flower in her hand, her exposed, withering breasts, and other elements make this a caricature of the old coquette who continues to woo men. She was possibly modelled on Erasmus's critique of ageing women in his highly popular *Praise of Folly*. Andrea Mantegna's *Virgin and Child* in the Museum of Fine Arts in Boston, to cite another example, has been described as an early representation of trisomy 21, or 'Down's syndrome'.[30] This diagnosis seems farfetched in the eyes of this author, who was trained in paediatric hospitals and worked as a physician himself. Its implications for our understanding of the painting seem outright absurd. If the child whom Mantegna used as a model truly had the characteristic features that we today associate with trisomy 21, then the artist would almost certainly have known that children with such facial features tended to be slow-witted. Should we truly believe that Mantegna intended to represent Jesus as dumb—the same Jesus whose reasoning, when he was still a child, proved superior to that of the 'Pharisees'? Hard to believe.

Historical diagnosis

As I have argued, there are some areas of historical enquiry in which a retrospective diagnosis may seem justified or indeed indispensable in spite of its inherent anachronism. In most cases, however, attempts at establishing a modern medical diagnosis retrospectively from textual or visual evidence contribute little or nothing to our historical understanding or are outright misleading. This should not be taken to mean, however, that historians and art historians, in particular, can avoid making a diagnosis altogether. It is sometimes crucial, in fact, that they do. It is a type of diagnosis, however, that is fundamentally different from retrospective diagnosis. It is not based on modern medical concepts and terminology but on the explanatory models and diagnostic categories that shaped the perception and understanding of the body and its diseases in the artist's time. In order to distinguish it from presentist retrospective diagnosis, I will call it 'historical diagnosis'.

There are numerous paintings, drawings, and sculptures by early modern artists that leave little doubt that the artist intentionally depicted sick or infirm bodies. In these cases, the historian faces two important questions. First, did the artist want to show just a general state of illness or infirmity, or did he seek to represent a certain, identifiable symptom or disease with its characteristic features? Second, if we arrive at the conclusion that the artist did intend to depict the physical appearance of a specific disease rather than a generalized sickly state, why did he do so? What meaning did he and his contemporaries attribute to that symptom or disease?

The answer to the first question is frequently quite easy. We can safely assume that an artist who sought to represent a specific symptom or type of disease would want ordinary contemporary viewers without a medical training to be able to identify them as such. In most cases, he would therefore focus on distinct, clearly visible pathological changes. Although an ontological understanding of diseases as distinct entities only gradually emerged in the Renaissance, physicians and laypersons alike distinguished and named a fair number of diseases. Since many of these diseases were not associated with characteristic changes on the outside of the body, however, it does not come as a surprise that the bodies of many sick and infirm people in early modern art look more or less healthy or just somewhat sickly in very general terms. The *tavolette votive* which Fredrika Jacobs has studied, for example, usually show the patient just lying in bed, often with his or her hands folded for prayer, without suggesting a particular disease. It is only from added textual elements or from other sources that describe, for example, the miracle in question that the nature of the disease emerges.

Moreover, as Jenni Kuuliala and John Henderson point out, artists—or their patrons—were reluctant to show drastic, repulsive signs of disease in public spaces. Explicit representations of the disfiguring effects of leprosy, as in *La Franceschina* (Figure 5.1), discussed by Diana Bullen Presciutti, or what clearly looks like an ulcer or a wound on the chest of a young woman reaching out for a God-sent healing potion in a fifteenth-century fresco of Santa Maria della Grazia in Milan are rare exceptions.[31] At the time, there were not only aesthetic but also medical reasons for this reluctance. According to the widely accepted notion of the power of imagination, pregnant women who saw a mole or some other morbid change on the skin risked giving birth to a child with a similar defect. Paintings or frescoes that showed disfiguring lesions of the skin constituted, from this perspective, a health hazard to female churchgoers and the unborn children in their wombs.[32]

For various reasons, then, the range of diseases that early modern artists represented by showing their visible symptoms was ultimately quite small. The large majority of artistic representations of distinct diseases was limited to showing goitres, plague buboes, leprosy, and rashes that could be depicted without appearing too repulsive and diseases that visibly changed the form and general appearance of the body, such as dropsy and paralysis or apoplexy.

Once we have ascertained that an artist purposely sought to depict a specific disease with its characteristic outward appearance, the major challenge of a historical, that is a historicizing rather than presentist, retrospective diagnosis is to inquire which meaning the artist and his or her contemporaries attributed to that disease and its symptoms. This will usually involve taking account of the more strictly medical aspects, from a contemporary point of view.

The early modern medical understanding of the nature and cause of diseases was more complex, varied, and changing than is often assumed, and it differed fundamentally from our modern one. Historical writings—and this includes even some recent textbooks of medical history—have often reduced early modern disease theory to the idea of humoral imbalance. According to this conventional account, diseases arose when one or two of the four natural humours in the body (blood, yellow and black bile, and phlegm) or one or two of the primary qualities (hot, cold, moist, and dry) associated with them was in excess. This is a very poor and inaccurate account of the principles of early modern disease theory, however. Medieval physicians still did resort to this model. It continued to be taught, to some degree, in the early modern universities, and the idea that people have different temperaments or complexions due to the dominance of one particular natural humour remained alive far into the modern era. In ordinary medical practice, however, early modern physicians hardly ever attributed diseases to an imbalance of the four natural humours and their qualities in the body. Physicians relied on an explanatory model that was fundamentally different, as we learn from their personal notebooks, journals recording their practice, thousands of case histories of individual patients that were published in the early modern period, and similar sources. In its own way, though, this model was also 'humoral', which has contributed to the confusion. Physicians attributed most illnesses not to an imbalance of humours or qualities in the body but to some unnatural, more or less specific, morbid, impure, or corrupted fluid matter that 'infected' the blood or accumulated in certain parts. The patients and their families widely shared this belief.[33]

This morbid matter was thought to have, above all, three sources. The first was an incomplete 'concoction' of food and drink, which was by definition foreign to the body and thus impure. The second was the corruption of natural humours in the body, especially when their flow was obstructed due, for example, to a hardening of the liver or the spleen. The third source was an insufficient evacuation of the natural excrements that inevitably arose in the process of 'concocting' and assimilating food and drink.

In the course of the early modern period, various new schools of thought emerged. Iatrochemistry, iatromechanics, and Stahlianism were the most influential ones. They maintained the fundamental belief, however, that most diseases resulted from preternatural, impure, corrupted, or otherwise morbid humours and called for a treatment that promoted the evacuation of these humours with the natural excretions and/or through additional artificial pathways, as in phlebotomy, cupping, and cauterization.

These notions were also at the heart of early modern medical conceptions of the skin and, thus, of most signs of disease that early modern artists could visually represent. For obvious reasons, visual representations of sickness in the living were largely limited to depicting changes in or under the skin. In some diseases, most notably plague, the changes were quite specific. In contrast to the plague bubo, rashes and petechiae, for example, were known to look very much the same in various diseases. After all, they were believed to serve the same purpose. According to the early modern understanding, skin changes were not so much a symptom of disease as the result of Nature's efforts to fight it. Nature—and this was common knowledge among medical practitioners and laypersons alike—sought to evacuate the preternatural matter that caused the disease through the skin via ulcers, bursting pustules, buboes, furuncles, and the like. At the very least, it sought to drive this matter towards the skin, where it could do less damage than when it was in closer proximity to the vital organs. This understanding of morbid changes in the skin was very different from our modern one, and it had far-reaching implications for the perception of rashes and other visible skin changes. The skin appeared, from this perspective, primarily as a site of excretion. The matter that issued forth from pustules, ulcers, and similar manifestations of disease was a kind of excrement, one that sometimes hardened on the surface of the skin in the form of scabs. Even cancer was understood in these terms; at the time, cancer could be diagnosed during the patient's lifetime only when it was close to the body's surface or orifices. Leading authors attributed cancer to burnt, aggressive yellow or black bile, which could consume the surrounding flesh and eat its way through the skin. Its typical manifestation was the cancerous ulcer, through which Nature sought to expel the cancerous matter.[34]

Skin changes were thus closely associated with notions of impurity. Depicting someone with morbid skin changes meant signifying the presence of impurities inside the body, which could also reflect a state of internal, spiritual impurity. Moreover, the impure excretions that issued from the skin in a range of diseases were known to be frequently contagious. It was widely accepted that diseases like leprosy, the plague, the French disease, and scabies, which all came with marked skin changes, could be transmitted from one person to another. Whoever introduced impure matter into his or her own body by touching or through the air risked contracting the same disease. Far into the nineteenth century, even the secretions from festering cancerous ulcers were frequently considered to be contagious. Those who could be seen taking care of patients with skin changes were thus implicitly shown as exposing themselves voluntarily to impurity and danger to the highest degree.

Quite possibly, the strong disgust and revulsion that skin diseases evoke among large parts of the population today are historically rooted in this close association with impurity and contagion. Certainly, the association with impurity helps us understand why early modern artists were reluctant to depict oozing ulcers and the like, while they did not shy away from visualizing more extreme disruptions of the body's surface that were not associated with excretions, such as the wounds and sores suffered by martyrs.

In the case of Michelangelo's *Night*, one could thus argue that this was the reason why the artist avoided showing the typical cancerous ulcer, even though it would have made it easier for contemporaries to recognize the disease. A group of oncologists has recently argued that Michele Tosini, in his later painting of the *Night*, accentuated the typical signs of breast cancer—bulging, swelling, and a retraction of the nipple—suggesting that some contemporaries at least were indeed able to identify the breast in Michelangelo's sculpture as cancerous. Jonathan Nelson, who is the only contributor to the present volume who engages in detail with the problem of retrospective diagnosis, endorses this diagnosis of breast cancer. Some serious doubts remain, however, not only on medical grounds. It is very difficult to distinguish with absolute certainty breast cancer from other diseases by just from the way it appears to the naked eye, and in particular from an inflammation of the breast. Even if Michelangelo, as historians have pointed out, did not seem particularly interested in having his iconography understood, one still wonders why he would resort to showing a deformity of the breast that was only perceptible at closer examination. If he wished to indicate a melancholic temperament, he had better options than breast cancer, which, at the time, was commonly attributed to pathological, burnt black or yellow bile rather than to the natural melancholic humour. Like Albrecht Dürer, Michelangelo could have drawn on the much more positive Neoplatonic notion of melancholy as a token of genius, which Marsilio Ficino had made famous a few decades earlier in the same city, Florence, where the *Night* is located.[35] And if he wanted to visualize consuming time, as Nelson argues based on Michelangelo's own poetic writing, a thin, consumed body rather than one with strikingly strong muscles would seem a much more obvious choice.

Pathological processes inside the body that did not result in the visible excretion of impure, morbid matter were explained within the same basic conceptual framework as those that came with skin changes, but often learned physicians also drew on additional explanatory elements and, at times, on highly sophisticated pathogenetic theories. The more complex and specific the contemporary medical understanding of a certain symptom or disease, the more it becomes important that we ask to what degree the artists (and their patrons) can be assumed to have been familiar with these ideas. Historians who seek to reconstruct 'the' medical understanding of a certain disease in the past tend to look at learned medical writings, including 'popular' medical works, which were often written by physicians or based on academic writing. Such printed works are easily accessible, but they may not always be our best guide. Ideally, we should draw on patient letters, personal diaries and correspondence, and similar sources that reflect the understanding of ordinary educated laypersons, such as artists and their patrons.

In some cases, learned contemporary medical theory may ultimately turn out to be largely irrelevant for our historical understanding. Dropsy, for example, was commonly attributed in learned medical writing to an insufficient transformation or 'concoction' of chyle into blood in the liver. When the liver was weak or obstructed, the theory ran, the blood would be very watery, and increasing amounts of fluid would make the belly and other parts of the body swell. This was hardly the theory, however, that Lanfranco had in mind or even knew of when he painted *St Luke Healing the Dropsical Child*. Like consumption and paralysis, dropsy was quite simply one of a handful of diseases that were widely considered incurable, certainly in their more advanced stages.[36] Markedly changing the shape of the body, dropsy was therefore an obvious choice when it came to visualizing a miraculous cure.

Haemoptysis, the coughing up or spitting out of blood, the one distinct symptom depicted on some of the votive paintings analysed by Fredrika Jacobs, is a similar case. In the early modern period, it was widely known and feared among ordinary folk, who perceived it as a sign of severe consumption. Learned medical writers commonly attributed haemoptysis to the corrosion of the walls of a vessel in the lungs by a particularly aggressive, acrimonious humour. They usually located the source of this humour in the brain, where noxious vapours, arising from the belly, were thought to condense and to then flow down into the airways. By all appearances, the painters of votive images and those who commissioned their works were interested in the dramatic, life-threatening loss of blood itself, however, not in the underlying disease process. The Virgin was praised not because she cured the patient's disease but because she saved his or her life. Tellingly, we find the same type of representation for patients whose heavy nose bleeding was stopped by saintly intercession without any suggestion of an underlying chronic condition.

Goitres, in Latin *strumae*, to cite a last example, were commonly attributed in learned medical writing to a gradual accumulation and hardening of slimy, viscous fluid inside the *glandulae* in the area of the neck. They were known to occur primarily in certain mountainous regions. According to Theodor Zwinger, people in these regions often drank icy, cold mountain water or cold water from wells. The frequent swallowing of cold fluid, he argued, caused the openings in these *glandulae* to constrict and make stagnating fluid harden into watery, cheesy, earthy matter. Shouting loud and pushing hard when giving birth or in defecation were further reasons.[37] However, this medical explanation is unlikely to have informed paintings that depicted people with distinctive goitres. More likely, the woman with the prominent goitre in Caravaggio's *Crucifixion of Saint Andrew* signalled general diseases of the neck. St Andrew was revered in Southern Italy as a patron saint of those who suffered from diseases of the neck, and goitre was the one disease of the neck that could most easily be depicted and recognized as such. Of course, this was only one of the various possible meanings of goitres in early modern art. When they combined with unusual or outright grotesque facial features, for example, as we find them in paintings of Christ's crucifixion and in artistic representations of the martyrdom of saints, they clearly indicated moral depravity.[38]

Conclusion

In this chapter, I have focused on the visual representation of bodily signs of disease. Of course, artists also had a range of other means at their disposition to indicate diseases that did not come with characteristic changes in outward appearance. Arrows raining down on a city were sufficient to indicate the plague to early modern Tuscans, and in the same way, seventeenth-century Dutch burghers understood that a young woman holding a letter, surrounded by erotic sculptures and images, and visited by a physician suffered from love-sickness.[39] Similarly, a patient who could be seen fumigated would immediately be recognizable as affected by the French disease. There are other examples. Lukas Cranach could indicate the disease *melancholia* (not to be confused with a melancholic temperament), which Martin Luther viewed as a *balneum diaboli*, by showing dark clouds with witches and other demonic figures. According to contemporary medical teaching, the blackish morbid vapours that ascended to the brain in *melancholia* could take such forms in the ventricles of the brain.[40]

When we consider how artists represented the actual bodily manifestations of a specific disease, it is essential that we engage with the contemporary—rather than the modern—medical understanding, if only to make sure that it was of little relevance for the ways in which the artist conceived his work and his contemporaries viewed it.

Notes

1 Daston and Park, *Wonders*.
2 See, for example, Gersdorff, *Feldtbuch*.
3 See the contributions by Paolo Savoia and Evelyn Welch to this volume.
4 See Benay, *Exporting Caravaggio*, and the contribution by Danielle Carrabino to this volume.
5 Borkowski, 'Mona Lisa'.
6 Adour, 'Solving the enigma'.
7 Keele, 'Genesis'.
8 Daley, 'Mona Lisa's enigmatic smile'.
9 Mehra and Campbell, 'Mona Lisa decrypted'.
10 Ashrafian, 'Hypothyroidism'.
11 Lazzeri and Nicoli, 'Goitrous Salting madonnas'.
12 Duqueker, 'Rheumatism'; Duqueker, 'Arthritis'; Duqueker, 'Siebrandus Sixtus'.
13 Roth, 'Arteriitis temporalis'.
14 Duqueker, 'Early evidence'.
15 Stark and Nelson, 'Breasts'; see the contribution by Jonathan Nelson to this volume.
16 Sterpetti, De Toma, and De Cesare, 'Thyroid swellings'.
17 Hales, *Mona Lisa*, 96.
18 Bianucci and others, 'Earliest evidence'; see Jonathan Nelson's contribution for other publications on the same issue.
19 Hales, *Mona Lisa*, 97.
20 See Cropper, 'On Beautiful Women' for the underlying aesthetic ideals.
21 Karenberg and Moog, 'Next emperor'; see also Probst, 'Reine Spekulation'; Leven, 'Krankheiten'; Cunningham, 'Identifying disease'.
22 Eckart and Jütte, *Medizingeschichte*, 329–31.
23 Stolberg, 'Möglichkeiten'; see also Arrizabalaga, 'Problematizing retrospective diagnosis' for a discussion of the pros and cons.
24 Stolberg and Walter, 'Martin Luthers viele Krankheiten'.
25 Dequeker, 'Polymyalgia'.
26 Dequeker, 'Paget's disease'.
27 www.nationalgallery.org.uk/paintings/quinten-massys-an-old-woman-the-ugly-duchess (15 November 2019).
28 Dequeker, 'Arthritis', 1205; Duqueker, 'Paget's disease', 1581.
29 The contributions by John Henderson, Jonathan Nelson, and Danielle Carrabino to this volume highlight this problem, each in its own way.
30 Stratford, 'Down's syndrome'.
31 Vaidya, 'Locally advanced breast cancer'; Vaidya's retrospective diagnosis is rather speculative. If the unknown artist had wanted to depict breast cancer, one would expect him to place the ulcer clearly in the bared breast—even the nipple can be seen—rather than close to the collar bone.
32 Zaun, Watzke, and Steigerwald, *Imagination*.
33 For a more detailed discussion of early modern professional and lay theories of disease, see Stolberg, '"You have no good blood"'; Stolberg, 'Post-mortems' in *Pathology in Practice*; and, for the English situation, see Wear, *Knowledge*, 133–46.
34 Stolberg, 'Metaphors'.

35 Ficino, *Three Books*.
36 Österreichische Nationalbibliothek Vienna, Cod. 11240, fol. 42r (manuscript notes by the Bohemian physician Georg Handsch, from the 1550s).
37 Zwinger, *Theatrum*, 473 74.
38 Merke, *History*, 288–317.
39 Petterson, *Amans amanti*.
40 Stolberg, 'Lukas Cranachs "Melancholia"-Darstellungen'.

Bibliography

Primary sources

Ficino, Marsilio, *Three Books on Life: A Critical Edition and Translation with Introduction and Notes*, ed., Carol V. Kaske and John R. Clark (Binghamton, NY: Medieval & Renaissance Texts & Studies, 1989).
Gersdorff, Johannes von, *Feldtbuch der Wundtartzney*, rev. edn (Strasbourg: Schott, 1528).
Zwinger, Theodor, *Theatrum praxeos medicae* (Basel: Brandmüller, 1710).

Secondary sources

Adour, K. K., 'Mona Lisa Syndrome: solving the enigma of the Gioconda smile', *Annals of Ontology, Rhinology & Laryngology*, 98 (1989), 196–99.
Arrizabalaga, Jon, 'Problematizing retrospective diagnosis in the history of disease', *Asclepio*, 54 (2002), 51–70.
Ashrafian, H[utan], 'Hypothyroidism in the "Arnolfini Portrait" (1434) by Jan Van Eyck (1390–1441)', *Journal of Endocrinological Investigation*, 41 (2018), 145–47.
Benay, Erin E., *Exporting Caravaggio: The Crucifixion of Saint Andrew* (London: Giles, 2017).
Bianucci, Raffaela and others, 'Earliest evidence of malignant breast cancer in Renaissance paintings', *The Lancet Oncology*, 19 (2018), 166–67.
Borkowski, Joseph E., 'Mona Lisa: the enigma of the smile', *Journal of Forensic Sciences*, 37 (1992), 1706–11.
Clark, Carol Z. and Orlo H. Clark, *The Remarkables: Endocrine Abnormalities in Art* (San Francisco: University of California Press, 2011).
Cropper, Elizabeth, 'On beautiful women, Parmigianino, Petrarchismo, and the vernacular style', *Art Bulletin*, 58 (1976), 374–94.
Cunningham, Andrew, 'Identifying disease in the past: cutting the Gordian knot', *Asclepio* (2002), 13–34.
Daley, Jason, 'Was Mona Lisa's enigmatic smile caused by a thyroid condition?', *Smithsonian Magazine* (10 September 2018), www.smithsonianmag.com/smart-news/mona-lisa-may-have-had-thyroid-disorder-180970245/.
Daston, Lorraine and Katharine Park, *Wonders and the Order of Nature 1150–1750* (New York: Zone Books, 1998).
Dequeker, Jan, 'Arthritis in Flemish paintings 1400–1700', *British Medical Journal* (1977), 1203–05.
Dequeker, Jan, 'Paget's disease in a painting by Quinten Metsys (Massys)', *British Medical Journal*, 299 (1989), 1579–81.
Dequeker, Jan, 'Polymyalgia rheumatica with temporal arteritis as painted by Jan Van Eyck in 1436', *Canadian Medical Association Journal*, 124 (1981), 1597–98.
Dequeker, Jan, 'Rheumatism in the art of the late Middle Ages', *Organorama*, 16 (1979), 9–16.

Dequeker, Jan, 'Siebrandus Sixtius: evidence of rheumatoid arthritis of the robust reactive type in a seventeenth century Dutch priest', *Annals of Rheumatic Diseases*, 51 (1992), 561–62.

Dequeker, Jan, Erik Muls, and Kathleen Leenders, 'Xanthelasma and lipoma in Leonardo da Vinci's *Mona Lisa*', *Israel Medical Association Journal*, 6 (2004), 505–06.

Dequeker, Jan, L. Vanopdenbosch, and A. Castill-Ojugas, 'Early evidence of scleroderma', *British Medical Journal*, 311 (1995), 1714–15.

Desneux, J., 'Un diagnostic dermatologique sur un tableau de Jean van Eyck (1436)', *Annales de dermatologie et de syphilographie*, 8° série 10 (1950), 153–56.

Eckart, Wolfgang Uwe and Robert Jütte, *Medizingeschichte. Eine Einführung* (Cologne, Weimar, and Vienna: Böhlau, 2007).

Hales, Dianne, *Mona Lisa: A Life Discovered* (New York: Simon & Schuster, 2014).

Harley, David, 'Rhetoric and the social construction of sickness and healing', *Social History of Medicine*, 12 (1999), 407–35.

Karenberg, Axel and Ferdinand Peter Moog, 'Next emperor, please! No end to retrospective diagnostics', *Journal of the History of the Neurosciences*, 13 (2004), 143–49.

Keele, Kenneth D., 'The genesis of Mona Lisa', *Journal of the History of Medicine and Allied Sciences*, 14 (1959), 135–59.

Leven, Karl-Heinz, 'Krankheiten—historische Deutung versus retrospektive Diagnose', in Norbert Paul and Thomas Schlich (eds), *Medizingeschichte. Aufgaben, Probleme, Perspektiven* (Frankfurt: Campus, 1998), 153–85.

Mehra, Mandeep R. and Hilary R. Campbell, 'Letter to the editor: the Mona Lisa decrypted: allure of an imperfect reality', *Mayo Clinic Proceedings*, 93 (2018), 1325–27.

Merke, Franz, *History and Iconography of Endemic Goitre and Cretinism* (Bern: Huber, 1984).

Petterson, Einar, *Amans amanti medicus. Das Genremotiv 'Der ärztliche Besuch' in seinem kulturgeschichtlichen Kontext* (Berlin: Gebr. Mann, 2000).

Probst, Christian, 'Reine Spekulation. Leserbrief zu einem Beitrag von Guido Kluxen, Sehstörungen des Apostels Paulus', *Deutsches Ärzteblatt*, series C 91 (1993), 561–62.

Roth, W. G., 'Arteriitis temporalis dargestellt an einem Gemälde des Reichsmuseums in Amsterdam', *Hautarzt*, 20 (1969), 320–32.

Stark, James J. and Jonathan K. Nelson, 'The breasts of *Night*: Michelangelo as Oncologist', *The New England Journal of Medicine*, 343 (2000), 1577–78.

Sterpetti, Antonio V., Giorgio De Toma, and Alessandro De Cesare, 'Thyroid swellings in the art of the Italian Renaissance', *American Journal of Surgery*, 210 (2015), 591–95.

Stolberg, Michael, 'Lukas Cranachs "Melancholia"-Darstellungen und die zeitgenössische Medizin', in Stefan Oehmig (ed.), *Medizin und Sozialwesen in Mitteldeutschland in der Reformationszeit* (Leipzig: Evangelische Verlagsanstalt, 2007), 249–71.

Stolberg, Michael, 'Metaphors and images of cancer in early modern Europe', *Bulletin of the History of Medicine*, 88 (2014), 48–74.

Stolberg, Michael, 'Möglichkeiten und Grenzen einer retrospektiven Diagnose', in Waltraud Pulz (ed.), *Zwischen Himmel und Erde. Körperliche Zeichen der Heiligkeit* (Stuttgart: Franz Steiner, 2012), 209–27.

Stolberg, Michael, 'Post-mortems, anatomical dissections and humoural pathology in the sixteenth and early seventeenth centuries', in Silvia De Renzi, Marco Bresadola, and Maria Conforti (eds), *Pathology in Practice: Diseases and Dissections in Early Modern Europe* (New York and London: Routledge, 2017), 79–95.

Stolberg, Michael, '"You have no good blood in your body". Oral communication in sixteenth-century physicians' medical practice', *Medical History* 59 (2015), 63–82.

Stolberg, Michael and Tilmann Walter, 'Martin Luthers viele Krankheiten. Ein unbekanntes Konsil von Matthäus Ratzenberger und die Problematik der retrospektiven Diagnose', *Archiv für Reformationsgeschichte*, 109 (2018), 126–51.

Stratford, Brian, 'Down's syndrome at the court of Mantua', *Maternal and Child Health*, 7 (1982), 250–54.

Vaidya, Jayant S., 'Locally advanced breast cancer in a 15th century painting in Milan', *The Breast*, 16 (2007), 102–03.

Vescia, Fernando G. and Lawrence Basso, 'Goiters in the Renaissance', *Vesalius*, 3, 1 (1997), 23–32.

Wear, Andrew, *Knowledge & Practice in English Medicine, 1550–1680* (Cambridge: Cambridge University Press, 2000).

Zaun, Stefanie, Daniela Watzke, and Jörn Steigerwald, eds, *Imagination und Sexualität. Pathologien der Einbildungskraft im medizinischen Diskurs der frühen Neuzeit* (Frankfurt: Klostermann, 2004).

INDEX

INDEX OF DISEASES

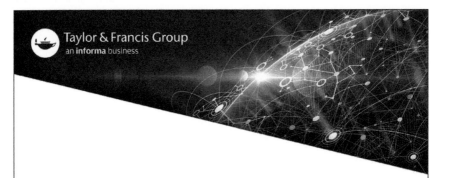

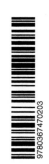

9780367470203